AMERICAN WOMEN

images and realities

AMERICAN WOMEN
Images and Realities

Advisory Editors
ANNETTE K. BAXTER
LEON STEIN

A Note About This Volume

Marie Elizabeth Zakrzewska (1829-1902) was born in Berlin. Her liberal-minded father had been dismissed from the Prussian army; her mother, descended from Lombardi gypsies, was compelled to put her to work learning domestic service at age 13. Five years later she obtained a job for her daughter in the charity hospital in which she worked. By the time she was 23, Marie was chief midwife and professor. The remainder of her life, spent in America, is a record of opposition overcome, of fierce dedication to medicine and the training of women doctors, of compassion tested among the poor in New York and in Boston, of the founding of two outstanding hospitals for women and children, and of steady battle against the ignorance, prejudice and poverty that shortened feminine life.

Agnes C. Vietor, a Boston surgeon, based this biography on material and letters given to her by Marie Zakrzewska.

A WOMAN'S QUEST

THE LIFE OF MARIE E. ZAKRZEWSKA, M.D.

EDITED BY

AGNES C. VIETOR

ARNO PRESS

A New York Times Company

New York • 1972

Reprint Edition 1972 by Arno Press Inc.

Reprinted from a copy in The Pennsylvania
State Library

American Women: Images and Realities
ISBN for complete set: 0-405-04445-3
See last pages of this volume for titles.

Manufactured in the United States of America

- - - - - - - - - - - -

Library of Congress Cataloging in Publication Data

Zakrzewska, Marie Elizabeth, 1829-1902.
  A woman's quest.

  (American women: images and realities)
  Bibliography: p.
  I. Vietor, Agnes Caecilia, ed. II. Title.
III. Series.
R154.Z3A3 1972   610'.92'4   72-2630
ISBN 0-405-04486-0

A WOMAN'S QUEST

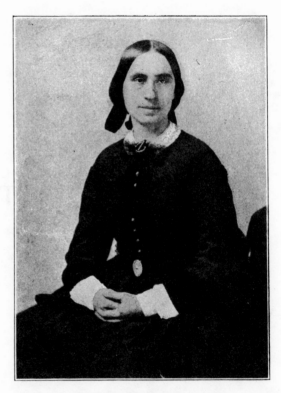

MARIE E. ZAKRZEWSKA, M.D.
(From a photograph thought to have been taken some time
in the '60's.)

A WOMAN'S QUEST

THE LIFE OF MARIE E. ZAKRZEWSKA, M.D.

EDITED BY

AGNES C. VIETOR, M.D., F.A.C.S,

FORMERLY INSTRUCTOR IN PHYSICAL DIAGNOSIS AND SURGERY, WOMAN'S
MEDICAL COLLEGE OF THE NEW YORK INFIRMARY; LATER ASSISTANT
SURGEON, NEW ENGLAND HOSPITAL FOR WOMEN
AND CHILDREN, BOSTON

D. APPLETON AND COMPANY
NEW YORK :: LONDON :: MCMXXIV

PRINTED IN THE UNITED STATES OF AMERICA

MARIE E. ZAKRZEWSKA, M.D. (1829-1902)

Accoucheuse en chef, Royal Hospital Charité, Berlin, Prussia; First Resident Physician, New York Infirmary for Women and Children, New York; Professor of Obstetrics and Diseases of Women and Children, and Founder and Attending Physician of the Clinical Department (Hospital), New England Female Medical College, Boston; Founder and First Attending Physician, New England Hospital for Women and Children, Boston.

DEDICATED TO
THE DEAR MEMORY OF A FRIEND
ELIZABETH BIGELOW CONANT

FOREWORD

Viewed impersonally, this story of Marie E. Zakrzewska (Zak-shef'ska) is one more document testifying to the Humanity of Woman. The fact that the individual urge for the expression of this humanity found vent along the line of Medicine, is a detail. It is also a detail that the story is interwoven with an interesting transitional period in American history and with the evolution of the American woman physician.

The essential interest lies in the fundamental human instinct asserting itself through the individual woman, dominating her and driving her to reach out into the world until, after migrations over thousands of miles and through various phases of civilization, she at last found an environment favorable for the development which her spirit so ardently demanded.

Eventually stretching across the Atlantic Ocean, this Polish-German branch of the Human Tree pushed through first one crevice and then another, with here and there a struggling blossoming and leafage, to find at last its best efflorescence and fruitage in the favoring sun and air of America.

Transpanted here, as are all the nations of mankind, her life finally found fulfillment through the creation of the New England Hospital for Women and Children, and though the influence which she exerted upon the lives of the numbers of women medical students, women physicians, women surgeons, and women nurses who have there, in turn, been helped to develop and to express *their* Humanity.

Stopping on her way to help in the birth of the *first* true "Woman's Hospital" in the history of the world (the New York Infirmary for Women and Children), to develop the short-lived *second* (Clinical Department of the New England Female Medical College), and to assist in the conception of the *third* (the Woman's Hospital of Philadelphia), her life reached its fullest expression in the evolution of the *fourth* (the New England Hospital for Women and Children).

Thus in no ordinary sense do the life and personality of Doctor Zakrzewska endure in America, and especially in Boston. Thence the inspiration of her life has extended throughout New England; throughout the United States; back across the Atlantic to Europe; and across the Pacific to the Orient.

Is there, then, any part of the earth reached by educated medical women where her living spirit does not penetrate, that unconquerable spirit made manifest through her unchanging ideal—reasoned human standards for women as for men.

It is a common habit of our people to abbreviate long or unfamiliar words and the American populace so generally declined to apply itself to the complete pronunciation of the word *Zakrzewska* that the name was characteristically shortened to the first syllable. Hence, "Doctor Zak" became the more familiar title, first of convenience and then of that personal and unceremonious aptitude for appropriation which we as a people display toward those whom we regard with admiration and affection.

The material for this biography was given to the editor by Dr. Zakrzewska to prepare for publication with what might be called one condition, and this has now been fulfilled. Circumstances which the editor could not control, and which it is unnecessary to discuss here, have delayed its appearance until now. The earlier chapters are autobiographical and most of them were written in the form of a letter to Miss Mary L. Booth, of New York, and were published in 1860 by Mrs. Caroline H. Dall under the title of "A Practical Illustration of 'Woman's Right to Labor'; or A Letter from Marie E. Zakrzewska, M.D., late of Berlin, Prussia."

Finally, the editor desires to express her appreciation of the assistance rendered by Miss Anne Sullivan, her secretary and synergetic critic.

AGNES C. VIETOR

CONTENTS

PART I

(1829–1862)

BERLIN

New York

Cleveland

New York

PART II
(1862–1902)

ILLUSTRATIONS

PART I

(1829—1862)

A WOMAN'S QUEST

CHAPTER I

Her reason for writing autobiography, to encourage average woman to determine and decide for herself to do whatever she can—Polish-German ancestry—Childhood in Berlin—Recollection of experience when nineteen months old—Walks nine miles when twenty-six months old. (Birth to five years of age: 1829-1834.)

I AM not a great personage, either through inherited qualifications or through the work that I have to show to the world; yet you may find, in reading this little sketch, that with few talents and very moderate means for developing them, I have accomplished more than many women of genius and education would have done in my place, for the reason that confidence and faith in their own powers were wanting.

And for this reason I know that this story may be of use to others, by encouraging those who timidly shrink from the field of action, though endowed with all that is necessary to enable them to come forth and do their part in life.

The fact that a woman of no extraordinary powers can make her way, by the simple determination that whatever she can do she will do, must inspire those who are fitted to do much, yet who do nothing because they are not accustomed to determine and decide for themselves.

3

I do not intend to weary you with details of my childhood, as I think that children are generally very uninteresting subjects of conversation to any except their parents, who naturally discover what is beautiful and attractive in them and appreciate what is said that corresponds to their own feelings. I shall therefore tell you only a few facts of this period of my life, which I think absolutely necessary to illustrate my character and nature.

I was born in Berlin, Prussia, on the 6th of September, 1829; and am the eldest of a family of five sisters and one brother.[1]

My early childhood passed happily, though heavy clouds of sorrow and care at times overshadowed our family circle. I was of a cheerful disposition, and was always in good humor, even when sick. I was quiet and gentle in all my amusements. My chief delight consisted in telling stories to my sister, one year younger than myself. She was always glad to listen to these products of my imagination, which were wholly original, for no stories were told me, nor had I any children's books.

My heroes and heroines were generally distinguished for some mental peculiarity—as kind or cruel, active or indolent—which led them into all sorts of adventures till it suited my caprice to terminate their career.

In all our little affairs I took the lead, planning and directing everything; and my playmates seemed to take it for granted that it was their duty to carry out my commands.

---

[1] The figures throughout the text refer to corresponding numbers in Notes, pages 483 to 498.

My memory is remarkable in respect to events that occurred at this time, but it always fails to recall dates and names.

When twenty years of age, I asked my father what sort of a festival he took me to once, in company with a friend of his who had only one arm. We walked through meadows where daisies were blossoming in millions and rode in carriages that went round continually until they were wound up.

My father answered, with much surprise, that it was a public festival of the cabinet-makers, which was celebrated in a neighboring village, and that I was, at that time, only nineteen months old. He was so much interested in my story that I related another of my memories.

One dark morning, my mother wakened me and hastened my dressing. After this was accomplished, she handed me a cup of something which I had never tasted before and which was as disagreeable as was asafœtida in later years. This was some coffee which I had to take instead of my usual milk.

Then I went with my father to the large park called "The Thiergarten," where we saw the sun rise. I began to spring about, looking at the big oaks which seemed to reach into the heavens, or stooping down to pluck a flower. Birds of all kinds were singing in chorus, while the flower-beds surrounding the statue of Flora scented the pure morning air with the sweetest of perfumes.

The sun ascended meanwhile, from the edge of a little pond covered with water-lilies. I was intoxicated with joy. The feeling of that morning is as fresh to-day as when I related this to my father. I know I walked till I got fairly tired, and we reached a solitary house beyond the park.

Probably fatigue took entire possession of me, for I remember nothing more till we were on our way home and the sun was setting. Then I begged for some large yellow plums which I saw in the stores. My father bought some, but gave me only a few. I had a desire for all and stole them secretly from his pockets, so that when we reached home, I had eaten them all.

I was sick after I went to bed, and remember taking some horrible stuff the next morning (probably rhubarb), thus ending the day which had opened so poetically in rather a prosaic manner.

When I repeated this, my parents laughed and said that I was only twenty-six months old when my father's pride in his oldest child induced him to take me on this visit, and that I walked the whole way—a distance of about *nine miles*.

These anecdotes are worth preserving only because they indicate an impressionable nature and great muscular endurance.

It is peculiar that between these two events and a third which occurred a year after, everything should be a blank.

A little brother was then born to me, and he lay undressed upon a cushion, while my father cried with sobs. I had just completed my third year and could not understand why, the next day, this little thing was carried off in a black box. From that time I remember almost every day's life.

I very soon began to manifest the course of my natural tendencies. Like most little girls I was well provided with dolls, and on the day after a new one came into my possession I generally discovered that the dear little thing was ill and needed to be nursed and doctored.

Porridges and teas were accordingly cooked on my little toy stove, and administered to the poor doll until the *papier mâché* was thoroughly saturated and broken, when she was considered dead and preparations were made for her burial—this ceremony being repeated over and over again.

White dresses were put on for the funeral; a cricket was turned upside down to serve as the coffin; my mother's flower pots furnished the green leaves for decoration; and I delivered the funeral oration in praise of the little sufferer while placing her in the tomb improvised of chairs.

I hardly ever joined the other children in their plays except upon occasions like these, when I appeared in the characters of doctor, priest and undertaker; generally improving the opportunity to moralize, informing my audience that Ann (the doll) had died in consequence of disobeying her mother by going out before she had recovered from the measles, etc.

Once I remember moving my audience to tears by telling them that little Ann had been killed by her brother who, in amusing himself with picking off the dry skin after she had had the scarlatina, had carelessly torn off the real skin over the heart, as they could see; thus leaving it to beat in the air and causing the little one to die. This happened after we had all had the scarlatina.

CHAPTER II

Begins school life—Her conduct already guided by habits of reasoning and self-government—Conflict between such guidance and the school rule of unquestioning obedience to authority—First friendship with a girl—First contact with an insane person; changes an intractable patient to a docile one—Allowed to assist nurse in hospital in care of blind cousin—Observation of defects in hospital care arouses desire to be some day a head nurse, so as to prevent such defects and have patients treated more kindly. (Five to nine years of age: 1834-1838.)

WHEN five years old, I was sent to a primary school. Here I became a favorite of the teacher of arithmetic, for which study I had quite a fancy. The rest of the teachers disliked me. They called me unruly because I would not obey arbitrary demands without being given some reason, and obstinate because I insisted on following my own will when I knew I was in the right.

I was told that I was not worthy to be with my playmates; and when I reached the highest class in the school, in which alone the boys and the girls were taught separately, I was separated from the latter and placed with the boys by way of punishment, receiving instructions with them from men, while the girls in the other class were taught by women.

Here I found many friends. I joined the boys in

all their sports, sliding and snowballing with them in winter, and running and playing ball in summer. With them I was merry, frank and self-possessed, while with the girls I was quiet, shy and awkward. I never made friends with the girls or felt like approaching them.

Once only, when I was eleven years old, a girl in the young ladies' seminary in which I had been placed when eight years of age won my affection. This was Elizabeth Hohenhorst, a child of twelve, remarkably quiet and disposed to melancholy.

She was a devout Catholic, and knowing that she was fated to become a nun, was fitting herself for that dreary destiny, which rendered her very sentimental. She was full of fanciful visions, but extremely sweet and gentle in her manners. My love for her was unbounded. I went to church in her company, was present at all the religious festivals, and accompanied her to receive religious instruction: in short, I made up my mind to become a Catholic and, if possible, a nun like herself. My parents, who were Rationalists, belonging to no church, gave me full scope to follow out my own inclinations, leaving it to my nature to choose for me a fitting path.

This lasted until Elizabeth went for the first time to the confessional. And when the poor innocent child could find no other sin of which to speak than the friendship which she cherished for a Protestant, the priest forbade her to continue this, until I too had become a Catholic, reminding her of the holiness of her future career. The poor girl conscientiously promised to obey.

When I came the next morning and spoke to her as usual, she turned away from me and burst into tears. Surprised and anxious, I asked what was the matter. In a voice broken with sobs, she told me the whole story and begged me to become a Catholic as soon as I was fourteen years old.

Never in my whole life shall I forget that morning. For a moment, I gazed on her with the deepest emotion, pitying her almost more than myself; then suddenly turned coldly and calmly away without answering a single word. My mind had awakened to the despotism of theology and the church had lost its expected convert. I never went near her again and never exchanged another word with her. This was the only friend I had during eight and a half years of uninterrupted attendance at school.

A visit that I paid to my maternal grandfather when seven or eight years old made a strong impression on my mind.

My grandfather, on his return from the war of 1813-1815 in which he had served, had received from the authorities of Prenzlau (the city in which he lived) a grant of a half-ruined cloister with about a hundred acres of uncultivated land attached, by way of acknowledgment of his services. He removed thither with his family, and, shortly after, invited the widows of some soldiers who lived in the city to occupy the apartments which he did not need. The habitable rooms were soon filled to overflowing with widows and orphans, who went to work with him to cultivate the ground.

It was not long before crippled and invalid soldiers arrived, begging to be allowed to repair the cloister and to find a shelter also within its walls. They were set to work making brick, the material for which my grandfather had discovered on his land: and in about five years an institution was built, the more valuable from the fact that none lived there on charity but all earned what they needed by cultivating the ground; having first built their own dwelling which at this time looked like a palace surrounded·by trees, grass and flowers. Here, in the evening, the old soldiers sang martial songs or told stories of the wars to the orphans gathered about them, while resting from the labors of the day.

I tell you of this institution so minutely to prove to you how wrong it is to provide charitable homes for the poor as we provide them, homes in which the charity always humiliates and degrades the individual. Here you have an instance in which poor crippled invalids and destitute women and children established and supported themselves under the guidance of a clear-headed, benevolent man, who said, "Do what you like, but work for what you need." He succeeded admirably, though he died a very poor man, his younger children becoming inmates of the establishment until they were adopted by their relatives.

When I visited my grandfather, the "convent," as he insisted on calling it—rejecting any name that would have indicated a charitable institution—contained about a hundred invalid soldiers, a hundred old women and two hundred and fifty orphans. One of the wings of the building was fitted up as a hospital and a few of the rooms were occupied by lunatics.

It was my greatest delight to take my grandfather's hand at noon as he walked up and down the dining room between the long tables around which were grouped so many cheerful, hearty faces; and I stood before him with an admiration that it is impossible to describe as he prayed, with his black velvet cap in his hand, before and after dinner. Though I could not comprehend why he should thank another person for what had been done, when every one there told me that all that they had they owed to my grandfather.

One afternoon, on returning from the dining room to his study, I spied on his desk a neatly written manuscript. I took it up and began to read. It was a dissertation on immortality, attempting by scientific arguments to prove its impossibility. I became greatly interested, and read on without noticing that my grandfather had left the room or that the large bell had rung to call the family to dinner.

My grandfather, a very punctual man who would never allow lingering, came back to call and to reprimand me; he suddenly started on seeing the paper in my hands and snatching it from me tore it in pieces, exclaiming, "That man is insane, and will make this child so too!" A little frightened, I went to the dinner table, thinking as much about my grandfather's words as about what I had read, without daring, however, to ask who this man was.

The next day, curiosity mastered fear. I asked my grandfather who had written that paper, and was told in reply that it was poor crazy Jacob. I then begged to see him, but this request my grandfather decidedly refused, saying that he was like a wild beast and lay without clothes upon the straw. I knew nothing of lunatics, and the idea of a wild man stimulated my curiosity to such an extent that from that time I teased my grandfather incessantly to let me see Jacob. He finally yielded to be rid of my importunity and led me to the cell in which he was confined. What a spectacle presented itself in the house that I had looked on as the abode of so much comfort! On a bundle of straw in a corner of the room, with no furniture save its bare walls, sat a man clad only in a shirt, with the left hand chained to the wall and the right foot to the floor. An inkstand stood on the floor by his side, and on his knee was some paper on which he was writing. His hair and beard were uncombed, and his fine eyes glared with fury as we approached him. He tried to rise, ground his teeth, made grimaces, and shook his fist at my grandfather, who tried in vain to draw me out of the room.

But, escaping from his grasp, I stepped towards the lunatic who grew more quiet when he saw me approach, and I tried to lift the chain which had attracted my attention. Then, finding it too heavy for me, I turned to my grandfather and asked, "Does not this hurt the poor man?" I had hardly spoken the words when his fury returned, and he shrieked:

"Have I not always told you that you were cruel to me? Must this child come to convince you of your barbarity? Yes, you have no heart."

I looked at my grandfather: all my admiration of him was gone, and I said, almost commandingly:

"Take off these chains! It is bad of you to tie this man!"

The man grew calm at once and asked imploringly to be set free, promising to be quiet and tractable if my grandfather would give him a trial. His chains were removed the same day, and Jacob was ever after not only harmless and obedient but a very useful man in the house.

I never afterwards accompanied my grandfather. I had discovered a side in his nature which repelled me. I spent the remainder of my visit in the work rooms and the sick room, always secretly fearing that I should meet with some new cruelty, but no such instance ever came to my view.

On my return from my grandfather's I found that a cousin had suddenly become blind. She was soon after sent to the ophthalmic hospital, where she remained for more than a year, and, during this time, I was her constant companion after school hours. I was anxious to be useful to her; and being gentler than the nurse, she liked to have me wash out the issues that were made in her back and arms. The nurse, who was very willing to be relieved of this duty, allowed me also to cleanse the eyes of the girl next my cousin; and thus these cares were soon made to depend on my daily visit.

Child as I was, I could not help observing the carelessness of the nurses and their great neglect of cleanliness. One day, when the head nurse had washed the floor and left pools of water standing under the beds, the under nurse found fault with it, and said, "I shall tell the doctor when he comes why it is that the patients always have colds." "Do," said the head nurse. "What do men understand of such matters? If they knew anything about them, they would long ago have taken care that the mattress upon which one patient dies should always be changed before another comes in.''

This quarrel impressed itself upon my memory, and the wish rose in my mind that some day I might be a head nurse to prevent such wrongs and to show kindness to poor lunatics.

CHAPTER III

School life continues—Her mother begins training for career of midwife—Because of eye trouble, Marie resides in hospital with her mother, and becomes protégée of Dr. Müller—First real knowledge of medicine as a career—Adventure in morgue and dissecting rooms—Begins to read medical books. (Nine to eleven years of age: 1838-1840.)

AT the end of the year, my cousin left the hospital. At the same time, trouble and constant sickness fell upon our family.

My father, who held liberal opinions and was of an impetuous temperament, manifested some revolutionary tendencies, which drew upon him the displeasure of the government and caused his dismissal, with a very small pension, from his position as military officer. This involved us in great pecuniary difficulties, for our family was large and my father's income too small to supply the most necessary wants, and to obtain other occupation was for the time out of the question.

In this emergency, my mother determined to petition the city government for admission to the school of midwives established in Berlin, in order in this manner to aid in the support of the family. Influential friends of my father secured her the election, and she was admitted to the school in 1839, I being at that time ten years of age.

The education of midwives for Berlin requires a two years' course of study, during six months of which, they are obliged to reside in the hospital to receive instructions from the professors together with the male students. My mother went there in the summer of 1840. I went to stay at the house of an aunt who wished my company, and the rest of the children were put out together, to board.

In a few weeks my eyes became affected with weakness so that I could neither read nor write, and I begged my mother to let me stay with her in the hospital. She applied for permission to the director and received a favorable answer.

I was placed under the care of one of the physicians (Dr. Müller), who took a great fancy to me and made me go with him wherever he went while engaged in the hospital. My eyes being bandaged, he led me by the hand, calling me his "little blind doctor." In this way, I was constantly with him, hearing all his questions and directions, which impressed themselves the more strongly on my mind from the fact that I could not see but had to gain all my knowledge through hearing alone.

One afternoon, when I had taken the bandage off my eyes for the first time, Dr. Müller told me that there was a corpse of a young man in the dead-house that had turned completely green in consequence of poison that he had eaten. I went there after my rounds with him, but finding the room filled with relatives who were busily engaged in adorning the body with flowers, I thought that I would not disturb them but would wait until they had gone before I looked at it; meanwhile I went through the adjoining rooms.

These were all freshly painted. The dissecting tables, with the necessary apparatus, stood in the center, while the bodies, clad in white gowns, were ranged on boards along the walls. I examined everything, came back, and looked to my heart's content at the poisoned young man, without noticing that, not only had the relatives left but the prosector had also gone away, after locking up the whole building.

I then went a second time to the other rooms, and looked again at everything there; and at last, when it became dark and I could not leave the house, sat down upon the floor and went to sleep, after knocking for half an hour at the door in the hope that some passer might hear.

My mother, who knew that I had gone with Dr. Müller, did not trouble herself about me until nine o'clock, when she grew uneasy at my stay; and, thinking that he might have taken me to his rooms, went there in search of me, but found that he was out and that the doors were locked. She then inquired whether the people in the house knew anything about me, and was told that they had last seen me going into the dead-house. Alarmed at this intelligence, my mother hastened to the prosector, who unwillingly went with her to the park in which the dead-house stood, assuring her all the way that I could not possibly be there; but, on opening the door, he saw me sitting close by on the floor fast asleep.

In a few days after this adventure, I recovered

the use of my eyes. As it was at this time the summer vacation in which I had no school tasks, I asked Dr. Müller for some books to read. He inquired what kind of books I wanted. I told him, "Books about history," upon which he gave me two huge volumes, the *History of Midwifery* and the *History of Surgery*. Both were so interesting that I read them through during the six weeks of vacation, which occupied me so closely that even my friend Dr. Müller could not lay hold of me when he went his morning and evening rounds.

From this time I date my study of medicine, for though I did not continue to read on the subject, I was instructed in the no less important branch of psychology by a new teacher whom I found on my return to school at the close of the summer vacation.

CHAPTER IV

Takes highest prizes at school—Helpful friendship with one of her men teachers—Begins to understand relation of public opinion to personal conduct—School life ends. (Eleven to fourteen years of age: 1840-1843.)

To explain better how my mind was prepared for such teaching, I must go back to my position in school. In both schools that I attended I was praised for my punctuality, industry and quick perception. Beloved I was in neither. On the contrary, I was made the target for all the impudent jokes of my fellow pupils, ample material for which was furnished in the carelessness with which my hair and dress were usually arranged, these being left to the charge of a servant who troubled herself very little about how I looked, provided I was whole and clean.

The truth was, I often presented a ridiculous appearance; and once I could not help laughing heartily at myself on seeing my own face by accident in a glass, with one braid of hair commencing over the right eye and the other over the left ear. I quietly hung a map over the glass to hide the ludicrous picture and continued my studies, and most likely appeared in the same style the next day.

My face, besides, was neither handsome nor even prepossessing, a large nose overshadowing the undeveloped features; and I was ridiculed for my ugli-

ness both in school and at home, where an aunt of
mine who disliked me exceedingly always said in
describing plain people, "Almost as ugly as Marie."

Another cause arose to render my position at
school still more intolerable. In consequence of the
loss of his position in the army, my father could no
longer afford to pay my school bills, and was about
to remove me from school, when the principal offered to retain me without pay. She disliked me
and did not hesitate to show it, nor to tell me whenever I offended her that she would never keep so
ugly and naughty a child *without being paid for it,*
were it not for the sake of so noble a father.

These conditions and harsh judgments made me a
philosopher. I heard myself called obstinate and
willful, only because I believed myself in the right
and persisted in it. I felt that I was not maliciously
disposed towards any one but wished well to all, and
I offered my services not only willingly, but cheerfully wherever they could be of the least use, and
saw them accepted, and even demanded, by those
who could not dispense with them, though they
shunned and ridiculed me the same as before. I
felt that they sought me only when they needed me;
this made me shrink still more from their companionship, and, when my sister did not walk home
from school with me, I invariably went alone.

The idea that I might not wish to attach myself
to playmates of this sort never occurred to any one,
but I was constantly reproached with having no
friends among my schoolfellows, and was told that
no one could love so disagreeable and repelling a
child. This was a severe blow to my affectionate

nature, but I bore it calmly, consoling myself with the thought that they were wrong, that they did not understand me, and that the time would come when they would learn that a great, warm heart was concealed beneath the so-called repulsive exterior.

But, however soothing all this was for the time, a feeling of bitterness grew up within me. I began to be provoked at my ugliness, which I believed to be excessive. I speculated why parents so kind and good as mine should be deprived of their means of support merely because my father would not consent to endure wrong and imposition. I was indignant at being told that it was only for my father's sake that I was retained in a school where I tried to do my best and where I always won the highest prizes; and I could not see why, at home, I should be forced to do housework when I wanted to read, while my brother who wished to work was compelled to study. When I complained of this last grievance, I was told that I was a girl and never could learn much, but was only fit to become a housekeeper.

All these things threw me upon my own resources and taught me to make the most of every opportunity, custom and habit to the contrary notwithstanding.

It was at this juncture that I found, on my return to school, the psychologic instructor of whom I have spoken, in a newly engaged teacher of history, geography and arithmetic, all of which were my favorite studies.

With this man I formed a most peculiar friendship, he being twenty years older than myself, and in every respect highly educated; I, a child of twelve, neglected in everything except my common-school education.

He began by calling my attention to the carelessness of my dress and the rudeness of my manners, and was the first one who ever spoke kindly to me on the subject.

I told him all my thoughts; that I did not mean to be disagreeable, but that every one thought that I could not be otherwise; that I was convinced I was good enough at heart; and that I had at last resigned myself to my position as something that could not be helped.

My new friend lectured me on the necessity of attracting others by an agreeable exterior and courteous manners, and proved to me that I had unconsciously repelled them by my carelessness, even when trying the most to please. His words made a deep impression on me. I thanked him for every reproach, and strove to do my best to gain his approbation.

Henceforth, my hair was always carefully combed, my dress nicely arranged, and my collar in its place; and as I always won the first prizes in the school, two of the other teachers soon grew friendly towards me and began to manifest their preference quite strongly.

In a few months, I became a different being. The bitterness that had been growing up within me gradually disappeared, and I began to have confidence in myself and to try to win the companionship of the other children.

But a sudden change took place in my schoolmates,

who grew envious of the preference shown me by the teachers. Since they could no longer ridicule me for the carelessness of my dress, they now began to reproach me for my vanity and to call me a coquette who only thought of pleasing through appearances.

This blow was altogether too hard for me to bear. I knew that they were wrong, for with all the care I bestowed on my dress, it was not half so fine as theirs, as I had but two calico dresses which I wore alternately, a week at a time, through the summer. I was again repelled from them; and at noon, when the rest of the scholars went home, I remained with my teacher-friend in the schoolroom, assisting him in correcting the exercises of the pupils.

I took the opportunity to tell him of the curious envy that had taken possession of the girls, upon which he began to explain to me human nature and its fallacies, drawing inferences therefrom for personal application. He found a ready listener in me. My inclination to abstract thought, combined with the unpleasant experience I had had in life, made me an attentive pupil and fitted me to comprehend his reasoning in the broadest sense.

For fifteen months, I thus spent the noon hour with him in the schoolroom, receiving lessons in logic and reasoning upon concrete and abstract matters that have since proved of far more psychologic value to me than ten years of reading on the same subjects.

A strong attachment grew up between us: he became a necessity to me, and I revered him like an oracle. But his health failed, and he left the school at the end of these fifteen months in a consumption.

Shortly after, he sent to the school for me one morning to ask me to visit him on his deathbed. I was not permitted to leave the class until noon; when, just as I was preparing to go, a messenger came to inform the principal that he had died at eleven.

This blow fell so heavily upon me that I wished to leave the school at once. I was forced to stay three weeks longer, until the end of the quarter, when I left the schoolroom on the first of April, 1843, at the age of thirteen years and seven months, and never entered it again.

CHAPTER V

Training in all details of housework—After mastering them, spends most of time reading in father's library —Gradually begins assisting mother in care of patients —Contact with the heights and depths of human nature, from dens to palaces—Nurses two aunts and keeps house for their family—Dr. Arthur Lutze guides her reading in homeopathy and mesmerism— Attack of "brain fever"—Father burns books from Dr. Lutze—Marie learns French, plain sewing, dressmaking and the management of the household, while continuing to assist in mother's practice. (Fourteen to eighteen years of age: 1843-1847.)

On the same day that I quitted my school, an aunt with whom I was a favorite was attacked with a violent hemorrhage from the lungs, and wished me to come to stay with her. This suited my taste. I went, and for a fortnight was her sole nurse.

Upon my return home, my father told me that, having quitted school, I must now become a thorough housekeeper of whom he might be proud, as this was the only thing for which girls were intended by nature. I cheerfully entered upon my new apprenticeship, and learned how to sweep, to scrub, to wash and to cook. This work answered very well as long as the novelty lasted, but as soon as this wore off, it became highly burdensome.

Many a forenoon when I was alone, instead of sweeping and dusting, I passed the hours in reading

26

books from my father's library, until it grew so late that I was afraid that my mother, who had commenced practice, would come home and scold me for not attending to my work, when I would hurry to get through, doing everything so badly that I had to hear daily that I was good for nothing and a nuisance in the world; and that it was not at all surprising that I was not liked in school, for nobody could ever like or be satisfied with me.

Meanwhile, my mother's practice gradually increased, and her generous and kindly nature won the confidence of hundreds who, wretchedly poor, found in her not only a humane woman but a most skillful practitioner.

The poor are good judges of professional qualifications. Without the aid that money can buy, without the comforts that the wealthy hardly need, and without friends whose advice is prompted by intelligence, they must depend entirely upon the skill and humanity of those to whom they apply. Their life and happiness are placed in the hands of the physician and they jealously regard the one to whom they intrust them.

None but a good practitioner can gain fame and praise in this class, which is thought so easily satisfied. It is often said, "Oh! those people are poor and will be glad of any assistance." Far from it! There is no class so entirely dependent for their subsistence upon their strength and health. These constitute their sole capital, their stock in trade; and when sick, they anxiously seek out the best physicians, for, if unskillfully attended, they may lose their all, their fortune and their happiness.

My mother went everywhere, both night and day, and it soon came to pass that when she was sent for and was not at home I was deputed to go in search of her. In this way, I gradually became a regular appendage to my mother, going with her in the winter nights from place to place and visiting those whom she could not visit during the day.

I remember that in January, 1845, my mother attended thirty-five women in childbed—the list of names is still in my possession—and visited from sixteen to twenty-five daily, with my assistance. I do not think that, during the month, we were in bed for one whole night. Two thirds of these patients were unable to pay a cent.

During these years, I learned all of life that it was possible for a human being to learn. I saw nobleness in dens, and meanness in palaces; virtue among prostitutes, and vice among so-called respectable women. I learned to judge human nature correctly, to see goodness where the world found nothing but faults, and also to see faults where the world could see nothing but virtue.

The experience thus gained cost me the bloom of youth; yet I would not exchange it for a life of everlasting juvenescence. To keep up appearances is the aim of every one's life; but to fathom these appearances and to judge correctly of what is beneath them ought to be the aim of those who seek to draw true conclusions from life or to benefit others by real sympathy.

One fact I learned, both at this time and afterwards, namely, that men always sympathize with fallen and wretched women, while women themselves are the first to raise and cast the stone at them.

Why is this? Have not women as much feeling as men? Why, women are said to be made up entirely of feeling. How does it happen then that women condemn where men pity? Do they do this in the consciousness of their own superior virtue? Ah, no! for many of the condemning are no better than the condemned.

The reason is that men know the world, that is, they know the obstacles in the path of life, and they know that they draw lines to exclude women from earning an honest livelihood while they throw opportunities in their way to earn their bread by shame. All men are aware of this; therefore, the good as well as the bad give pity to those who claim it.

It is my honest and earnest conviction that the reason that men are unwilling for women to enter upon public or business life is not so much the fear of competition or the dread lest women should lose their gentleness, and thus deprive society of this peculiar charm, as the fact that they are ashamed of the foulness of life which exists outside of the house and home. The good man knows that it is difficult to purify it; the bad man does not wish to be disturbed in his prey upon society.

If I could but give to all women the tenth part of my experience, they would see that this is true, and would see, besides, that only faith in ourselves and in each other is needed to work out a reformation.

Let woman enter fully into business with its serious responsibilities and duties; let it be made as honorable and as profitable to her as to men; let her have an equal opportunity for earning competence and comfort—and we shall need no other purification of society. Men are no more depraved than women, or rather, the total depravity of mankind is a lie.

From the time of my leaving school until I was fifteen years old, my life was passed as I have described, in doing housework, attending the sick with my mother, and reading a few books of a scientific and literary character. At the end of this time, a letter came from an aunt of my mother's, who was ill and whose adopted daughter (who was my mother's sister) was also an invalid, requesting me to visit and nurse them. I went there in the fall.

This was probably the most decisive event of my life. My great-aunt had a cancer that was to be taken out. The other was suffering from a nervous affection which rendered her a confirmed invalid. She was a most peculiar woman, and a clairvoyant and somnambulist of the most decided kind. Though not ill-natured, she was full of caprices that would have exhausted the patience of the most enduring of mortals.

This aunt of mine had been sick in bed for seven years with a nervous derangement which baffled the most skillful physicians who had visited her. Her senses were so acute that one morning she fell into convulsions from the effect of distant music which she heard. None of us could perceive it, and we fully believed that her imagination had produced this result. But she insisted upon it, telling us that the music was like that of the Bohemian miners

who played nothing but polkas. I was determined
to ascertain the truth, and really found that in a
public garden one and a half miles from her house
such a troop had played all the afternoon. No public music was permitted in the city because the
magistrate had forbidden it on her account.

She never was a Spiritualist, though she frequently went into what is now called a trance.
She spoke, wrote, sang and had presentiments of
the finest kind while in this condition, far better
than I have ever seen here in America in the case
of the most celebrated mediums.

She even prescribed for herself with success, yet
she was not a Spiritualist. She was a somnambulist, and, though weak enough when awake, threatened several times to pull the house down by her
violence while in this condition. She had strength
like a lion and no man could manage her. I saw the
same thing in the hospital later.

This aunt is now healthy; not cured by her own
prescriptions or the magnetic or infinitesimal doses
of Dr. Arthur Lutze, but by a strong emotion which
took possession of her at the time of my great-
aunt's death. She is not sorry that she has lost all
these strange powers, but heartily glad of it.

When she afterwards visited us in Berlin, she
could speak calmly and quietly of the perversion to
which the nervous system may become subject if
managed wrongly; and she could not tell how glad
she was to be rid of all the emotions and notions she
had been compelled to dream out. Over-care and
over-anxiety had brought this about, and the same
causes could again bring on a condition which the

ancients deemed holy and which the psychologist treats as one bordering on insanity.

The old aunt was extremely suspicious and avaricious. Eight weeks after my arrival, she submitted to an operation. The operating surgeon found me so good an assistant that he intrusted me often with the dressing of the wound.

For six weeks, I was the sole nurse of the two, going from one room to the other both night and day, and attending to the household matters besides, with no other assistant than a woman who came every morning for an hour or two to do the rough work, while an uncle and a boy cousin were continually troubling me with their torn buttons, etc.

I learned in this time to be cheerful and lighthearted under all circumstances, going often into the anteroom to have a healthy, hearty laugh. My surroundings were certainly anything but inspiring. I had the sole responsibility of the two sick women —the one annoying me with her caprices, the other with her avarice. In one room, I heard fanciful forebodings; in the other, reproaches for having used a teaspoonful too much sugar. I always had to carry the key of the storeroom to the old aunt in order that she might be sure that I could not go in and eat bread when I chose. At the end of six weeks she died, and I put on mourning for the only time in my life, certainly not through grief.

In connection with the illness of my aunt I have mentioned Dr. Arthur Lutze. He was a disciple of Hahnemann, and I think a doctor of philosophy— certainly not of medicine. Besides being an infinitesimal homeopathist, this man was a devotee of

mesmerism. He became very friendly towards me
and supplied me with books, telling me that I would
not only make a good homeopathic physician but
also an excellent medium for mesmerism, magnetism, etc.

At all events, I was glad to get the books, which
I read industriously, and he constantly supplied me
with new ones so that I had quite a library when he
left the place, which he did before my return. He,
too, lived in Berlin, and inquired my residence, promising to visit me there and to teach me the art he
practiced.

I remained with my aunt until late in the spring,
when my health failed and I returned home. I was
very ill for a time with brain fever, but at last recovered and set to work industriously to search for
information in respect to the human body.

Dr. Lutze kept his word: he visited me at my
home, gave me more books, and directed my course
of reading. But my father, who had become reconciled to my inclination to assist my mother, was
opposed to homeopathy and especially opposed to
Dr. Arthur Lutze. He even threatened to turn him
out of the house if I permitted him to visit me again,
and burned all my books except one that I snatched
from the flames.

From this time, I was resolved to learn all that
I could about the human system. I read all the
books that I could get on the subject, and tried besides to educate myself in other branches.

My father was satisfied with this disposition, and
was glad to hear me propose to have a French
teacher in the house, both for my sake and for that

of the other children. I studied in good earnest by myself; at the same time, going through the usual discipline of German girls. I learned plain sewing, dressmaking and the management of the household, but was allowed to use my leisure time as I pleased.

When my sisters went skating, I remained at home to study; when they went to balls and theaters, I was thought the proper person to stay to watch the house. Having become so much older, I was now of great assistance to my mother in her business. No one complained any longer of my ugliness or my rudeness. I was always busy, and, when at liberty, always glad to do what I could for others; and though these years were full of hardships, I consider them among the happiest of my life. I was as free as it was possible for any German girl to be.

CHAPTER VI

*Decides to qualify herself as midwife—Meets great dif-
ficulties due to being unmarried and too young—
Studies privately under Dr. Schmidt—History and
organization of the School for Midwives: first school
established through Justina Ditrichin (obstetric surgeon and writer about 1735); after her death, owing
to the opposition of medical men, educated women
withdrew from the profession which then deterio-
rated; it became legally standardized in 1818 with the
present school, and women of the higher classes returned to the profession—Marie being refused for the
third time, Dr. Schmidt obtains an order from the
King for her admission to the school—Becomes assistant teacher under Dr. Schmidt—Receives diploma of
highest degree, and the class which she taught makes
the highest known record. (Eighteen to twenty-two
years of age: 1847-1851.)*

My household duties, however, continued distasteful to me, much to the annoyance of my father who
still contended that this was the only sphere for
woman. From being so much with my mother, I
had lost all taste for domestic life—anything out of
doors was preferable to the monotonous routine of
the household.

I at length determined to follow my inclinations
by studying, in order to fit myself to become a practitioner of midwifery, as is usual in Berlin.

My father was satisfied and pleased with this
idea, which opened the way to an independent, re-

spectable livelihood, for he never really wished to have us seek this in marriage.

My mother did not like my resolution at all. She practiced, not because she liked the profession, but because in this way she obtained the means of being independent and of aiding in the education of the children.

I persisted, however, in my resolution, and immediately took measures to carry it into effect by going directly to Dr. Joseph Hermann Schmidt, the Professor of Midwifery in the University and the School for Midwives, and Director of the Royal Hospital Charité; while my father, who for several years held the position of a civil officer, made the application to the city magistrates for me to be admitted as a pupil to the School for Midwives, in which my mother had been educated.

In order to show the importance of this step, it is necessary to explain more fully the history and organization of the school.

About 1735, Justina Ditrichin (the wife of Siegemund, a distinguished civil officer of Prussia) was afflicted with an internal disease which baffled the skill of the midwives, who had pronounced her pregnant, and none of whom could define her disorder. After many months of suffering, she was visited by the wife of a poor soldier, who told her what ailed her; in consequence of which, she was cured by her physicians.

This circumstance awakened in the mind of the lady an intense desire to study midwifery, which she did; and afterwards practiced it with such success that, in consequence of her extensive practice, she was obliged to confine herself solely to irregular cases. She performed all kinds of operations with masterly skill and wrote the first book on the subject ever published in Germany by a woman. She was sent for from all parts of Germany, and was appointed body-physician to the Queen and ladies of the court of Prussia and Mark Brandenburg.

Through her influence, schools were established in which women were instructed in the science and the art of obstetrics. She also taught many herself, and a very successful and respectable practice soon grew up among women. After her death, however, this was discountenanced by the physicians, who brought it into such disrepute by their ridicule that the educated class of women withdrew from the profession. This left it in the hands of ignorant pretenders who continued to practice it until 1818. At this time, public attention was called to the subject and strict laws were enacted by which women were required to call in a male practitioner in every irregular case of confinement, under penalty of from one to twenty years of imprisonment and the forfeiture of the right to practice.

These laws still continue in force. A remarkable case is recorded by Dr. Schmidt of a woman who, feeling her own competence to manage a case committed to her care, *did not* send for a male physician as the law required. Although it was fully proved that she had done everything that could have been done in the case, her penalty was imprisonment for twenty years. Two other cases are quoted by Dr. Schmidt, in which male practitioners were summoned before a legal tribunal. It was proved that

they *had not* done that which was necessary, yet
their penalty was no heavier than that inflicted on
the woman who had done exactly what she ought.

At this time (1818), it was also made illegal for
any woman to practice who had not been educated.
This brought the profession again into repute
among women of the higher classes. A school for
midwives, supported by the government, was established in Berlin, in which women have since continued to be educated for practice in this city and
in other parts of Prussia. Two midwives are elected
each year, by a committee, from the applicants, to
be educated for practice in Berlin. And as they
have to study two years, there are always four of
these students in the school, two graduating every
year. The remainder of the students are from the
provincial districts.

To be admitted to this school is considered a
stroke of good fortune, as there are generally more
than a hundred applicants, many of whom have to
wait eight or ten years before they are elected.
There is, besides, a great deal of favoritism, those
women being generally chosen who are the widows
or wives of civil officers or physicians, to whom this
chance of earning a livelihood is given in order that
they may not become a burden on the government.
Though educated apart from the male students
while studying the theory of midwifery, they attend
the accouchement ward together, and receive clinical or practical instruction in the same class from
the same professor.

The male students of medicine are admitted to the
university at the age of eighteen, having first been

required to go through a prescribed course of collegiate study and to pass the requisite examination. Here they attend the lectures of various professors, often of four or five upon the same subject, in order to learn how it is treated from different points of view. Then, after having thus studied for a certain length of time, they present themselves for an examination by the professors of the university, which confers upon them the title of *M.D.*, without the right to practice. They are then obliged to prepare for what is called the State's examination, before a Board of the most distinguished men in the profession appointed to this place by the government; these also constitute the medical court. Of this number, Dr. Schmidt was one.

Dr. Schmidt approved my resolution and expressed himself warmly in favor of it. He also recommended to me a course of reading, to be commenced at once as a kind of preliminary education. And although he had no influence with the committee of the city government who examined and elected the pupils, he promised to call upon some of them and urge my election. But despite his recommendation and my father's position as civil officer, I received a refusal, on the grounds that I was much too young (being only eighteen) and that I was unmarried.

The latter fault I did not try to remove; the former I corrected daily; and when I was nineteen, I repeated my application and received the same reply.

During this time, Dr. Schmidt became more and more interested in me personally. He promised

that he would do all in his power to have me chosen
the next year and urged me to read and study as
much as possible in order to become fully acquainted
with the subject.

As usual, I continued to assist my mother in visiting her patients, and thus had a fine opportunity
for explaining to myself many things which the mere
study of books left in darkness. In fact, these years
of preliminary practical study were more valuable
to me than all the lectures that I ever listened to
afterwards. Full of zeal and enthusiasm and stimulated by a friend whose position and personal ac-
quirements inspired me with reverence and devotion, I thought of nothing else than how to prepare
myself in such a way that I should not disappoint him nor those to whom he had commended
me.

Dr. Schmidt was consumptive and almost an invalid, often having to lecture in a reclining position.
The author of many valuable medical works and
director of the largest hospital in Prussia (the
Charité of Berlin), he found a most valuable assistant in his wife—one of the noblest women that
ever lived. She was always with him except in
the lecture room, and almost all of his works
are said to have been written by her from his
dictation.

This had inspired him with the highest possible
respect for women. He had the utmost faith in their
powers when rightly developed, and always declared their intellectual capacity to be the same with
that of men. This belief inspired him with the desire to give me an education superior to that of the

common midwives; and at the same time, to reform the school of midwives by giving to it a professor of its own sex.

To this position he had in his own mind already elected me. But before I could take it, I had to procure a legitimate election from the city to the school as pupil, and during my attendance, he had to convince the government of the necessity of such a reform, as well as to bring over the medical profession. This last was not so easily done, for many men were already waiting for Dr. Schmidt's death in order to obtain this very post which was considered valuable.

When I was twenty, I received my third refusal. Dr. Schmidt, whose health was failing rapidly, had exerted himself greatly to secure my admission. The medical part of the committee had promised him that they would give me their vote, but some theological influence was set to work to elect one of the deaconesses in my stead, so that she might be educated for the post of superintendent of the lying-in ward of the hospital which was under Dr. Schmidt's care. She also was rejected in order not to offend Dr. Schmidt, but for this he would not thank them.

No sooner had I carried him the letter of refusal than he ordered his carriage and, proceeding to the royal palace, obtained an audience with the king, to whom he related the refusal of the committee to elect me on the ground that I was too young and unmarried, and entreated of him a cabinet order which should compel the city to admit me to the school, adding that he saw no reason why

Germany as well as France should not have and be proud of a Lachapelle.

The king, who held Dr. Schmidt in high esteem, gave him at once the desired order, and I became legally the student of my friend. His praise, however, procured me intense vexation, for my name was dropped entirely and I was only spoken of as Lachapelle the Second, which would by no means have been unpleasant had I earned the title, but to receive it sneeringly in advance before having been allowed to make my appearance publicly, was indeed unbearable.

On the third day after his visit to the king, Dr. Schmidt received me into the class and introduced me to it as his future assistant teacher. This announcement was as surprising to me as to the class, but I took it quietly, thinking that if Dr. Schmidt did not consider me fit for the place, he would not risk being attacked for it by the profession *en masse,* by whom he was watched closely.

On the same day, a little incident occurred which I must mention. In the evening, instead of going alone to the class for practical instruction, I accompanied Dr. Schmidt at his request. We entered the hall where his assistant, the chief physician, had already commenced his instructions. Dr. Schmidt introduced me to him as his private pupil to whom he wished him to give particular attention, ending by giving my name. The physician hurriedly came up to me and grasped my hand, exclaiming, "Why, this is my little blind doctor!" I looked at him and recognized the very Dr. Müller with whom I used to make the rounds of the hospital when I was twelve years old, and who had since risen to the position of chief physician. This *rencontre* and the interest that he manifested afterwards greatly relieved Dr. Schmidt who had feared that he would oppose me instead of giving me any special aid.

During this winter's study, I spent the most of the time in the hospital, being almost constantly at the side of Dr. Schmidt. I certainly made the most of every opportunity, and I scarcely believe it possible for any student to learn more in so short a time than I did during this winter. I was continually busy, acting even as nurse whenever I could learn anything by it. During the following summer, I was obliged to reside wholly in the hospital, this being a part of the prescribed education. Here I became acquainted with all the different wards and had a fine opportunity to watch the cases by myself.

In the meantime, Dr. Schmidt's illness increased so rapidly that he feared he might die before his plans in respect to me had been carried out, especially as the state of his health had compelled him to give up his position as Chief Director of the Hospital Charité. His intention was to make me chief accoucheuse in the hospital, and to surrender into my hands his position as professor in the School for Midwives, so that I might have the entire charge of the midwives' education.

The opposition to this plan was twofold. First, the theological influence that sought to place the deaconess (Sister Catherine) in the position of house-midwife; and, second, the younger part of the profession, many of whom were anxious for the post of professor in the School for Midwives, which never would have been suffered to fall into the hands of Sister Catherine. Dr. Schmidt, however, was determined to yield to neither. Personal pride demanded that he should succeed in his plan, and several of the older and more influential members of the profession took his part, among whom were Johannes Müller, Busch, Müller, Kilian, etc.

During the second winter, his lecturing in the class was only nominal, often nothing more than naming the heads of the subjects while I had to give the real instruction. His idea was to make me feel the full responsibility of such a position, and at the same time to give me a chance to do the work that he had declared me preëminently capable of doing. This was an intrigue, but he would not have it otherwise. He did not intend that I should perform his duty for his benefit, but for my own. He wished to show to the government the fact that I had done the work of a man like himself and had done it well; and that, if he had not told them of his withdrawal, no one would have recognized his absence from the result.

At the close of this term, I was obliged to pass my examination at the same time with the fifty-six students who composed the class. Dr. Schmidt invited some of the most prominent medical men to be present, besides those appointed as the examining committee. He informed me of this on the day before the examination, saying, "I want to convince them that you can do better than half of the young men at *their* examination."

The excitement of this day I can hardly describe. I had not only to appear before a body of strangers of whose manner of questioning I had no idea, but also before half a dozen authorities in the profession, assembled especially for criticism.

Picture to yourself my position: standing before the table at which were seated the three physicians composing the examining committee, who questioned in the most perplexing manner, while four other physicians of the highest standing were seated on each side, making eleven in all; Dr. Schmidt, a little way off, anxious that I should prove true all that he had said in praise of me, and the rest of the class in the background, filling up the large hall. It was terrible. The trifling honor of being considered capable was rather dearly purchased.

I went through the whole hour bravely, without missing a single question, until finally the clock struck twelve, when everything suddenly grew black before my eyes, and the last question sounded like a humming noise in my ear. I answered it—how, I know not—and was permitted to sit down and rest for fifteen minutes before I was called to the practical examination on the manikin. I gave satisfaction to all, and received the diploma of the first degree.

This by no means ended the excitement. The students of the year were next examined. This examination continued for a week, after which the diplomas were announced, when it was found that never before had there been so many of the first degree and so few of the third. Dr. Schmidt then made it known that this was the result of my exertions, and I was pronounced *a very capable woman.*

CHAPTER VII

Dr. Schmidt urges Marie's appointment as Chief of the School, including the surrender to her of his own position as professor—Violent medical and diplomatic opposition, becoming a controversy over "Woman's Rights"—Marie's father refuses his consent and insists that she marry a man she has never even seen— Eventually, Dr. Schmidt wins and Marie receives her appointment—Triumph immediately turned to tragedy by sudden death of Dr. Schmidt on the same day. (Twenty-two years of age: 1851-1852.)

THE acknowledgment that I was a very capable woman having been made by the medical men present at the examination, Dr. Schmidt thought it would be an easy matter to get me installed into the position for which I had proved myself capable. But such could not be the case in a government ruled by hypocrisy and intrigue. To acknowledge the capability of a woman did not by any means say that she was at liberty to hold a position in which she could exercise this capability.

German men are educated to be slaves to the government: positive freedom is comprehended only by a few. They generally struggle for a kind of negative freedom, namely, for themselves. For each man, however much he may be inclined to show his subserviency to those superior in rank, thinks himself the lord of creation and, of course, regards woman only as his appendage. How can this lord

46

of creation, being a slave himself, look upon the
free development and *demand for recognition* of
his appendage otherwise than as a nonsense or a
usurpation of his exclusive rights?

And among these lords of creation, I heartily dis-
like that class which not only yield to the influence
brought to bear upon them by the government but
who also possess an infinite amount of narrowness
and vanity united to an infinite servility to money
and position. There is not ink and paper enough in
all the world to write down the contempt I feel for
men in whose power it is to be free in thought and
noble in action, and who yet act to the contrary to
feed their ambition or their purses. I have learned,
perhaps, too much of their spirit for my own
good.

You can hardly believe what I experienced in respect to intrigue within the few months following
my examination. All the members of the medical
profession were unwilling that a woman should take
her place on a level with them.

All the diplomatists became fearful that Dr.
Schmidt intended to advocate the question of
"Woman's Rights"; one of them exclaiming one
evening, in the heat of discussion, "For Heaven's
sake! the Berlin women are already wiser than all
the men of Prussia: what will become of us if we
allow them to manifest it?"

I was almost forgotten in the five months during
which the question was debated: it became more
than a matter of personal intrigue. The real question at stake was, "How shall women be educated,
and what is their true sphere?" And this was dis-

cussed with more energy and spirit than ever has been done here in America.

Scores of letters were written by Dr. Schmidt to convince the government that a woman could really be competent to hold the position in question, and that I had been pronounced so by the whole faculty.

The next objection raised was that my father was known as holding revolutionary principles; and to conquer this cost a long discussion, with many interviews of the officials with my father and Dr. Schmidt.

The next thing urged was that I was much *too young;* that it would be necessary, in the course of my duties, to instruct the young men also, and that there was danger in our thus being thrown together. In fact, this reason, read to me by Dr. Schmidt from one of the letters written at this time (all of which are still carefully preserved), runs thus, "To give this position to Miss M. E. Zakrzewska is dangerous. She is a prepossessing young lady, and from coming in contact with so many gentlemen must necessarily fall in love with some one of them, and thus end her career." To this, I have only to reply that I am sorry that I could not have found *one* among them that could have made me follow the suggestion.

This objection, however, seemed for a while the most difficult to be met, for it was well known that, when a student myself, I had stood on the most friendly terms with my fellow students. And that they had often taken my part in little disturbances that naturally came up in an establishment where no one was permitted to enter or to leave without giving a reason. Even my private patients were

sometimes sent away at the door because I did not
know of their coming and for this reason could not
announce to the doorkeeper the name and residence
of those who might possibly call.

That this difficulty was finally conquered, I have
to thank the students themselves. My relation with
these young men was of the pleasantest kind. They
never seemed to think that I was not of their sex,
but always treated me like one of themselves. I
knew of their studies and their amusements; yes,
even of the mischievous pranks that they were planning both for college and for social life. They often
made me their confidante in their private affairs,
and were more anxious for my approval or forgive-
ness than for that of their relatives. I learned during this time how great is the friendly influence of
a woman even upon fast-living and licentious young
men; and this has done more to convince me of the
necessity that the two sexes should live together
from infancy, than all the theories and arguments
that are brought to convince the mass of this fact.

As soon as it became known among the students
that my youth was the new objection, they treated
it in such a manner that the whole thing was transformed into a ridiculous bugbear, growing out of
the imagination of the *virtuous* opposers.

Nothing now seemed left in the way of my attaining to the position, when suddenly it dawned
upon the mind of some that I was irreligious, that
neither my father nor my mother attended church,
and that, under such circumstances, I could not of
course be a church-goer.

Fortunately, I had complied with the requirements of the law, and could therefore bring my certificate of confirmation from one of the Protestant churches. By the advice of Dr. Schmidt, I commenced to attend church regularly, and continued until a little incident happened which I must relate here.

One Sunday, just after the sermon was over, I remembered that I had forgotten to give instructions to the nurse in respect to a patient and I left the church without waiting for the end of the service. The next morning, I was summoned to answer to the charge of leaving the church at an improper time. The inquisitor (who was one of those who had accused me of irreligion), being vexed that I contradicted him by going to church regularly, was anxious to make me confess that I did not care for the service. But I saw through his policy as well as his hypocrisy, and simply told him the truth, namely, that I had forgotten important business and therefore thought it excusable to leave as soon as the sermon was over.

Whether he sought to lure me on to further avowals, I know not; but whatever was his motive, he asked me in reply whether I believed that he cared for the humdrum custom of church-going, and whether I thought him imbecile enough to consider this as anything more than the means by which to keep the masses in check, adding that it was the duty of the intelligent to make the affair respectable by setting the example of going themselves, and that he only wished me to act on this principle, when all accusations of irreligion would fall to the ground.

I had always known that this man was not my

friend, but when I heard this, I felt disenchanted with the whole world. I had never thought him more than a hypocrite, whereas I now found him the meanest of men both in theory and in practice. I was thoroughly indignant, the more so, since I felt guilty myself in going to church simply to please Dr. Schmidt.

I do not remember what answer I gave, but I know that my manners and words made it evident that I considered him a villain. He never forgave me for this, as all his future acts proved to me. For, in his position of chief director of the hospital, he had it in his power, more than any one else, to annoy me, and that he did so you will presently see.

The constant opposition and attendant excitement, together with the annoyances which my father, as civil officer, had to endure, made him resolve to present a declaration to the government that I should never, with his consent, enter the position. He had become so tired of my efforts to become a public character in my profession that he suddenly conceived the wish to have me married.

Now, take for a moment into consideration the facts that I was but twenty-two years of age, full of sanguine enthusiasm for my vocation, and strong in the friendship of Dr. Schmidt. He had inspired me with the idea of a career different from the common routine of domestic life.

My mother, overcoming her repugnance to my entering my profession, had been my best friend, encouraging me steadily; while my father, yielding to the troubles that it involved, had become disgusted with it, and wished me to abandon my career. He was stern, and would not take back his word. I could do nothing without his consent; while Dr. Schmidt had finally overcome all difficulties and had the prospect of victory if my father would but yield.

A few weeks of this life were sufficient to drive one mad, and I am sure that I was near becoming so. I was resolved to run away from home or to kill myself, while my father was equally resolved to marry me to a man whom I had never seen.

Matters finally came to a crisis through the illness of Dr. Schmidt, whose health failed so rapidly that it was thought dangerous to let him be longer excited by the fear of not realizing his favorite scheme. Some of his medical advisers influenced the government to appeal to my father to withdraw his declaration, which, satisfied with the honor thus done him, he did on the 1st of May, 1852.

On the 15th of May, I received my legal installment to the position for which Dr. Schmidt had designed me. The joy that I felt was great beyond expression. A youthful enthusiast of twenty-two, I stood at the height of my wishes and expectations. I had obtained what others could obtain only after the protracted labor of half a lifetime, and already I saw myself in imagination occupying the place of Dr. Schmidt's aspirations—that of a German *Lachapelle*.

No one who has not passed at the same age through the same excitement can comprehend the fullness of my rejoicing, which was not wholly selfish, for I knew that nothing in the world would please Dr. Schmidt so much as this victory. The wildest joy of an accepted suitor is a farce com-

pared to my feelings on the morning of that 15th of
May. I was reconciled to my bitterest opponents,
I could even have thanked them for their opposition, since it had made the success so much the
sweeter.

Not the slightest feeling of triumph was in my
heart; all was happiness and rejoicing. And it was
in this condition of mind and heart that I put on
my bonnet and shawl to carry the good news to Dr.
Schmidt. Without waiting to be announced, I
hastened to his parlor, where I found him sitting
with his wife upon the sofa. I did not walk, but
flew, towards them and threw the letter upon the
table, exclaiming, "There is the victory!"

Like a conflagration, my joy spread to Dr. Schmidt
as well as to his wife, who thought that she saw in
these tidings a cup of new life for her husband. I
stayed only long enough to accept their congratulations. Dr. Schmidt told me to be sure to come the
next morning to enter legally upon my duties at
his side. He saw that I needed the open air, and
felt that he too must have it to counteract his joy.
I went to tell my father and several friends, and
spent the day in blissful ignorance of the dreadful
event that was transpiring.

The next morning at seven o'clock, I left home to
go to my residence in the hospital. I had not slept
during the night; the youthful fire of enthusiasm
burnt too violently to allow me any rest.

The old doorkeeper opened the door for me, and
gazed at me with an air of surprise. "What is the
matter?" I asked. "I am astonished to see you so
cheerful," said he. "Why?" I asked with aston-

ishment. "Don't you know that Dr. Schmidt is dead?" was the answer. Dr. Schmidt dead! I trembled; I staggered; I fell upon a chair.

The beautiful entrance hall, serving also as a greenhouse during the winter, filled in every place with flowers and tropical fruit, faded from my eyes; and in its stead I saw nothing but laughing faces, distorted with scorn and mockery.

A flood of tears cooled the heat of my brain, and a calmness like that of death soon took possession of me. I had fallen from the topmost height of joy and happiness to the profoundest depth of disappointment and despair. If there was nothing else to prove the strength of my mind, the endurance of this sudden change would be sufficient.

I went at once to Dr. Schmidt's residence in the Hospital Park, where I met him again, not as I had expected an hour before ready to go with me to the hospital department which I was henceforth to superintend, but as a corpse.

After I had left the day before, he had expressed a wish to go into the open air, his excitement nearly equaling mine. Mrs. Schmidt ordered the carriage, and they drove to the large park. He talked constantly and excitedly about the satisfaction he felt in this success until they arrived, when he wished to get out of the carriage and walk with his wife. Mrs. Schmidt consented, but they had taken only a few steps when he sank to the ground, and a gush of blood from his mouth terminated his existence.

CHAPTER VIII

Death of Dr. Schmidt opens doors for hosts of office-seek-
ers and for Marie's opponents—Hostilities of latter
nullified by her methods, and by her continued pro-
fessional success with patients and with both men and
women students—After six months' struggle with un-
abated animosities and intrigue, she resigns her po-
sition in the hospital. (Twenty-three years of age:
1852.)

I LEFT Dr. Schmidt's house, and entered alone into
the wards, where I felt that I was without friendly
encouragement and support. During the three days
that intervened before the burial of Dr. Schmidt, I
was hardly conscious of anything, but moved about
mechanically like an automaton.

The next few days were days of confusion, for the
death of Dr. Schmidt had left so many places vacant
that some fifty persons were struggling to obtain
some one of his offices. The eagerness, servility and
meanness which these educated men displayed in
striving to conquer their rivals was more than dis-
gusting. The serpents that lie in wait for their
prey are endurable, for we know that it is their nature to be cunning and relentless; but to see men of
intellect and education sly and snaky, ferocious yet
servile to the utmost, makes one almost believe in
total depravity. The most of these men got what
they deserved, namely, nothing. The places were

filled temporarily with others, and everything went on apparently as before.

My position soon became very disagreeable. I had received my installment, not because I was wanted by the directors of the hospital, but because they had been commanded by the government to accept me, in the hope of thus prolonging the life of Dr. Schmidt.

Young and inexperienced in petty intrigue, I had now to work without friendly encouragement and appreciation, in an establishment where three thousand people were constantly at war about each other's affairs; with no one about me in whom I had a special interest, while every one was regretting that the installment had been given me before Dr. Schmidt's death which might have happened just as well from some other excitement. I surveyed the whole arena, and saw very well that, unless I practiced meanness and dishonesty as well as the rest, I could not remain there for any length of time, for scores were ready to calumniate me whenever there was the least thing to be gained by it.

I was about to commence a new period of life. I had a solid structure as a foundation, but the superstructure had been built up in so short a time that a change of wind would suffice to cast it down. I resolved, therefore, to tear it down myself and to begin to build another upon the carefully laid basis. I waited only for an opportunity to manifest my intention. This opportunity soon presented itself.

Sister Catherine, the deaconess of whom I have spoken, who had been allowed to attend the School for Midwives after my election, through the influ-

ence of her theological friends upon Dr. Schmidt
(the city magistrates having refused her because
I was already the third accepted pupil), had as yet
no position. These friends now sought to make her
the *second accoucheuse,* I having the first position,
with the additional title of Chief.

This she would not accept. She, the experienced
deaconess, who had been a Florence Nightingale
in the typhus epidemic of Silesia, was unwilling to
be under the supervision of a woman who had nothing to show but a thorough education, and who was
besides eight years younger than herself.

Her refusal made my enemies still more hostile.
Why they were so anxious for her services I can
only explain by supposing that the directors of the
hospital wished to annoy Pastor Fliedner, the originator of the Kaiserswerth Sisterhood. For, in placing Sister Catherine in this position, they robbed
him of one of the very best nurses that he had ever
had in his institution.

My desire to reconcile the government of the hospital, in order that I might have peace in my position to pursue my development and education so as
to realize and manifest to the people the truth of
what Dr. Schmidt had affirmed of me, induced me
to go to one of the directors and propose that Sister
Catherine should be installed on equal terms with
me, offering to drop the title of Chief and to consent that the department should be divided into two.

My proposition was accepted nominally, and Sister Catherine was installed but with a third less
salary than I received, while I had to give the daily
reports, etc., and to take the chief responsibility of

the whole. Catherine was quite friendly to me, and I was happy in the thought that there was now one at least who would stand by me should any difficulties occur. How much I was mistaken in the human heart! This pious, sedate woman, towards whom my heart yearned with friendship, was my greatest enemy, though I did not know it until after my arrival in America.

A few weeks afterwards, the city petitioned to have a number of women instructed in the practice of midwifery. These women were all experienced nurses who had taken the liberty to practice this art to a greater or less extent from what they had learned of it while nursing; and to put an end to this unlawful practice, they had been summoned before an examining committee, and the youngest and best educated were chosen to be instructed as the law required. Dr. Müller, the pathologist, was appointed to superintend the theoretical, and Dr. Ebert, the practical, instruction. Dr. Müller, who never had given this kind of instruction before, and who was a special friend of mine, immediately surrendered the whole into my hands; while Dr. Ebert, whose time was almost wholly absorbed in the department of the diseases of children, appointed me as his assistant. Both gentlemen gave me certificates of this when I determined to emigrate to America.

The marked preference for my wards that had always been shown by the male students was shared by these women when they came. Sister Catherine was neither ambitious nor envious, yet she felt that she was the second in place. Drs. Müller and Ebert never addressed themselves to her; neither did they impress the nurses and the servants with the idea that she was anything more than the head nurse. All these things together made her a spy; and though nothing happened for which I could be reproved, all that I said and did was watched and secretly reported.

Under a despotic government, the spy is as necessary as the corporal. The annoyance of this reporting is that the secrecy exists only for the one whom it concerns, while the subaltern officers and servants receive hints that such a person is kept under constant surveillance.

When it was found that no occasion offered to find fault with me, our administrative inspector was removed and a surly old corporal put in his place, with the hint that the government of the hospital thought that the former inspector did not perform his duty rightly, since he never reported disturbance in a ward that had formerly been notorious as being the most disorderly.

[Marie's method in transforming this ward and consequently its reputation is evidently described in the "Introduction" written by Mrs. Dall for these earlier chapters.

In the autumn of 1856, Marie was addressing a physiological institute in Boston. Mrs. Dall says:

She spoke to them of her experience in the hospital at Berlin, and showed that the most sinning, suffering woman never passed beyond the reach of a woman's sympathy and help.

Mrs. Dall then quotes from the address:

Soon after I entered the hospital [said Marie], the nurses called me to a ward where sixteen of the most forlorn objects had begun to fight with each other. The inspector and the young physician had been called to them, but dared not enter the *mêlée*. When I arrived, pillows, chairs, footstools and vessels had deserted their usual places; and one stout little woman, with rolling eyes and tangled hair, had lifted a vessel of slops which she threatened to throw all over me, as she exclaimed, "Don't dare to come here, you green young thing!"

I went quietly towards her, saying gently, "Be ashamed, my dear woman, of your fury."

Her hands dropped. Seizing me by the shoulder, she exclaimed, "You don't mean that you look on me as a woman?"

"How else?" I answered. She retreated to her bed while all the rest stood in the attitudes into which passion had thrown them.

"Arrange your beds," I said; "and in fifteen minutes, let me return and find everything right." When I returned, all was as I had desired, every woman standing at her bedside. The short woman was missing, but bending on each a friendly glance I passed through the ward, which never gave me any more trouble.

When, late at night, I entered my room, it was fragrant with violets. A green wreath surrounded an old Bible and a little bouquet rested on it. I did not pause to speculate over this sentimentality, but threw myself weary upon the bed when a light tap at the door startled me. The short woman entered and humbling herself on the floor, since she would not sit in my presence. entreated to be heard.

"You called me a woman," she said, "and you pity us. Others call us by the name the world gives us. You would help us, if help were possible. All the girls love you and are ashamed before you; and therefore *I* hated you—no: I will not hate you any longer. There was a time when I might have been saved—I, and Joanna, and Margaret, and Louise. We were not bad. Listen to me. If *you* say there is any hope, I will yet be an honest woman."

She had had respectable parents; and, when twenty years old, was deserted by her lover who left her three months pregnant. Otherwise kind, her family perpetually reproached her with her disgrace and threatened to send her away. At last, she fled to Berlin, keeping herself from utter starvation by needlework. In the hospital to which she went for confinement, she took the smallpox. When she came out, with her baby in her arms, her face was covered with red blotches. Not even the lowest refuge was open to her, her appearance was so frightful. With her baby dragging at her empty breast, she wandered through the streets. An old hag took pity on both, and carefully nursed till health returned, her good humor and native wit made those about her forget her ugly face. She was in a brothel, where she soon took the lead. Her child died, and she once more attempted to earn her living as a seamstress. She was saved from starvation only by her employer, who received her as his mistress. Now her luck changed. She suffered all that a woman could, handled poison and the firebrand. "I thought of stealing," she said, "only as an amusement; it was not exciting enough for a trade." She found herself in prison, and was amused to be punished for a trifle, when nobody suspected her crime. It was horrible to listen to these details; more horrible to witness her first repentance.

When I thanked her for her violets, she kissed my hands, and promised to be good.

While she remained in the hospital, I took her as my servant and trusted everything to her, and when finally discharged she went out to service. She wished to come with me to America. I could not bring her, but she followed, and when I was in Cleveland, inquired for me in New York.]

The truth was that in my innocence of heart I had been striving to gain the respect and friendship of my enemies by doing my work better than any before me had done. To go to bed at night regularly was a thing unknown to me. Once, I was not undressed for twenty-one days and nights; superintending and giving instructions on six or eight confinement cases in every twenty-four hours; lecturing three hours every afternoon to the class of midwives; giving clinical lectures to them twice a week for an hour in the morning; superintending the case of some twenty infants who were epidemically attacked with purulent ophthalmia; and having, besides, the general supervision of the whole department.

But all this could not overcome the hostility of my enemies, the chief cause of which lay in the mortification at having been vanquished by my appointment.

On the other hand, I was happy in the thought that Mrs. Schmidt continued to take the same interest in me as before, and was glad to hear of my partial success. The students, both male and female, were

devoted to me, and manifested their gratitude
openly and frankly. This was the greatest compensation that I received for my work.

The women wished to show their appreciation by
paying me for the extra labor that I performed in
their instruction, not knowing the fact that I did it
simply in order that they might pass an examination which should again convince the committee that
I was in the right place. I forbade all payment as I
had refused it to the male students when they wished
to pay me for their extra instruction on the manikin.
But in a true womanly way, they managed to learn
the date of my birthday, when two or three, instead
of attending the lecture, took possession of my room
which they decorated with flowers, while on the table
they displayed presents to the amount of some hundred and twenty dollars which the fifty-six women
of the class had collected among themselves.

This was, of course, a great surprise to me and
really made me feel sad, for I did not wish for things
of this sort. I wished to prove that unselfishness
was the real motive of my work, and thought that
I should finally earn the crown of appreciation from
my enemies for which I was striving. This gift
crossed all my plans. I must accept it, if I would
not wound the kindest of hearts, yet I felt that I
lost my game by so doing. I quietly packed everything into a basket and put it out of sight under
the bed, in order that I might not be reminded of
my loss.

Of course, all these things were at once reported.
I saw in the faces of many that something was in
agitation, and I waited a fortnight in constant ex-

pectation of its coming. But these people wished
to crush me entirely. They knew well that a blow
comes hardest when least expected, and they therefore kept quiet week after week until I really began to ask their pardon in my heart for having done
them the wrong to expect them to act meanly about
a thing that was natural and allowable.

In a word, I became quiet and happy again in the
performance of my duties; then suddenly, six weeks
after my birthday, I was summoned to the presence
of Director Horn (the same who had reprimanded me
for leaving the church). He received me with a face
as hard and stern as an avenging judge, and asked
me whether I knew that it was against the law to
receive any other payment than that given me by the
hospital. Upon my avowing that I did, he went on
to ask how it was then that I had accepted gifts on
my birthday.

This question fell upon me like a thunderbolt, for
I had never thought of looking upon these as a payment. If these women had paid me for the instruction that I gave them beyond that which was prescribed, they ought each one to have given me the
value of the presents. I told him this in reply and
also how disagreeable the acceptance had been to
me and how ready I was to return the whole at his
command, since it had been my desire to prove not
only my capability but my unselfishness in the work.

The man was ashamed—I saw it in his face as he
turned it away from me; yet he saw in me a proof
that he had been vanquished in intrigue, and he was
resolved that the occasion should end in my over-
throw.

Much more was said about the presents and their significance, and I soon ceased to be the humble woman and spoke boldly what I thought, in defiance of his authority, as I had done at the time of the religious conversation (by the way, I never attended church again after that interview).

The end was that I declared my readiness to leave the hospital.

He wished to inflict direct punishment on me and forbade me to be present at the examination of the class which was to take place the next day. This was really a hard penalty to which he was forced for his own sake. For if I had been present, I should have told the whole affair to men of a nobler stamp who would have opposed, as they afterwards did, my leaving a place which I filled to their entire satisfaction.

CHAPTER IX

She begins private practice—Mrs. Schmidt and many physicians plan to establish a Maternity Hospital for her—Her father renews his insistence that she should marry—Recollections of a report of the Female Medical College of Pennsylvania, located in Philadelphia, and of Dr. Schmidt's comment on it, turn her thoughts to America, and she decides to emigrate—She receives official acknowledgment of her work at the Hospital, together with a gift of money—Accompanied by a younger sister, she arrives in New York. (Twenty-four years of age: 1852-1853.)

I MADE my preparations to leave the hospital on the 15th of November, 1852. What was I to do? I was not made to practice quietly, as is commonly done; my education and aspirations demanded more than this. For the time, I could do nothing more than inform my patients that I intended to practice independently.

My father again wished that I should marry, and I began to ask myself whether marriage is an institution to relieve parents from embarrassment. When troubled about the future of a son, parents are ready to give him to the army; when in fears of the destiny of a daughter, they induce her to become the slave of the marriage bond. I never doubted that it was more unendurable and unworthy to be a wife without love than a soldier without a special calling for that profession, and I never could think of marriage as the means to procure a shelter and bread. I had so many schemes in my head that I would not listen to his words. Among these was especially the wish to emigrate to America.

The Pennsylvania Female Medical College had sent its first report to Dr. Schmidt, who had informed me as well as his colleagues of it and had advocated the justice of such a reform. It was in March, 1852, that he spoke of this, saying to those present, "In America, women will now become physicians, like the men; this shows that only in a republic can it be proved that science has no sex."

This fact recurred to my memory, and I decided to go to America to join in a work open to womanhood on a larger scale; and for the next two months, I did nothing but speculate how to carry out my design of emigration.

I had lived rather expensively and lavishly, without thinking of laying up any money; and my whole fortune, when I left the Charité, consisted of sixty dollars.

One thing happened in connection with my leaving the hospital which I must relate here. Director Horn was required to justify his conduct to the minister to whom the change had to be reported, and a committee was appointed to hear the accusation and to pass judgment upon the affair. As this was done in secrecy and not before a jury, and as the accuser was a man of high rank, I knew nothing of it until Christmas Eve when I received a document stating that, "as a gratification for my services for the benefit of the city of Berlin" in instructing the class of midwives, a compensation was decreed me of fifty dollars.

This was a large sum for Berlin, such as was given only on rare occasions. I was also informed that Director Horn was instructed to give me, should I ever demand it, a first-class certificate of what my position had been in the hospital, with the title of Chief attached.

For whatever I had suffered from the injustice of my enemies, I was now fully recompensed. I inquired who had taken my part so earnestly against Director Horn as to gain this action, and found that it was Dr. Müller the pathologist, backed by several other physicians. Director Horn, it was said, was greatly humiliated by the decision of Minister von Raumer, who could not see the least justice in his conduct in this matter, and had I not left the hospital so readily, I should never have stood so firmly as after this secret trial.

It was done, however, and I confidently told my mother of my design to emigrate. Between my mother and myself there existed not merely the strongest relation of maternal and filial love, but also a professional sympathy and peculiar friendship, which was the result of two similar minds and hearts, and which made me stand even nearer to her than as a child I possibly could have done. She consented with heart and soul, encouraged me in all my plans and expectations, and asked me at once at what time I would leave.

I next told my father and the rest of the family of my plan. My third sister (Anna), a beautiful, joyous young girl, exclaimed, "And I will go with you!'' My father, who would not listen to my going alone, at once consented to our going together. But I thought differently. In going alone, I risked only my own happiness; in going with her, I risked hers too, while I should be constantly restricted in my adventurous undertakings by having her, who knew nothing of the world save the happiness of a tranquil family life, with me.

The next day I told them that I had changed my mind and should not go away, but should establish myself in Berlin. Of course, I received a torrent of gibes on my fickleness, for they did not understand my feelings in respect to the responsibility that I feared to take for my younger sister.

I began to establish myself in practice. Mrs. Schmidt, who was anxious to assist me in my new career, suggested to those physicians who were my friends the establishment of a private hospital which should be under my care. She found them strongly in favor of the plan, and had I not been constantly speculating about leaving for America, this scheme would have been realized.

But Dr. Schmidt's words after reading the first report of the Philadelphia Female Medical College recurred to me again and again. I had resolved to emigrate, and I took my measures accordingly. I went secretly to Drs. Müller and Ebert and procured certificates attesting my position in respect to them in the hospital. I then obtained the certificate from Director Horn, and I carried them all to the American Chargé d'Affaires (Theodore S. Fay) to have them legalized in English, so that they would be of service to me in America.[2]

When I told Drs. Ebert and Müller and Mrs. Schmidt of my intention to emigrate, they pronounced me insane. They thought that I had the best field of activity open in Berlin and could not comprehend why I should seek greater freedom of person and of action.

Little really is known in Berlin about America, and to go there is considered as great an undertaking as to seek the river Styx in order to go to Hades. The remark that I heard from almost every quarter was, "What! you wish to go to the land of barbarism, where they have negro slavery and where they do not know how to appreciate talent and genius?"

But this could not prevent me from realizing my plans. I had idealized the freedom of America and especially the reform of the position of women, to such an extent that I would not listen to their arguments. After having been several years in America, very probably I would think twice before undertaking again to emigrate, for even the idealized freedom has lost a great deal of its charm when I consider how much better it could be.

Having put everything in order, I told my father of my conclusion to leave. He was surprised to hear of it the second time, but I showed him my papers in readiness for the journey and declared that I should go as soon as the ship was ready to sail, having a hundred dollars, just money enough to pay my passage.

He would not give his consent unless my sister Anna accompanied me, thinking her, I suppose, a counterpoise to any rash undertakings in which I might engage in a foreign land. If I wished to go, therefore, I was forced to have her company, of which I should have been very glad had I not feared the moral care and responsibility.

We decided to go in a fortnight. My father paid her passage and gave her a hundred dollars in cash, just enough to enable us to spend a short time in New York, after which he expected either to send us more money or that we would return; and, in case we did this, an agreement was made with the shipping merchant that payment should be made on our arrival in Hamburg.

On the 13th of March, 1853, we left the paternal roof, to which we should never return. My mother bade us adieu with tears in her eyes, saying, "*Au revoir* in America!" She was determined to follow us.

Here ends my Berlin and European life, and I can assure you that this was the hardest moment I ever knew. Upon my memory is forever imprinted the street, the house, the window behind which my mother stood waving her handkerchief. Not a tear did I suffer to mount to my eyes in order to make her believe that the departure was an easy one, but a heart beating convulsively within punished me for the restraint.

My father and brothers accompanied us to the depot, where the cars received us for Hamburg. On our arrival there, we found that the ice had not left the Elbe and that the ship could not sail until the river was entirely free. So we were forced to remain three weeks in Hamburg.

We had taken staterooms in the clipper ship *Deutschland*. Besides ourselves, there were sixteen passengers in the first cabin, people good enough in their way, but not sufficiently attractive to induce us to make their acquaintance. We observed a dead silence as to who we were, where we were going, or what was the motive of our emigrating to America. The only person that we ever spoke to was a Mr. R. from Hamburg, a youth of nineteen, who like ourselves had left a happy home in order to try his strength in a strange land.

The voyage was of forty-seven days' duration, excessively stormy but otherwise very dull, like all voyages of this kind, and had it not been for the expectations that filled our hearts, we should have died of *ennui*. As it was, the days passed slowly, made worse by the inevitable seasickness of our fellow-passengers, and we longed for the hour that should bring us in sight of the shores of the New World.

And now commences my life in America.

CHAPTER X

*First impressions of New York—Marie takes walk alone
the next day—Experience with a white slave agent—
Confronted with her ignorance of the English language, she postpones proceeding to Philadelphia—Begins housekeeping in a small apartment with her sister Anna—Astounded by hearing that "female physicians" have no professional standing in New York,
she puts out a sign and seeks private practice, as she
did in Berlin—While waiting for patients, she builds
up a business in making fancy worsted goods, Anna
works for a dressmaker, and they soon become self-
supporting. (Twenty-four years of age: 1853.)*

"DEAR Marie, best Marie! make haste to come
up on deck to see America! Oh, how pleasant it is
to see the green trees again! How brightly the sun
is gilding the land you are seeking—the land of
freedom!"

With such childlike exclamations of delight, my
sister Anna burst into my cabin to hasten my appearance on deck on the morning of the 22d of May,
1853. The beautiful child of nineteen summers was
only conscious of a heart overflowing with pleasure
at the sight of the charming landscape that opened
before her eyes after a tedious voyage of forty-
seven days upon the ocean.

We had reached the quarantine at Staten Island.
The captain, the old pilot, every one, gazed at her
as she danced joyously about the deck, with a

73

mingled feeling of sadness and curiosity, for our reserve while on shipboard had surrounded us with a sort of mystery which none knew how to unravel.

As soon as I had dressed for going on shore and had packed up the things that we had used on our voyage in order that they might not be stolen during this time of excitement, I obeyed the last call of my impatient sister to come at least to see the last rays of sunrise and went on deck, where I was at once riveted by the beautiful scene that was spread before my eyes.

It was a warm, glorious day. And the green sloping lawns with which the white cottages formed such a cheerful contrast; the trees clad in their first foliage, and suggesting hope by their smiling blossoms; the placid cows feeding quietly in the fields; the domestic chickens just visible in the distance; and the friendly barking of a dog—all seemed to greet me with a first welcome to the shores of this strange country; while the sun shining brightly from an azure sky strewn with soft white clouds mellowed the whole landscape, and so deeply impressed my soul that tears sprang to my eyes and a feeling rose in my heart that I can call nothing else than devotional, for it bowed my knees beneath me and forced sounds from my lips that I could not translate into words for they were mysterious to myself.

A stranger in a strange wide land, not knowing its habits and customs, not understanding its people, nor its workings and aims, yet my mind was not clouded with loneliness. I was happy. Had it not been my own wish that had made me leave the home of a kind father and of a mother beloved beyond all

earthly beings. I had succeeded in safely reaching
the shores of America. Life was again open before
me.

With these thoughts, I turned from the beautiful
landscape and finding the captain, a noble-hearted
sailor, inquired of him how long it would take us
to reach the port of New York. "That is New
York," said he, pointing to a dark mass of buildings
with here and there a spire towering in the air. "We
shall reach there about eight o'clock, but it is Sunday and you will have to stay on board till to-morrow." With this he turned away, calling his men
to weigh anchor, as the physician whose duty it was
to inspect the cargo of men, like cattle, had just left
in his boat.

On we went, my sister still dancing and singing for
joy; and Mr. R. and myself sitting somewhat apart,
he looking despondently into the water, and I with
my head firmly raised in the air, happy in heart, but
thoughtful in mind and trusting in my inward
strength for the future.

I took my breakfast on deck. No one seemed to
have any appetite, and I felt somewhat reproved
when I heard some one near me say, "She seems to
have neither head nor heart—see how tranquilly she
can eat at such a time as this!" These words were
spoken by one of the cabin passengers, a young man
who was exceedingly curious to know why I was
going to America and had several times tried to
make the rest of the passengers believe that it must
be in consequence of an unhappy love. The poor
simpleton! he thought that women could enter into
life only through the tragedy of a broken heart.

A bell sounded. We were opposite Trinity Church whose bell had just tolled eight. On our right were masses of brick houses and tall chimneys surrounded by a forest of masts; on our left were the romantic shores of New Jersey. Islands and projecting points of land, clad in the brilliant green of the fresh spring foliage, greeted the eye; ferryboats, like monstrous white swans, glided to and fro from the shores; rowboats plied everywhere, the white or red shirts of the oarsmen giving a bright touch of color to the ever-changing panorama. Such was the scene which gave us our first impressions of this new country, seeming to proclaim as its welcome freedom and hospitality to all newcomers.

This new civilization was utterly different from what we had been taught about the United States. Indeed, I think many of the passengers expected to see a *half-civilized* community who, under a rather anarchical state of government called a "republic," did just as each individual pleased, and who would greet every newcomer with an enthusiastic joy, inviting him to come and partake of all the good the country could offer.

Such, or similar, were the vague ideas which many passengers of the good ship *Deutschland* entertained no matter whether in the cabin or steerage. The captain had done his best to rectify these false expectations but with very little success, I am sure.

Therefore, the picture that unrolled itself as we approached slowly from the quarantine to the dock, while arousing the old enthusiasm that started the emigrants from their homes, brought also a kind of disappointment—a surprise to see a well-built and well-regulated "brick-house" city with all the accessories of a large commercial port; a city, in fact, to all appearances not very much unlike European cities. But the admiration with which I had gazed upon Staten Island was gone as I stood before this beautiful scene; the appreciation of nature was mastered by another feeling, a feeling of activity that had become my ideal.

I had come here for a purpose—to carry out the plan which a despotic government and its servile agents had prevented me from doing in my native city. I had to show to those men who had opposed me so strongly because I was a woman that, in this land of liberty, equality and fraternity, I could maintain that position which they would not permit to me at home. My talents were in an unusual direction. I was a physician, and, as such, had for years moved in the most select circles of Berlin. Even my enemies had been forced to give me the highest testimonials, and these were the only treasure that I brought to this country, for I had given my last dollar to the sailor who brought me the first news that land was in sight.

I looked again upon New York, but with a feeling that a great mystery was lying before my eyes—a feeling that was confirmed by the men who came off to the ship in small boats speaking a language that seemed like a chaos of sounds.

Then, though standing before the promised land of freedom and in spite of all youthful enthusiasm and vigor, a sadness overcame me, especially one which bordered very closely on homesickness, even before my foot had been once more planted on *terra firma.*

As I turned, I saw my sister coming slowly up from the cabin with a changed air; and I asked her with surprise what was the matter. "O Marie!" said she, "most of the passengers are called for. Mr. R.'s brother has just come to take him on shore. He was so glad to see him (for he thought he was in New Orleans), that I think he will forget to say good-by. I am afraid that we shall have to stay here all alone, and——" "Are the Misses Zakrzewska on board?" called a voice from a little boat by the side of the ship. We looked down in surprise but did not recognize the man, who spoke as if he were an acquaintance. The captain answered, "Yes." Upon which the same voice said, "Mr. G. requests them to wait; he will be here in a moment."

This announcement surprised us the more that it came from a totally unexpected quarter. An acquaintance of ours, who had emigrated to New York a few years before and had shortly after married a Mr. G. had heard from her brother in Berlin of our departure for America in the ship *Deutschland,* and these good people, thinking that they could be of use to us in a new country, had been watching for its arrival.

No one on board dared ask a question as to who our friends were, so reserved had we been in regard to our plans. Only the young man who had accused me of having neither head nor heart said, half aside, "Ah ha! Now we know the reason why Miss Marie ate her breakfast so calmly, while her sister danced for joy. They had beaus who were expecting them." "Simpleton!" thought I, "must women always have beaus in order to be calm about the future?"

Mr. G. came on board in a few minutes, bringing us from his wife an invitation of welcome to her house. I cannot express in words the emotion awakened in my heart by the really unselfish kindness that had impelled these people to greet us in this manner; and this was increased when we reached their very modest dwelling, consisting of a large shop in which Mr. G. carried on his business of manufacturing fringes and tassels, one sitting room, a bedroom and a small kitchen. My strength left me, and my composure dissolved in a flood of tears. The good people did all that they could to make us feel at home, and insisted that we should occupy the sitting room until we had decided what to do further. Of course, I determined that this should be for as short a time as possible, and that we would immediately look out for other lodgings. But for the moment, nothing but pleasure was in our hearts. Questions and answers concerning friends and relations at home filled every minute, and joy and thankfulness to be safe and sound on land quickened the heart beats.

One-half of this first day was spent in talking about home; the other, in making an excursion to Hoboken. This visit we would gladly have dispensed with, so exhausted were we by the excitement that we had passed through since sunrise, but our friends were bent on entertaining us with stories and sights of the New World, and we followed them rather reluctantly. I have since been glad that I did so, **for** my mind was in a state that rendered it far more impressible than usual and therefore better fitted to observe much that would have been lost to me in a less-excited condition.

Here I first saw the type of common German life on Sunday in America, and I saw enough of it on that one Sunday afternoon to last a whole lifetime. My friends called on several of their acquaintances. Everywhere that we went, I noticed two peculiarities—comparative poverty in the surroundings and apparent extravagance in the manner of living. For in every house we found an abundance of wine, beer, cake, meat, salad, etc., although it was between the hours of meals; and every one was eating, although no one seemed hungry. At nine o'clock in the evening, the visit was concluded by going to a hotel, where a rich supper was served up to us; and at eleven at night we returned home.

My work in America had already commenced. Was it not necessary for a stranger in a new country to observe life in all its phases before entering upon it? It seemed so to me, and I had already planned while on shipboard to spend the first month in observations of this kind. I had made a fair beginning, and when I saw many repetitions of this kind of life among my countrymen, I feared that this was their main purpose in this country and their consolation for the loss of the entertainments and recreations which their fatherland offered to them.

But as soon as I got opportunity to make my observations among the educated classes, I found my fear ungrounded; and I also found that the Americans had noticed the impulse for progress and higher development which animated these Germans. The German mind, so much honored in Europe for its scientific capacity, for its consistency regarding principles and for its correct criticism, is not dead here. But it has to struggle against difficulties too numerous to be detailed here, and therefore it is that the Americans do not know of its existence, and the chief obstacle is their different languages. A Humboldt must remain unknown here unless he chooses to Americanize himself in every respect— and could he do this without ceasing to be Humboldt, the cosmopolitan genius?

It would be a great benefit to the development of this country if the German language were made a branch of education and not simply an accomplishment. Only then would the Americans appreciate how much has been done by the Germans to advance higher development and to diffuse the true principles of freedom. It would serve both parties to learn how much the Germans aid in developing the reason and in supporting progress in every direction. The revolution of 1848 has been more serviceable to America than to Germany, for it has caused the emigration of thousands of men who would have been the pride of a free Germany. America has received the German freemen, whilst Germany has retained the *subjects*.

The next morning, I determined to return to the ship to look after my baggage. As Mr. and Mrs. G. were busy in their shop, there was no one to accompany me. I therefore had either to wait until they were at leisure or to go alone. I chose the latter, and took my first walk in the city of New York

on my way to the North River where the ship was
lying. The noise and bustle everywhere about me
absorbed my attention to such a degree that instead
of turning to the right, I went to the left and found
myself at the East River, in the neighborhood of
Peck Slip. Here I inquired after the German ship
Deutschland and was directed, in my native tongue,
down to the Battery and thence up to Pier 13, where
I found the ship discharging the rest of her passengers and their baggage. It was eleven o'clock
when I reached the ship; I had, therefore, taken a
three hours' walk. I had now to wait until the cus-
tom-house officer had inspected my trunk, and afterwards for the arrival of Mr. G., who came at one
o'clock with a cart to convey the baggage to his
house.

While standing amidst the crowd, a man in a light
suit of clothes of no positive color and with a complexion of the same sort, came up to me and asked
in German whether I had yet found a boarding-place.
The man's smooth face instinctively repelled me,
yet the feeling that I was not independently established made me somewhat indefinite in my reply.
On seeing this, he at once grew talkative and friendly
and speaking of the necessity of finding a safe and
comfortable home, said that he could recommend
me to a hotel where I would be treated honestly; or
that, if I chose to be in a private family, he knew
of a very kind, motherly lady who kept a boarding
house for ladies alone, not to make money but for
the sake of her countrywomen.

The familiarity that he mingled in his conversation while trying to be friendly made me thoroughly

indignant. I turned my back upon him, saying that I did not need his services.

It was not long before I saw him besieging my sister Anna, who had come with Mr. G., being nervous lest I might not have found the ship. What he said to her, I do not know. I only remember that she came to me, saying, "I am afraid of that man; I wish that we could go home soon."

This meeting with a man who makes friendly offers of service may seem a small matter to the mere looker-on, but it ceases to be so when one knows his motives. And since that time, I have had but too many opportunities to see for what end these offers are made.

Many an educated girl comes from the Old World to find a position as governess or teacher who is taken up in this manner and is never heard from again or is found only in the most wretched condition. It is shameful that the most effective arrangements should not be made for the safety of these helpless beings who come to these shores with the hope of finding a Canaan.

To talk with our friends about the future and the cause of my arrival in New York became now a necessity. So I related how the information of 1852, concerning a medical school for women, in Philadelphia, had inspired me to offer my assistance as a practical instructor and to assist in organizing a hospital.

My good friends not only showed dismay in face and manner as I proceeded, but they expressed it in words, telling me that they had never heard of any "female physicians" except those of a very dis-

reputable character who advertised in all newspapers and carried on criminal practices.

Confronted with my ignorance of the English language, as I now realized myself, I postponed starting for the medical school in Philadelphia, and,
having letters of introduction to well-stationed people in New York, I decided to settle in a two-room
home of my own as soon as this could be found,
we having concluded to commence housekeeping on
a small scale in order to be more independent and
to save money.

The week was mostly spent in looking for apartments. On our arrival, I had borrowed from my
sister the hundred dollars which my father had given
her on our departure from Berlin and which was to
be my capital until I had established myself in business. I succeeded in finding a suite of rooms with
windows facing the street, in the house of a grocer;
and having put them in perfect order, we moved
into them on the sixth of June, paying eleven dollars as our rent for two months in advance.

My sister took charge of our first day's housekeeping, while I went to deliver my letters of introduction. I went first to Dr. Reisig, in Fourteenth
Street. My mother, who had employed him when he
was a young man and we were small children, had
spoken of him kindly, and for this reason I had
confidence in him. I found him a very friendly man,
but by no means a cordial one.

He informed me that female physicians in this
country were of the lowest rank and that they did
not hold even the position of a good nurse. He said
that he wished to be of service to me if I were will-

ing to serve as nurse, and as he was just then in need of a good one, he would recommend me for the position. I thanked him for his candor and kindness, but refused his offer as I could not condescend to be patronized in this way.

Depressed in hope but strengthened in will, I did not deliver any more of my letters, since they were all to physicians and I could not hope to be more successful in other quarters. I went home, therefore, determined to commence practice as a stranger.

The result of my experiment discouraged my sister greatly. After meditating for some time, she suddenly said, "Marie, I read in the paper this morning of a dressmaker who wanted some one to sew for her. I know how to sew well; I shall go there, and you can attend to our little household. No one here knows me, and I do not think there is anything wrong in my trying to earn some money."

She was determined, and went. I put up my sign, and spent my time in attending to the household duties and in reading in order to gain information of the country and of the people. Occasionally I took walks through different parts of the city to learn from the houses and their surroundings the character of life in New York. I am sure that, though perhaps I appeared idle, I was not so in reality, for during this time I learned the philosophy of American life.

But our stock of money was becoming less and less. To furnish the rooms had cost us comparatively little as we had brought a complete set of household furniture with us, but paying the rent and completing the arrangements had not left us more than enough to live upon, in the most economical manner, until the first of August.

My sister obtained the place at the dressmaker's; and after working a week from seven in the morning until twelve (when she came home to dinner), then from one in the afternoon until seven in the evening, she received two dollars and seventy-five cents as the best sewer of six. She brought home the hard-earned money with tears in her eyes, for she had expected at least three dollars for the week's work. She had made each day a whole muslin dress, with the trimmings. And this was not all—the dressmaker often did not pay on Saturday nights, because, as she said, people did not pay her punctually, and the poor girls received their wages by six or eight shillings at a time. For the last two weeks of my sister's work, she received her payment seven weeks after she had left.

We lived in this manner until the middle of July, when I lost patience, for practice did not come as readily as I wished nor was I in a position for making money in any other way. My sister, usually so cheerful and happy, grew grave from the unusual work and the close confinement. One of these nights on lying down to sleep, she burst into tears and told me of her doubts and fears for the future. I soothed her as well as I could, and she fell asleep. For myself, I could not sleep but lay awake all night meditating what I could possibly do. Should I write home, requesting help from my father? He certainly would have given it, for two weeks before we had received a letter offering us all desirable aid.

No! All my pride rebelled against it. "I must help myself," I thought, "and that to-morrow."

The next morning my sister left me as usual. I went out and walked through the city to Broadway, turning into Canal Street, where I had formed an acquaintance with a very friendly German woman by purchasing little articles at various times at her store. I entered without any particular design and exchanged a few commonplaces with her about the weather.

Her husband stood talking with a man about worsted goods, and their conversation caught my ear. The merchant was complaining because the manufacturer did not supply him fast enough, upon which the man answered that it was very difficult to get good hands to work and that besides he had more orders than it was possible to fill, naming several merchants whose names I had seen in Broadway who were also complaining because he did not supply them.

After he had left, I asked carelessly what kind of articles were in demand and was shown a great variety of worsted fancy goods. A thought entered my brain. I left the store and, walking down Broadway, asked at one of the stores that had been mentioned for a certain article of worsted goods in order to learn the price. Finding this enormous, I did not buy it, and I returned home, calculating on my way how much it would cost to manufacture these articles and how much profit could be made in making them on a large scale. I found that two hundred per cent profit might be made by going to work in the right way.

My sister came home as usual to dinner. I sat down with her, but could not eat. She looked at me anxiously, and said, "I hope you are not sick again. Oh, dear! What shall we do if you ξ et sick?" I had been ill for a week and she feared a relapse. I said nothing of my plan, but consoled her in respect to my health.

As soon as she had left, I counted my money. But five dollars remained. If I had been dependent upon money for cheerfulness, I should certainly have been discouraged. I went to John Street and entering a large worsted store, inquired of a cheerful-looking girl the wholesale price of the best Berlin wool, how many colors could be had in a pound, etc. The pleasant and ready answers that I received in my native tongue induced me to tell her frankly that I wanted but a small quantity at that time, that I intended to make an experiment in manufacturing worsted articles; and if successful, I would like to open a small credit, which she said they generally would do when security was given.

I purchased four and a half dollars' worth of worsted, so that fifty cents were left in my pocket when I quitted the store. I then went to the office of a German newspaper, where I paid twenty-five cents for advertising for girls who understood all kinds of knitting.

When my sister came home at night, the worsted was all sorted on the table in parcels for the girls who would come the next morning, while I was busily engaged in the experiment of making little worsted tassels. I had never been skillful in knitting, but in

this I succeeded so well that I could have made a
hundred yards of tassels in one day.

My sister turned pale on seeing all this, and hurriedly asked, "How much money have you spent?"
"All, my dear Anna," answered I, "all, except
twenty-five cents, which will be sufficient to buy a
pound of beefsteak and potatoes for to-morrow's
dinner. Bread, tea and sugar, we have still in the
house; and to-morrow night you will bring home
your twenty-two shillings." "May you succeed,
Marie! That is all I have to say," was her reply.
She learned of me that evening how to make the
tassels, and we worked till midnight, finishing a
large number.

The next day was Saturday, and some women
really came to get work. I gave them just enough
for one day, keeping one day's work in reserve. The
day was spent busily in arranging matters, so that
on Monday morning, I might be able to carry a
sample of the manufactured articles to those stores
that I had heard mentioned as not being sufficiently
supplied.

In the evening, my sister came home without her
money—the dressmaker had gone into the country
in the afternoon without paying the girls. She was
more than sad, and I felt a little uncomfortable, for
what was I to do without money to provide for the
next two days or to pay those girls on Monday with
whose work I might not be satisfied? What was to
be done? To go down to our landlord, the grocer,
and ask him to advance us a few dollars? No! He
was a stranger and had no means of knowing that
we would return the money. Besides, I did not

wish the people in the house to know of our condition.

My resolution was taken. I proposed to my sister to go to the market with me to buy meat and fruit for the morrow. She looked at me with blank astonishment, but without heeding it I said calmly, taking from the bureau drawer the chain of my watch, "Anna, opposite the market there is a pawnbroker. No one knows us, and by giving a fictitious name we can get money without thanking any one for it." She was satisfied, and taking a little basket, we went on our errand. I asked six dollars of the pawnbroker under the name of Müller, and received the money, after which we made our purchases and went home in quite good spirits.

On Monday morning, the knitters brought home their work. I paid them, and gave them enough for another day, after which I set about finishing each piece, completing the task about two in the afternoon. This done, I carried the articles to Broadway, and leaving a sample in a number of stores, received orders from them for several dozens. Here, I have to remark that not being able to speak English, I conducted my business at the different stores either in German or in French, as I easily found some employees who could speak one of these languages.

I then went to the worsted store in John Street, where I also obtained orders for the manufactured articles together with ten dollars' worth of worsted on credit, having first given my name and residence to the bookkeeper, with the names of the stores from which I had received orders.

In the evening when my sister came home, I was,

therefore, safely launched into a manufacturing business. The news cheered her greatly, but she could not be induced to quit her sewing. The new business had sprung up so rapidly and pleasantly that she could not trust in the reality of its existence.

CHAPTER XI

*Social relations largely limited to learning the lives of her
employees and helping them by work, by sympathy and
by friendliness, and sometimes by taking them into
her house to tide over an emergency. (Twenty-four
years of age: 1853.)*

I MUST tell you here something of the social life
that we led. We had brought a number of friendly
letters with us from our acquaintances in Berlin to
their friends and relatives in America; all of which
upon our arrival we sent by post, with the exception
of two—the one sent by a neighbor to his son, Albert C., the other to a young artist, both of whom
called for their letters.

About four weeks after we were settled in New
York, we received a call from some young men whose
sisters had been schoolmates of my sisters in Berlin, who came to inquire of us where to find Mr. C.
We could give them no information, as we had not
seen him since he called for his letter; neither did
we now see anything of the G.'s. But the acquaintance thus formed with these young men was continued, and our solitude was now and then enlivened
by an hour's call from them. Soon after I had commenced my new business, they came one day in company with Mr. C., whom they had met accidentally
in the street, and, on his expressing a wish to see
us. had taken the liberty to bring him to our house.

My business continued to prosper, and by constantly offering none but the best quality of goods for sale, in a very short time I had so much to do that my whole time in the day was occupied with out-door business, and I was forced to sit up at night with my sister to prepare work for the knitters.

At one time, we had thirty girls constantly in our employ, and in this way I became acquainted with many of those unfortunates who had been misled and ruined on their arrival by persons pretending friendship. Two of these in particular interested me greatly.

One, the granddaughter of a famous German and bearing his name, was the daughter of a physician. She had come to this country hoping to find a place as governess. Poor girl! She was a mere wreck when I found her, and all my efforts to raise her up were in vain. She was sick and in a terrible mental condition. We took her into our house, nursed her and cared for her. When she recovered, we supplied her with work for which we paid her so well that she always had three dollars a week, which paid for her board and washing. It was twice as much as she could earn, yet not enough to make her feel reconciled with life.

At one time, she did not come to us for a whole week. I went to see her, and her landlady told me that she was melancholy. I persuaded her to come and stay with us for a few days, but in spite of all my friendly encouragement, I could not succeed in restoring her to cheerfulness. She owned that she could not work merely to live; she did not feel the pangs of hunger, but she felt the want of comforts to which she had been accustomed and which in our days are regarded as necessities.

She attempted to find a situation as governess, but her proficiency in music, French and drawing counted as nothing. She had no city references, and though having been two years in New York, dared not name the place to which she had been conducted on her arrival. She left us at last in despair after having been a week with us. She never called again and I could not learn from her landlady where she had gone.

Three months afterwards, I heard from one of the girls in our employ that she had married a poor shoemaker in order to have a home, but I never learned whether this was true. About a year later, I met her in the Bowery, poorly but cleanly dressed. She hastily turned away her face on seeing me, and I only caught a glimpse of the crimson flush that overspread her countenance.

The other girl that I referred to was a Miss Mary ——, who came with her mother to this country, expecting to live with a brother. They found the brother married and unwilling to support his sister, while his wife was by no means friendly in her reception of his mother. The good girl determined to earn support for her mother, and a pretended friend offered to take care of their things until she could find work and rent lodgings. After four weeks' search, she found a little room and bedroom in a rear building in Elizabeth Street at five dollars a month, and was preparing to move when her "friend" presented a bill of forty dollars for his services. She could only satisfy his rapacity by selling everything that she could possibly spare, after which she commenced to work, and as she embroidered a great deal besides working for me (for which I paid her six dollars a week), for a time she lived tolerably well.

After some time, her mother fell ill, and she had to nurse her and attend to the household as well as to labor for their support. It was a trying time for the poor girl. She sought her brother, but he had moved to the West. I did all that I could for her, but this was not half enough. And after I had quitted the manufacturing business and left the city, my sister heard that she had drowned herself in the Hudson, because her mother's corpse was lying in the house while she had not a cent to give it burial or to buy a piece of bread unless she sold herself to vice.

Are not these two terrible romances of New York life? And many besides did I learn among these poor women, so many indeed that I forget the details of them all. Stories of this kind are said to be without foundation, but I say that there are more of them in our midst than it is possible to imagine.

Women of good education but without money are forced to earn their living. They determine to leave their home, either because false pride prevents their seeking work where they have been brought up as ladies, or because this work is so scarce that they cannot earn by it even a life of semi-starvation, while they are encouraged to believe that in this country they will readily find proper employment.

They are too well educated to become domestics,

better educated indeed than half the teachers here, but modesty, and the habit of thinking that they must pass through the same legal ordeal as in Europe, prevent them from seeking places in this capacity. They all know how to embroider in the most beautiful manner, and knowing that this is well paid for in Europe, they seek to find employment of this kind in the stores.

Not being able to speak English, they believe the stories of the clerks and proprietors, are made to work at low wages, and are often swindled out of their money. They feel homesick, forlorn and forsaken in the world. Their health at length fails them, and they cannot earn bread enough to keep themselves from starvation. They are too proud to beg, and the consequence is that they walk the streets or throw themselves into the river.

I met scores of these friendless women. Some I took into my house; for others I found work and made myself a sort of guardian; while to others I gave friendship to keep them morally alive. It is a curious fact that these women are chiefly Germans. The Irish resort at once to beggary or are inveigled into brothels as soon as they arrive, while the French are always intriguing enough either to put on a white cap and find a place as *bonne,* or to secure a *private* lover.

I am often in despair about the helplessness of women, and the readiness of men to let them earn money in abundance by shame while they are ground down to the merest pittance for honorable work.

Shame on society, that women are forced to surrender themselves to an abandoned life and to death when so many are enjoying wealth and luxury in extravagance! I do not wish the rich to divide their estates with the poor—I am no friend to communism in any form. I only wish institutions that shall give to women an education from childhood that will enable them, like young men, to earn their livelihood. These weak women are the last to come forth to aid in their emancipation from inefficient education. We cannot calculate upon these; we must educate the children for better positions, and leave the adults to their destiny.

How many women marry only for a shelter or a home! How often have I been the confidante of girls who the day before, arrayed in satin, had given their hands to rich men before the altar, while their hearts were breaking with suppressed agony! And this, too, in America, this great free nation, which, notwithstanding, lets its women starve.

It is but lately that a young woman said to me, "I thank Heaven, my dear doctor, that you are a woman, for now I can tell you the truth about my health. It is not my body that is sick, but my heart. These flounces and velvets cover a body that is sold —sold legally to a man who could pay my father's debts."

Oh! I scorn men, sometimes, from the bottom of my heart. Still, this is wrong, for it is the fault of the woman—of the mother—in educating her daughter to be merely a beautiful machine fit to ornament a fine establishment; not gaining this, there is nothing left but wretchedness of mind and body.

Women, there is a connection between the Fifth Avenue and the Five Points! Both the rich and the wretched are types of womanhood, both are linked together forming one great body, and both have the same part in good and evil. I can hardly leave this subject, though it may seem to have little to do with my American experience, but a word spoken from a full heart not only gives relief but may carry a message to at least one listening ear with far-reaching results.

CHAPTER XII

*Her former rival (and later her successor), Sister Cather-
ine, comes from Berlin to New York to ask her aid—
Marie is joined also by a second sister and a brother
—She is robbed of all her savings—The end of her
first year in America finds her profoundly depressed
because, though successful in business, she has found
no opening in her profession—Her hopes are suddenly
renewed by hearing of Dr. Elizabeth Blackwell upon
whom she calls. (Twenty-four years of age: 1853-
1854.)*

I MUST now return to my new enterprise. The
business paid well, and, although I was often forced
to work with my sister till the dawn of morning, we
were happy, for we had all that we needed, and I
could write home that the offered assistance was
superfluous.

Here I must say that I had resolved, on leaving
Berlin, never to ask for aid, in order that I might
be able with perfect freedom to carry out my plans
independently of my family. How this was ever to
be done, I did not yet see, though I had a good opportunity to learn, from life and from the papers,
what I had to expect here. But this mode of instruction, though useful to one seeking to become a
philosopher, was very unsatisfactory to me.

The chief thing that I learned was that I must acquire English before I could undertake anything.
And this was the most difficult point to overcome.

I am not a linguist by nature; all that I learn of languages must be obtained by the greatest perseverance and industry, and for this my business would not allow me time.

Shortly after I had fairly established myself in the manufacturing business, I received news from Berlin that Sister Catherine had left the Hospital Charité and was intending to join me in America, in order to aid me in carrying out my plan for the establishment of a hospital for women in the New World. The parties interested in her had finally succeeded in placing her in the wished-for position, thus disconnecting her from the sisterhood. But, after my departure, the position became greatly modified in rank and inferior in character. Private reasons, besides, made it disagreeable for her to remain there any longer, and in this moment she remembered my friendship towards her. And in the unfortunate belief which she shared with many others that all that I designed to do I could do, she at once resolved to come to me and offer her assistance.

She joined us on the 22d of August, and was not a little disappointed to find me in the tassel business instead of in the medical line. The astonishment with which her acquaintances in Berlin heard her announce her intention of going to seek help from a person to whom she had been less than a friend could not be expressed in words. And she told me that the annoyance they manifested was really the chief stimulus that decided her to come at last. She arrived without a cent. Having always found enough friends ready to supply her with money whenever she wished to establish a temporary hospital, it had never occurred to her that she should need any for private use beyond just enough to furnish the simple blue merino dress of the sisterhood, which had often been provided for her by the Kaiserswerth Institute.

But here she was, and she very soon learned to understand the difficulties which must be overcome before I could enter again into my profession. She became satisfied, and lived with us, sharing equally in whatever we had ourselves. There is a peculiar satisfaction in showing kindness to a person who has injured us even though unconsciously, but in her case, she was not entirely unconscious of the harm she had done me. While in America she confessed to me that her acquaintance had been courted by all those who had opposed my appointment and that they sought every opportunity to annoy me.

On the 18th of September, a sister, one year younger than myself, joined us, having been tempted by our favorable accounts to try a life of adventure. We were now four in family.

But Catherine gradually grew discontented. Having been accustomed to the comforts afforded in large institutions and to receiving attentions from the most aristocratic families of Prussia, the monotonous life that we led was endurable to her only so long as the novelty lasted. This soon wore off, and she became anxious for a change.

She had heard her fellow-passengers speak of a Pastor S., who had been sent to America as a missionary, and she begged me to seek him out and take her to him that she might consult him as to what she had best do. I did so, and she soon became acquainted with his family. Mr. S. exerted himself in her behalf and secured her a place as nurse in the Home for the Friendless, where she had charge of some thirty children.

This was a heavy task, for though none was under a year old, she was constantly disturbed through the night and could get but a few consecutive hours of sleep. Besides, she could not become reconciled to washing under the hydrant in the morning and to being forced to mingle with the commonest Irish girls. She was in every respect a lady and had been accustomed to having a servant at her command, even in the midst of the typhus fever epidemic in the desolate districts of Silesia, while here she was not treated even with humanity.

This soon grew unbearable, and she returned to us on the 16th of October, after having been only ten days in the institution. So eager was she to make her escape that she did not even ask for the two dollars that were due her for wages. But we could not receive her, for we had taken another woman in her place who was as friendless and as penniless as she.

Besides, a misfortune had just fallen upon us. During the night before, our doors had been unlocked, our bureau drawers inspected, and all our money, amounting to fifty-two dollars, carried off. And when Catherine arrived, we were so poor that we had to borrow the bread and milk for our breakfast. Fortunately, the day before, I had refused the payment due me for a large bill of goods, and this came now in a very good time.

I did not feel justified, however, in increasing the family to five after our loss, nor did she claim our assistance, but went again to Pastor S. who had invited her to visit his family. With his assistance, she obtained some private nursing, which maintained her until the congregation had collected money enough to enable her to return to Berlin, which she did on the 2d of December. Having many friends in the best circles of that city, she immediately found a good practice again and she is now, as she says, enjoying life in a civilized manner.

We moved at once from the scene of the robbery and took a part of a house in Monroe Street, for which we paid two hundred dollars a year. Our business continued good, and I had some prospect of getting into practice. But with the spring (1854), the demand for worsted goods ceased, and as my practice brought me work but no money, I was forced to look for something else to do.

By accident, I saw in a store a coiffure made of silk in imitation of hair, which I bought. But I found on examination that I could not manufacture it as it was machine work. I went, therefore, to Mr. G. and proposed to him the establishment of a business in which he should manufacture these coiffures, while I would sell them by wholesale to the merchants with whom I was acquainted.

Mr. G. had completely ruined himself during the winter by neglecting his business and meddling with Tammany Hall politics, which had wasted his money and his time. He had not a single workman in his shop when I called, and he was too much discouraged to think of any new enterprise; but on my tell-

ing him that I would be responsible for the first outlay, he engaged hands and in less than a month had
forty-eight persons busily employed. In this way,
I earned money during the spring and freed myself
from the obligations which his kindness in receiving us the spring before had laid upon us.

My chief business now was to sell the goods manufactured by Mr. G. Our worsted business was very
small, and the prospect was that it would cease entirely, and also that the coiffure that we made would
not long continue in fashion. Some other business,
therefore, had to be found, especially as it was impossible for us to lay up money.

Our family now consisted of myself and two sisters, the friend that was staying with us, and a
brother, nineteen years of age, who had just joined
us during the winter and who, though an engineer
and in good business, was, like most young men,
thoughtless and more likely to increase than to
lighten our burdens. Our friend Mr. C., who had
become our constant visitor, planned at this time a
journey to Europe, so that our social life seemed
also about to come to an end.

On the 13th of May, 1854, as I was riding down
to the stores on my usual business, reveries of the
past took possession of my mind. Almost a year in
America, and not one step advanced towards my
purpose in coming hither! It was true that I had
a comfortable home, with enough to live on, and
had repaid to my sister the money that I had borrowed from her on our arrival; yet what kind of
life was it that I was leading, in a business foreign
both to my nature and to my inclinations, and with-

out even the prospect of enlarging this? These reflections made me so sad that when I reached the
store, the bookkeeper, noticing my dejection, told
me by way of cheering me that he had another order
for a hundred dollars' worth of goods, etc., but this
did not relieve me.

I entered the omnibus again, speculating constantly on what I should do next. Everywhere, my
inquiries about women physicians were received
with a pitiful shrug of the shoulders, and I could
obtain no information concerning the Philadelphia
Female Medical College whose report I had read in
Berlin. I had finally consulted the newspapers in
spite of all the warnings against so doing, and I was
almost at the point of calling upon a Mr. and Mrs.
B. who advertised their private lying-in hospital
(Mrs. B., after becoming a widow, resumed the name
of her first husband and became the originator of
the homeopathic medical college for women), when
a thought suddenly dawned upon me.

Might not the people in the Home for the Friendless be able to give me advice? I had hardly conceived the idea, when I determined to ride directly
up there instead of stopping at the street in which
I lived. I thought, besides, that some employment
might be found for my sister Anna where she could
learn the English language for which she had
evinced some talent, although I had decided that I
could never become master of it.

I had once seen the matron, Miss Goodrich, when
I had called there on Catherine S. She had a humane face, and I was persuaded that I should find
a friend in her. I was not mistaken. I told her of

my plans in coming here and of our present mode of life and prospects, and confided to her my disappointment and dejection as well as my determination to persevere courageously. She seemed to understand and to enter into my feelings and promised to see Dr. Elizabeth Blackwell, whom she advised me to call upon at once.

I went home full of the hope and inspiration of a new life—the happiness of that morning can hardly be comprehended. I was not suffering, it is true, for the necessaries of life, but what was far worse, I suffered from the feeling that I lived for no purpose but to eat and to drink. I had no friends who were interested in the pursuits towards which my nature inclined, and I saw crowds of arrogant people about me to whom I could not prove that I was their equal in spite of their money. My sisters had not seen me so cheerful since our arrival in America and they thought that I had surely discovered the philosophers' stone. I told them of what I had done and received their approbation,

CHAPTER XIII

*Learns that Dr. Blackwell is working for the same purpose
that brought her (Marie) to America, that is, to establish a Hospital for Women; and that she (Dr. Blackwell) has already progressed as far as opening a dispensary (the New York Infirmary for Indigent
Women and Children)—Dr. Blackwell invites Marie
to assist her in the dispensary, gives her lessons in
English, and urges her to acquire the degree of M.D.
—Elizabeth Blackwell first English-speaking woman
to receive such degree—Italian, German and French
women her only predecessors in this respect—Since beginning of the race, women have instinctively practiced
obstetrics and general medicine but their education
has been opposed—Marie's business goes out of fashion—She substitutes a new one which pays very poorly
and is complicated by frequent suggestions for irregular sex life with employers—Refusal leads to loss of
work—She is compelled to draw on her savings—In
the autumn with a balance of fifty dollars, she sets
out for Cleveland to enter the Medical Department
of the Western Reserve College. (Twenty-five years
of age: 1854.)*

On the morning of the 15th of May, 1854—the anniversary of the death of Dr. Schmidt, the day of
my greatest joy and my greatest misery—we received a call from Miss Goodrich who told us that
she had seen Dr. Elizabeth Blackwell, and that she
thought she had also procured a suitable place for
my sister. She gave us the addresses of Dr. Blackwell and of Miss Catherine Sedgwick.

We called first upon the latter, who was extremely kind, and although she had quite misunderstood our wishes—having exerted herself to procure a place for my sister in a way that manifested the belief that we had neither a home nor the means to live— yet her friendliness and readiness to assist us made us forever grateful to her. At that time we did not know her standing in society and looked upon her merely as a benevolent and wealthy woman. We soon learned more of her, however, for though unsuccessful in her first efforts, she shortly after sent for my sister, having secured for her a place in Mr. Theodore Sedgwick's family, which was acceptable inasmuch as it placed her above the level of the servants. She remained there for seven weeks and then returned home.

On the same morning, I saw Dr. Elizabeth Blackwell—and from this call of the 15th of May, 1854, I date my new life in America. She spoke a little German and understood me perfectly when I talked. I gave her all my certificates for inspection, but said nothing to her of my plans in coming to America. It would have seemed too ludicrous for me in my position to tell her that I entertained the idea of interesting the people in the establishment of a hospital for women. I hardly know what I told her, indeed, for I had no other plan of which to speak, and therefore talked confusedly like an adventurer. I only know that I said that I would even take the position of nurse if I could enter one of the large hospitals, in order to learn the manner in which they were managed in this country.

I cannot comprehend how Dr. Blackwell could

ever have taken so deep an interest in me as she manifested that morning, for I never in my life was so little myself. Yet she did take this interest, for she gave me a sketch of her own experience in acquiring a medical education and explained the requirements for such in this country and the obstacles that are thrown in the way of women who seek to become physicians.

She told me of her plan of founding a hospital—the long-cherished idea of my life—and said that she had opened a little dispensary on the 1st of May, two weeks before (the New York Infirmary for Indigent Women and Children), which was designed to be the nucleus for this hospital, and she invited me to come and assist her.

She insisted that first of all I should learn English, and she offered to give me lessons twice a week and also to make efforts to enable me to enter a college to acquire the title of "M.D.," which I had not the right to attach to my name. I left her after several hours' conversation, and we parted friends.

[Dr. Blackwell, in her autobiography, tells of writing to her sister, Dr. Emily, giving her impression of this interview: "I have at last found a student in whom I can take a great deal of interest, Marie Zakrzewska, a German about twenty-six. . . . There is true stuff in her, and I shall do my best to bring it out. . . . She must obtain a medical degree."]

I found Dr. Elizabeth Blackwell a rather short but stately lady, blonde with wavy hair, very dignified, kindly in speech, and very deliberate and wise in her remarks.

The cordiality with which she welcomed me as a

co-worker, I can never describe nor forget. It aroused all my sunken hopes and energies and directed them again to the field of work which I had cultivated and which I had almost given up in despair. Now, I was finding the welcome and the beginning of which I had dreamed, and all the many days of disappointment were instantly forgotten.

I met in Dr. Elizabeth Blackwell no eccentric person who wanted to bring about the millennium for women, for I soon learned from her of the great obstacles which were to be overcome in the social stratum. Soon, indeed, I learned that social prejudices, habits and customs can be as strong barriers to intellectual development as those placed in the way of reform by a despotic German government.

However, behind this social barrier, a number of high-minded and intellectually advanced women were ready to enter upon a struggle for greater freedom of action. They were especially inspired by the Anti-Slavery movement, which was then fully established and which appealed so strongly to the emotional nature of women. The paths these women trod were full of thorns and thistles yet they bore everything patiently, for, knowing their country and its people, they foresaw all the possibilities for good which could be achieved.

Dr. Elizabeth Blackwell, while not the first woman practitioner of medicine even in America, was yet the pioneer in the movement which insisted that medical women should be educated so as to stand equal with men physicians in medical knowledge and in legalized position. Hence, she began her medical life not by practicing her art but by working for

the degree of "M.D." from one of the regularly constituted medical colleges, this meaning at that time
a medical college established exclusively for men.

In this course, she followed the example of at least
three Italian women who had, near the end of the
eighteenth century and in the beginning of the nineteenth, taken the medical degree at the Universities
of Florence and Bologna. But her autobiography
is well entitled, *Pioneer Work in Opening the Medical Profession to Women,* because nothing of this
kind had been undertaken by an English-speaking
woman. Exceptionally, women have, here and there,
received the same training as men, as evidenced by
ancient histories. And early in this nineteenth century, two German women had received the medical
degree at the University of Giessen. And the
French obstetrician, Madame Boivin, had the medical degree conferred on her by the University of
Marburg before she died in 1841.

From the earliest history of the human race,
women have been the practitioners of obstetrics,
and thence, naturally, the practitioners in the diseases of women and children.

But even such women suffered from the subjection which was inflicted upon all their sex. Hence,
as the science of medicine became organized, and as
systematized instruction in both the science and the
art became established, opportunities for study and
advanced practice were more and more monopolized
by men; and women were more and more hindered
from exercising and developing their instinctive
tendencies in these directions.

But the monopoly has never been secure. Always,

large numbers of people, especially of women, have
persisted in the desire to be advised medically by
women; and always, a certain number of women
have responded to their instincts and have prepared
themselves as best they could to give medical advice
and help, especially to women and children.

Thus even at this date all over the world large
numbers of women continued to practice obstetrics,
largely as "midwives." But a considerable number of women also practiced general medicine, especially where they did not come in conflict with
medical or civil laws, which were designed to exclude all except the practitioners of the dominant
medical group. The passage of laws regulating the
practice of medicine is undoubtedly actuated by a
sincere desire to raise the standard of medical practice throughout the community, but only too frequently these laws give power to a group of medical
oligarchs, a fact which I was many times to observe
later.

The best known of the last class of women just
described is Dr. Harriot K. Hunt, who was at this
date preparing for publication her autobiography
which appeared under the title of *Glances and
Glimpses.*

Dr. Blackwell was graduated from the Geneva
(New York) Medical College, in 1849, and she then
went to Europe to obtain the clinical experience
which was denied to women in America, returning
to see her sister Emily also become a regular M.D.
(1854).

The two sisters procured a charter from the New
York Legislature to establish the New York Infir-

mary for Indigent Women and Children, both feeling the absolute necessity for continued clinical experience before offering their services to suffering humanity at large. Dr. Emily then went to Europe for special clinical study and she was still there. Dr. Blackwell said to me, "My sister has just gone to Europe to finish what she began here, and you have come here to finish what you began in Europe."

And here I am obliged to give a short statement of the mode of study in the medical profession at that time.

The young student had to find a "preceptor," a physician of good standing, with whom he studied the preliminaries necessary for entering a medical college or school. He also visited patients with this preceptor and assisted the latter in every way possible. The student thus became familiar with the details of practice even before matriculating regularly in a medical college. I have met young men who had been for years such assistants to physicians, and who later entered college merely to become legally qualified.

Any student who could bring certificates from an acceptable preceptor could easily procure a diploma by attending the medical school of any college for two short successive winter sessions, often of only sixteen weeks' duration.

This method of clinical experience in private practice made hospital attendance by the student seem almost unnecessary. Even opportunities for attendance at dispensaries, when such existed in the larger cities, were not much sought after by the young men, they feeling that they could gain all the required knowledge by attaching themselves to preceptors.

Society, and indeed civilization in general, was in a primitive stage of development, in spite of material elegance, yes, even of luxury and refined manners. It would take a long time to describe the great change which has taken place in the educational and intellectual development of the people in the United States and the increased facilities which they have for the higher and deeper studies.

The time which it would take with a monarchically limited people to advance any social improvement or reform would require generations, while under free, unlimited social laws, months instead of years will serve to bring about the desired evolution.

Under these conditions, I became the student of Dr. Elizabeth Blackwell, she assuming the rôle of medical preceptor, as well as most patient instructor in the English language.

In consequence of her having obtained a charter for a hospital, a few high-minded and progressive friends had contributed sufficient money to open one room for dispensary purposes in a very poor quarter of the East Side of New York. Here poor women and children came three afternoons a week, from three to five o'clock, for medical advice and such simple medicines as Dr. Blackwell could dispense without assistance, until I became her pupil.

The beneficiaries were by no means always grateful; on the contrary, they often considered themselves as important patrons of the women doctors. An incident will illustrate this.

One day, in the hall of the Dispensary, the few

settees were filled with patients waiting for our arrival, and two old and decrepit women had taken seats on the curbstone of the sidewalk, also waiting for us. It unavoidably happened that we were fifteen minutes behind the regular time for opening the Dispensary.

As these two old women saw us turning around the corner of Second Avenue, one of them called to those within hearing in the hall, "There come the Dispensary women now!"

And to us, she said, reproachfully, "Those ladies in the hall have been waiting a whole hour already."

I continued my work at home, going regularly to Dr. Blackwell to receive lessons in English and to assist her in the Dispensary. As we grew better acquainted, I disclosed more to her of the fact that I had a fixed plan in coming to this country, which increased her interest in me.

She wrote in my behalf to the different colleges, and at length succeeded in obtaining admission for me to the Cleveland Medical College (Western Reserve) on the most favorable terms, credit being given me on the lecture fees for an indefinite time.

Here I must stop to tell you why this credit was necessary. The articles that I had manufactured had gone out of fashion in May, and I could not invent anything new, partly because I no longer felt the same interest as before, knowing that I should soon go to a medical college, and partly because the articles then in fashion were cheaper when imported.

We had to live for a little while on the money that we had laid up, until I procured a commission for embroidering caps. It is perfectly wonderful into what kinds of business I was forced, all foreign to my taste.

And here let me tell you some secrets of this kind of business, in which hundreds of women starve and hundreds more go down to a life of infamy.

Cap-making (the great business of Water Street of New York) gives employment to thousands of unfortunates. For embroidering caps, the wholesale dealer pays seven cents each; and for making up, three cents. To make a dozen a day, one must work for sixteen hours.

The embroidering is done in this wise: I received the cut cloth from the wholesale dealer; drew the pattern upon each cap; gave them with three cents' worth of silk to the embroiderer, who received three cents for her work; then pressed and returned them; thus making one cent on each for myself.

By working steadily for sixteen hours, a girl could embroider fifteen in a day. I gave out about six dozen daily, earning like the rest fifty cents a day; unless I chose to do the stamping and pressing at night and to embroider a dozen during the day, in which case I earned a dollar. One can live in this way for a little while until health fails or the merchant says that the work has come to an end.

You will think this terrible again. Oh, no! This is not terrible. The good men provide another way.

They tell every woman of a prepossessing appearance that it is wrong in her to work so hard, that many a man would be glad to care for her, and that many women live quite comfortably with the help of a "friend." They say, further, that it is lonely to live without ever going to church, to the concert and theater, and that if these women would only permit the speakers to visit them and to attend them to any of these places, they would soon find that they would no longer be obliged to work so hard.

This is the polished talk of gentlemen who enjoy the reputation of piety and respectability and who think it a bad speculation to pay women liberally for their work. So it would be, in truth, for these poor creatures would not be so willing to abandon themselves to a disreputable life if they could procure bread in any other way.

During the summer of 1854, I took work on commission from men of this sort. While in Berlin, I had learned from the prostitutes in the hospital in what manner educated women often became what they then were.

The average story was always the same. Love, even the purest, made them weak; their lover deceived and deserted them; their family cast them off by way of punishment. In their disgrace, they went to bury themselves in large cities, where the work that they could find scarcely gave them their daily bread. Their employers, attracted by their personal appearance and the refinements of their speech and manners, offered them assistance in another way, in which they could earn money without work. In despair, they accepted the proposals and sank gradually step by step to the depths of degradation, as depicted by Hogarth in the *Harlot's Progress*.

In New York, I was thrown continually among men who were of the stamp that I described before, and I can say, even from my own experience, that no man is ever more polite, more friendly or more kind than one who has impure wishes in his heart. It is really so dangerous for a woman of refined nature to go to such stores that I never suffered my sister to visit them; not because I feared that she would listen to these men, but because I could not endure the thought that so innocent and beautiful a girl should come in contact with them or even breathe the same atmosphere.

When fathers are unwilling that their daughters shall enter life as physicians, lawyers, merchants, or in any other public capacity, it is simply because they belong to the class that so contaminates the air that none can breathe it but themselves; or because, from being thrown constantly in contact with such men, they arrive at the same point at which I then stood, and say to themselves, "*I* can afford to meet such men. I am steeled by my knowledge of mankind and supported by the philosophy that I have learned during years of trial. It cannot hurt *me;* but by all means, spare the young and beautiful the same experience!"

I dealt somewhat haughtily with the merchants whom I have described, in a manner that at once convinced them of my position. But the consequence was that the embroidery commission which had commenced so favorably, suddenly ceased, "because the Southern trade had failed"; in truth, because I would not allow any of these men to say any more to me than was absolutely necessary in our business.

My income became less and less, and we were forced to live upon the money that we had laid up during the year. I did not look for any new sources of employment for I was intending to go to Cleveland in October. My next sister had business of her own, and Anna was engaged to be married to our friend Mr. C. My brother was also with them, and my mother's brother, whom she had adopted as a child, was on his way to America.

After having settled our affairs, fifty dollars remained as my share, and with this sum I set out for Cleveland, on the 16th of October, 1854. Dr. Elizabeth Blackwell had supplied me with the necessary medical textbooks, so that I had no other expenses than those of my journey and the matriculation fees which together amounted to twenty dollars, leaving thirty dollars in my possession.

CHAPTER XIV

Attends the medical course at Cleveland, learning English at the same time—Is befriended by the Dean, Dr. John J. Delamater, and by Mrs. Caroline M. Severance—Some professors and students object to women as students—Students petition faculty to exclude women—Petition by Harvard medical students against admission of Dr. Harriot K. Hunt to lecures in 1851— No minister would offer prayer at early Commencements of Female Medical College of Pennsylvania— Philadelphia County Medical Society not only refused to admit women as members but issued an edict of excommunication against any of its members who should teach in the woman's medical college, or who should consult with women physicians or even with the male teachers of the medical women—Edict approved by Pennsylvania State Medical Society—Mrs. Mary A. Livermore witnesses on Chestnut St., Philadelphia, male students mobbing women students and pelting them with mud—Similar mobbing and pelting with mud of women medica' students at the gates of the University of Edinburgh—Dr. Blackwell writes she is obliged to close her dispensary for lack of funds and assistance—Marie and her roommate ostracized at the table and in the parlor by the other boarders. (Twenty-five years of age: 1854.)

I DO not believe that many begin the study of medicine with so light a purse and so heavy a heart as did I. My heart was heavy for the reason that I did not know a single sentence of English. All of my

120

study with Dr. Blackwell had been like raindrops falling upon stone; I had profited nothing.

The lectures I did not care for, since there was more need of my studying English than medicine, but the subjects were well known to me, and I therefore reasoned that by hearing familiar things treated of in English, I must learn the language—and the logic held good.

I have already told you that the faculty had agreed to give me credit for my lecture fees. Dr. Blackwell had written also to a lady in Cleveland, who had called upon her some time before in the capacity of president of a Physiological Society which, among other good things, had established a small fund for the assistance of women desirous of studying medicine. This lady (Mrs. Caroline M. Severance) replied in the most friendly manner, saying that I might come directly to her house, and that she would see that my board for the winter was secured by the Physiological Society over which she presided.

The journey to Cleveland was a silent but a pleasant one. Through a mishap, I arrived on Saturday night instead of in the morning, and being unwilling to disturb Mrs. Severance at so late an hour, I went first to a hotel. But what trials I had there! No one could understand me, until at last I wrote on a slate my own name and that of Mrs. Severance, with the words, "A carriage" and "to-morrow." From this, the people inferred that I wished to stay at the hotel all night and to have a carriage to take me to Mrs. Severance's the next day, as was the case. A waiter took my carpet-bag and conducted me to a room. I could not understand his directions to the supper-room, neither could I make him understand that I wanted some supper in my own room; and the consequence was that I went to bed hungry, having eaten nothing all day but a little bread and an apple for luncheon.

As soon as I was dressed the next morning, I rang the bell furiously, and on the appearance of the waiter, exclaimed, "Beefsteak!" This time he comprehended me, and went laughingly away to bring me a good breakfast. I often saw the same waiter afterwards at the hotel, and he never saw me without laughing and exclaiming, "Beefsteak!"

In the course of the forenoon, I was taken in a carriage to the house of Mrs. Severance, but the family was not at home. I returned to the hotel somewhat disheartened and disappointed. Although I should have supposed that death was not far off if some disappointment had not happened to me when I least expected it, yet this persistent going wrong of everything in Cleveland was really rather dispiriting. But a bright star soon broke through the clouds in the shape of Mr. Severance, who came into the parlor directly after dinner, calling for me in so easy and so cordial a manner that I forgot everything and was perfectly happy.

This feeling, however, lasted only until I reached the house. I found four fine children, all full of childish curiosity to hear me talk, but who, as soon as they found that I could not make myself understood by them, looked on me with that sort of contempt peculiar to children when they discover that a person cannot do as much as they themselves can. Mr. Severance, too, was expecting to find me accomplished in music "like all Germans," and had to learn that I had neither voice nor ear for the art. Mrs. Severance understood a little German, yet not half enough to gain any idea of how much or how little I was capable of doing, and therefore looked upon me with a sort of uncertainty as to what was my real capacity. This position was more provoking than painful—there was even something ludicrous in it, and when not annoyed, I often went into my room to indulge in a hearty laugh by myself.

[Mrs. Severance tells of this first meeting:

I had gone to take her to our home in response to a letter from Dr. Blackwell commending her to our care. The letter had come late the night before, and I had not realized the forlornness to her of being in a hotel over night in a strange city.

How condemned I felt for this thoughtlessness as I looked into the tearful eyes of the lonely foreigner who did not feel at home in English, and who had found no one to greet her in her own language until I ventured my crude German! Her eyes kindled into smiles at that and our years of close friendship were begun.]

I met with a most cordial reception in the college. The dean (Dr. John J. Delamater) received me like a father, and from the first day I felt perfectly at home. All was going on well. I had a home at Mrs. Severance's, and despite my mutilated English I found many friends in the college, when suddenly circumstances changed everything.

Some changes occurred in Mr. Severance's business and he was forced in consequence to give up housekeeping. At that time I did not know that the Physiological Society was ready to lend me money, and I was therefore in great distress.

I never experienced so bitter a day as that on which Mrs. Severance told me that I could stay with her no longer. It was but five weeks after my arrival, and I was not able to make myself understood in the English language, which was like chaos to me. On the same day I well remember that for the first time in my life I made an unsuccessful attempt to borrow money; and because it was the first and the last time, it was the more painful to me to be refused. I envied the dog that lived and was happy without troubling his brain; I envied the kitchenmaid who did her work mechanically and seemed to enjoy life far more than those fitted by nature for something higher.

Mrs. Severance secured a boarding place for me for the rest of the winter and paid my board, amounting to thirty-three dollars, from the funds of the society. I lived quietly by myself; studied six hours daily at home, with four dictionaries by me; attended six lectures a day, and went in the evening for three hours to the dissecting rooms.

[Dr. Blackwell, again writing to her sister Emily on November 13th, says: A pleasant circumstance occurred to my German, Dr. Zakrzewska. I arranged a Cleveland course for her, and she entered two weeks ago. She met a very friendly reception, and found that Dr. Kirtland is in correspondence with Professor Müller of Berlin, and he had mentioned her in some of his letters in such high terms that the faculty told her that if she would qualify herself for examination in surgery and chemistry and write an English thesis, they would graduate her at the end of this term. Of course, she is studying with might and main, and will, I have no doubt, succeed; so we may reckon on a little group of three next year. That will be quite encouraging.]

I never conversed with any one at the boarding house, nor even asked for anything at the table, but was supplied like a mute. This silence was fruitful to me. About New Year, I ventured to make my English audible; when, lo! every one understood me perfectly. From this time forward, I sought to make acquaintances, to the especial delight of good old Dr. Delamater who had firmly believed that I was committing gradual suicide.

My stay in that congenial family, the Severances, was meant to be only temporary, until a suitable boarding house could be obtained. Alas, nobody wanted to take a "female medical student!" For several weeks, Mrs. Severance hunted for such a place until she found a New England woman, Mrs. Shepard, who was willing to brave the criticism of neighborhood and church connections and take me and another female medical student who was in the same dilemma to board for the winter, the Association mentioned making themselves responsible for the expense.[3]

Being now well-housed, we trotted unconcernedly by neighbors staring from behind half-shut blinds, twice a day, to and from our college. And there being four women among a couple of hundred young men, we had our box seat to ourselves, unmolested by the tobacco-chewing and spitting Æsculapians in embryo. My three companions were Mrs. Chadwick who was my roommate, Miss Cordelia A. Greene, now practicing in her own institution in Castile, N. Y., and Miss Elizabeth Grissell, now a practicing physician in Salem, Ohio.[4]

In the college, we had nothing of which we could complain; the young men did not like our presence; some of the professors acted as if we did not exist, while others favored us in many ways; and one, the most eminent, Dr. Delamater, offered to be my preceptor and gave me good practical advantages.

On the whole, life was made quite pleasant in the college, although we were told that a strong petition was circulated by the male students to exclude women after that winter's term. The faculty refused to consent to this request because they had given the four women the promise of an opportunity to graduate. However, the assurance was given to the men that the college would not again admit women, especially as the faculty considered that the little Pennsylvania Medical College for Women was prospering and giving fully as good an education as the Western Reserve Medical College.

We did not see a copy of the petition of the men students, but as there was never any variety in the objections made to the study of medicine by women, it was undoubtedly similar to the one which the medical students at Harvard College presented against the admission of Dr. Harriot K. Hunt, in 1850, and which she published in *Glances and Glimpses*.

As it is interesting because showing the weakness

of the forces which everywhere opposed us, I will cite it here.

After quoting a communication which approved of her conduct and disapproved of that of the men students, and which appeared in the *Boston Evening Transcript,* July 5, 1851, Dr. Hunt adds: "This article brought out the resolutions of the students which I had endeavored to obtain in vain."

THE FEMALE MEDICAL PUPIL.—Mr. Editor: As an article, in some respects imaginative, appeared in the *Transcript* on Wednesday evening over the signature of *E. D. L.,* who professes to be "well informed" respecting the application of a female to the Medical Lectures, and the "insubordination" with which the intelligence was received by the students, allow me to correct any erroneous impression by claiming space for an insertion of the following series of resolutions passed at a meeting of the medical class with but *one* dissenting vote, and afterwards respectfully presented to the Faculty of the Medical College.

WHEREAS, it has been ascertained that permission has been granted to a female to attend the Medical Lectures of the present winter, therefore,

Resolved, That we deem it proper both to testify our disapprobation of said measure, and to take such action thereon as may be necessary to preserve the dignity of the school, and our own self-respect.

Resolved, That no woman of true delicacy would be willing in the presence of men to listen to the discussion of the subjects that necessarily come under the consideration of the student of medicine.

Resolved, That we object to having the company

of any female forced upon us, who is disposed to
unsex herself, and to sacrifice her modesty, by appearing with men in the medical lecture room.

Resolved, That we are not opposed to allowing
woman her rights, but do protest against her appearing in places where her presence is calculated
to destroy our respect for the modesty and delicacy
of her sex.

Resolved, That the medical professors be, and
hereby are, respectfully entreated to do away forth-
with with an innovation expressly at variance with
the spirit of the introductory lecture, with our own
feelings, and detrimental to the prosperity, if not to
the very existence of the school.

Resolved, That a copy of these resolutions be
presented to the Medical Faculty.

SCALPEL.

We women in Cleveland were fortunate that we
had to contend only with ostracism and petitions,
for in Philadelphia and in Edinburgh, women medical students suffered grievously at the hands of the
male medical students, as well as from other groups
in the community.

For instance, at the commencement exercises of
the Pennsylvania Female Medical College, prayer
was offered by a layman because no minister in
Philadelphia could be found who would take part
in the services.[5]

And the Philadelphia County Medical Society not
only refused to admit women physicians as members,
but, in 1859, it pronounced an edict of excommunication against any of its members who should teach
in the Pennsylvania Female Medical College, or
who should consult with women physicians or with

the male teachers of the women. And this edict of excommunication was approved, in 1860, by the Pennsylvania State Medical Society. As a leading member of both societies, Dr. Atlee, expressed it, "By the rules of our medical association, I dare not consult with the most highly educated female physician, and yet I may consult with the most ignorant masculine ass in the medical profession."

Again, in *The Business Folio*, Boston, March, 1895, Mrs. Mary A. Livermore tells of a personal observation which she made during the earlier days of this college. Speaking to a relative, she says:

Before you were born, and you are now nearly twenty-eight years old, my husband and myself went to Philadelphia to make your father and mother a visit.

One day, we were walking up Chestnut Street when suddenly we became aware that something unusual was the matter. Before us was a group of women hurrying along in great confusion; they were well dressed, but their clothing was then in a very dilapidated condition.

We wondered what had happened, and as we looked this way and that a chunk of mud flew by, perilously near my face, and hit one of the women who was then not far from us.

With a startled cry, the woman with the others ran into the wide-open doors of a large store. They were followed by a company of young men seemingly intent only upon reaching them. The proprietor and clerks sprang to the rescue of the young women, and, with the help of my husband and his brother, grabbed the unmannerly cubs by the napes of their necks and threw them into the street.

We then learned that the company of young women had entered one of the medical colleges in Philadelphia, and these young men from another college in another part of the city had determined that if they could prevent it no women should study medicine.

This Philadelphia episode suggests the mobbing and pelting with mud which Sophia Jex-Blake and her fellow women students received from the male medical students at the gates of the University of Edinburgh as late as 1870, but it lacks the compensating feature of the Edinburgh occurrence when "the decent male medical students" came to the rescue of the women and formed a protecting and chivalrous escort for them, continuing this gentlemanly course till the "rowdies" accepted the presence of women students. Though this "presence" was only short-lived.[14]

Meanwhile, I exchanged letters pretty regularly with Dr. Elizabeth Blackwell, telling her the details of my college life, and she telling me that she was obliged to close the little dispensary. One reason for this was the lack of funds to meet the expense, while another was the lack of such assistance as I had rendered, Dr. Emily Blackwell being in Europe, studying, and there being no other medical woman to avail herself of the opportunity for such practice. She also wrote me that the practice she sought increased but slowly while expenses were high, so she had decided to enter upon the new speculation of buying a house on Fifteenth Street and reducing her own expenses by sharing its rooms with friends.

The first three months of college life were rather

dull for me, as my imperfect knowledge of the English language excluded me from taking part in the comradeship of the few male students who rather enjoyed the presence of the women, and who had taken no part in the petition of objection to us.

After college hours, my roommate and I spent our time chiefly in our room as the other boarders would retire as soon as we entered the parlor; and at table would politely but decidedly manifest their intention to ignore us. On Sundays, we went to "Meeting," as it was called, sometimes under the auspices of our good hostess, Mrs. Shepard, who was a strict orthodox Presbyterian. More often, however, I went to a hall where a small society known as that of the Liberal Christians was addressed by Rev. A. D. Mayo. He was a humanitarian and belonged in the ranks of the Abolitionists. He was also interested in various other social reforms, among which was the Woman's Rights movement.

CHAPTER XV

*Marie's contact with "transcendentalism" and the Know-
Nothing movement—Meets Dr. Harriot K. Hunt, of
Boston—Why Harriot and her sister began to study
medicine in 1830—In 1847, Harriot applies to Harvard
for permission to attend medical lectures and is refused
—In 1850, she renews her application and receives permission—Harvard medical students send two petitions
of protest to the faculty: one against admission of
negro men students; one against admission of women
students—The faculty requests Harriot to withdraw
her application—Marie's father opposes her study of
medicine, denounces her leaving "woman's sphere"
and demands her return to New York or to Germany.
(Twenty-five years of age: 1854-1855.)*

RETRACING these later steps for a moment, I wish
to add that the years 1840 to 1860 form the period of
what is now called the "transcendentalism of New
England." What has given rise to this mode of
thinking and acting of the people has been explained
by many an able writer. I, arriving in America in
1853, experienced the effect of this phase of spiritual
life when it was on the wane; when phalansteries
had been tried and had failed; when social reforms
were discussed in all parts of the country by those
who led the van from Boston, New York, Philadelphia, and Cleveland.

Groups of reformers existed in the churches and
schools as well as in political and social circles.

Women, still timid and under the pressure of social propriety, hailed every one who dared to give expression to their wishes and longings for a sphere beyond that of domesticity.

The broader religious preaching of William Ellery Channing and of Theodore Parker encouraged many to join these men in their efforts, while transcendental thinking and reading had prepared their minds to accept any new theory of life and its aims, for the individual woman as well as for the whole sex.

The first impressions received from the few acquaintances I had, after arriving, were depressing in the highest degree; for I found that the life of the New World had not only confirmed my countrymen in their Old World prejudices but it had even a reactionary result upon their mode of thinking, leading them to ridicule the American ways and modes in social, religious and political forms of life.

The Know-Nothing party had just been established; and those immigrants who were exiled after the revolutionary efforts of the years following 1848, created a prejudice among themselves against the English-speaking people of New York, especially against all reformers, which included the Know-Nothings.

And, yet, it was through the accidental acquaintance of these Know-Nothings that I was introduced to the so-called reformers; and, strange to say, the family giving firm adherence to the Know-Nothing principles was of German birth, their parents having emigrated after the year 1830, when exiled following the student revolt.

This family opened the path to the first acquaintance to whom I could show my credentials, verified by letters from the American Secretary of Legation at Berlin, Theodore S. Fay.[2]

A new world seemed to appear before my eyes when I was first introduced to the different circles of reformers. It seemed to me then as if the whole social and religious life was undermined, and that a labyrinth of ways ran confusedly in all sorts of directions. All that education, habit and custom had nurtured in my perception of life seemed to crumble into pieces.

That negro slavery was still in full force I soon learned, and that women declared their incapability to speak freely and openly against it shocked me beyond comprehension. On the other hand, I was shocked that a Mrs. Wright and others had demanded the emancipation of women. That a Woman's Rights Convention was held in New York State seemed to me so ridiculous that I found the expression in one of the New York papers, "The hens which want to crow," quite appropriate.

However, I had tried to crow as hard as any of these women without realizing it, for I had been quite enthusiastic when I received the news that ways and means had been found through the efforts of Dr. Elizabeth Blackwell for me to enter the medical school of the Western Reserve College, at Cleveland. It was not a week after my arrival when through a visit from Dr. Harriot Kezia Hunt to the house of my hostess and protector, Mrs. Caroline M. Severance, I learned to my great astonishment that the "crowing hens" of Cleveland had taken me under their wings to shelter me and to promote my efforts.[6]

[As Marie became better acquainted with the "woman's rights" question her logical mind was impressed by the arguments in favor of the movement, and she eventually accepted it and became associated with its ardent advocates, though never herself taking the position of a militant suffragist.]

A few details regarding Dr. Hunt will be of interest here. Harriot Kezia Hunt and her sister, Sarah Augusta, had their minds withdrawn from their profession of teaching and turned towards medicine, in 1830, by the prolonged illness of Sarah and her ineffective treatment by the regular medical profession. "After forty-one weeks of sickness and one hundred and six professional calls, my sister was roused to more thought on this subject. We talked it over together; she obtained some medical works; and finally, she came to the conclusion that her case was not understood."

The sisters continued the study of medicine by themselves, and Harriot first thought of *woman* as a *physician* when, in 1833, Mrs. Mott and her husband, two irregular practitioners who had come to Boston from England, were called to see if they could in any way help Sarah. As Harriot writes: " . . . it did not occur to us that to die under regular practice, and with medical etiquette, was better than any other way."

Sarah soon began to improve and Harriot then decided to become a physician, giving up her teaching so that she might have more time to study. Sarah's new treatment eliminated the rather drastic

use of drugs then prevalent in medical practice, and
confined itself principally to attention to the somewhat neglected laws of hygiene, combined with
cheering assurances of a cure. As her health became established, Sarah joined in the study, and in
October, 1835, the two sisters formally began practice by advertising the fact in the daily papers.
Sarah later married and became the mother of six
children, gradually withdrawing from the practice
which Harriot continued alone.

Harriot persevered in her studies while building
up a very successful practice in Boston, and, in 1847,
she applied to Harvard College for permission to
attend medical lectures but was refused. In 1850,
she renewed her application and this time she received the desired permission, five of the seven members of the Faculty voting in the affirmative.

Of the two men who voted in the negative (Drs.
James Jackson and Jacob Bigelow), it was Dr.
Jackson who had introduced into Boston the midwife, Mrs. Janet Alexander. "Thus," comments
Dr. Putnam-Jacobi, "it would seem that his objection was not to women but to *educated* women who
might aspire to rank among regularly educated men
physicians."

But again Dr. Hunt's hopes met disappointment
for, as noted in a previous chapter, the men students
sent to the Faculty two petitions of remonstrance
—one against the admission of negro men students,
and one against the admission of women students.

The Faculty referred these petitions to a committee of which Dr. Jacob Bigelow (one of the two
members originally voting against Dr. Hunt's ad-

mission) was chairman. This committee reported the following votes regarding the petition against women students (and this report was accepted):

Voted, that the Faculty are at all times anxious to promote the gratification and welfare of the members of the medical class so far as their duty and the great interests of medical education permit.

Voted, that the female student who had applied for liberty to attend the lectures having by advice of the Faculty withdrawn her petition, no further action on this subject is necessary.

In 1853, Dr. Hunt received the honorary degree of M.D. from the Female Medical College of Pennsylvania, in Philadelphia.

I found among those whom Mrs. Severance had interested in my behalf, kind and intelligent as well as sympathizing friends who were willing to assist me even financially in my studies. These good people, I saw well, pitied my benightedness concerning the emancipation of women, without trying to proselyte, but leaving me in good faith that I would work out my own salvation and see the righteousness of their demands for a larger sphere for women.

Another tie of sympathy soon became apparent, namely, the religious tendency which was prevailing in the Severance circle of acquaintances. Mr. and Mrs. Severance were the leading spirits of a small Universalist congregation who held their meetings in the only public hall which Cleveland then possessed. This assembly was inspired by Rev. A. D. Mayo who had recently been called by them. They were adverse to Calvinism as well as to Episcopalianism, yet they felt the want and need of some form of church union.

This congregation was the most heterogeneous imaginable. Most of the people were in a transition stage from the darkest orthodoxy to atheism, neither of these extremes satisfying their ideals. There were also reformers in other directions dissatisfied with all existing codes of religion and law who sought refuge in the companionship of malcontents. Thus, we had not only Unitarians and Universalists to meet, but also Spiritualists, Magnetists, Fourierists, Freelovers, Women's Rights advocates, Abolitionists—in fact, followers of all kinds of *isms* then existing.

Every theory had its representatives and advocates when a couple of dozen men and women gathered in alternate houses, socially or for discussing problems in general. A woman medical student was a new element and was welcomed by all the factions. Fortunately, I could not speak the English language, so I belonged to the class of patient listeners. I thus received attention from all groups, learning a great deal of what was agitating the intelligent and thinking ones, and being befriended by many in the expectation of swelling their numbers by one more in support of their specific beliefs or theories.

However, as these people seemed to be the only group of human beings who were not afraid of female medical students, I decided to avail myself of the customary opportunity of calling on New Year's Day, 1855, at the house of Mr. Mayo, Mrs. Severance having inspired me with the courage to do so. To my great surprise, after arriving there I found that I could speak English well enough to be understood.

[At a later date Mr. Mayo writes of this call:
Among my visitors at my home in Cleveland, at the New Year's reception of 1855, was a young woman whose face I recognized as a bright presence in the Sunday congregations that waited on my ministry.

Despite her impossible Polish name and her picturesque pronunciation of the English language, she became at once the notable guest of the evening. Her cheerful voice, reinforced by her magnetic womanhood, sent every sentence to the right place and won our hearts.]

My roommate and fellow student, Mrs. Chadwick, refused to accompany me on this New Year's call. Mr. Mayo was too liberal for her. Such is the inconsistency of human nature; she herself did not hesitate to don the robe of a reformer as medical student, yet she did not dare to speculate on new theories in the realm of thought.

Thus the new year began very promisingly, as it opened to me the chance of entering somewhat into social relations which to my nature were absolutely necessary in order to keep up my hopes and aspirations. Besides, this connection gave me the opportunity to observe the habits and customs of this new life, both in the intellectual and the domestic spheres, during the little time that I could spare from my studies.

In the autumn of 1854, after deciding to go to

Cleveland to resume my medical studies, I wrote to my parents to tell them of my hopes and aims. These letters were not received with the same pleasure with which they had been written.

My father, who had encouraged me before my entrance upon a public career, was not only grieved by my return to my old mode of life but greatly opposed to it, and manifested this in the strongest words in the next letter that I received from him. My mother, on the contrary, who had not been at all enthusiastic in the beginning, was rather glad to receive the news.

As I had left many good friends among the physicians of Berlin, my letters were always circulated, after their arrival, by one of their number who stood high in the profession; and, though I did not receive my father's approbation, he sent me several letters from strangers who approved my conduct, and who, after hearing my letters, had sent him congratulations upon my doings in America.

How he received the respect thus manifested to him, you can judge from a passage in one of his letters, which I will quote to you:

I am proud of you, my daughter; yet you give me more grief than any other of my children. If you were a young man, I could not find words in which to express my satisfaction and pride in respect to your acts; for I know that all you accomplish you owe to yourself: but you are a woman, a weak woman; and all that I can do for you now is to grieve and to weep. O my daughter! return from this unhappy path. Believe me, the temptation of living

for humanity *en masse,* magnificent as it may appear
in its aim, will lead you only to learn that all is
vanity; while the ingratitude of the mass for whom
you choose to work will be your compensation.

Letters of this sort poured upon me; and when
my father learned that neither his reasoning nor his
prayers could turn me from a work which I had begun with such enthusiasm, he began to threaten;
telling me that I must not expect any pecuniary
assistance from him; that I would contract debts in
Cleveland which I should never be able to pay, and
which would certainly undermine my prospects;
with more of this sort.

My good father did not know that I had vowed
to myself, on my arrival in America, that I would
never ask his aid; and besides, he never imagined
that I could go for five months with a single cent
in my pocket. Oh, how small all these difficulties
appeared to me, especially at a time when I began
to speak English! I felt so rich that I never thought
money could not be had whenever I wanted it in good
earnest.

But with the closing of the term, which occurred
early in March, the financial assistance in paying
for my board ceased, and further provision had to
be made for my support.

Shortly before this period, a letter was received
from my father denouncing my leaving my sisters,
my despising the sphere of woman, and my entering
upon a field which so entirely belonged to men; he
demanded my return to New York or to Germany

and he utterly refused me any financial aid. After reading this letter to Mrs. Severance and asking her counsel, I retired to my room almost in despair.

That same evening, I attended a meeting which had been announced from all the pulpits and which was being held for the purpose of discussing how to aid the Cherokee Indians. Representatives of this tribe were sojourning in Cleveland on the way to Washington in order to see the Great White Father and to implore his help in their troubles.

During this meeting, I resolved to follow my father's advice and give up man's sphere, and offer myself as one of the missionaries to the Indians for which the leader pleaded as so necessary to civilize the squaws. Thus would I carry the working out of woman's sphere to the wilderness of the Indian Territory. The next morning I told my decision to Mrs. Shepard, to my fellow students and to Mr. Mayo; and in the evening I began a letter to my sisters who were now well established, my sister Anna having married a very estimable young man whose parents were friends and neighbors of ours in Berlin.

If I had not been visited in the morning of the next day by Dr. Seelye, a friend of my fellow student, Miss Greene, and an hour later by Mrs. Severance, my fate as an Indian missionary would have been decided by the arrival of the afternoon hour appointed for the meeting of all those interested in the Indian troubles. However, these two friends not only dissuaded me from any such change, but promised to provide in some way or other, means for my continuing my studies.

Dr. Seelye insisted on my first writing to Dr. Elizabeth Blackwell, showing me that I was under special obligation to her. The Indians had to leave before I received her reply. She was indignant at my proposition and requested me to return to New York immediately after my graduation the middle of the next March.

CHAPTER XVI

*During vacation months, Marie teaches German—Becomes
working guest in family of Rev. A. D. Mayo—Meets
many noted men and women—Her mother dies on the
voyage to New York and is buried at sea—Marie returns to New York, visits Dr. Blackwell, and finds the
Infirmary is still closed—She goes to Boston to visit
Dr. Hunt—Meets the Grimké sisters—Learns of the
New England Female Medical College—Meets William
Lloyd Garrison, Theodore Parker, Wendell Phillips,
and other noted people—Returns to Cleveland and
becomes the guest of Mrs. C. Vaughan for her closing
term at college—Meets Lyceum speakers, professors,
political and social leaders, and literary men and
women from various parts of the country. (Twenty-six
years of age: 1855.)*

WITHIN a few days, there were found some pupils
to whom I might teach German. There also came a
proposition from Mrs. Mayo who was expecting her
first baby within a very short time. The proposition
was that I should become a general member of the
family, attending to her needs as well as aiding in
the housekeeping, etc., till the arrival of her mother
later in the spring.

In April, I removed my possessions into that hospitable house which offered its little to me who had
less. Both Mr. and Mrs. Mayo were really nervous
invalids, and the troubles and trials of their position as anti-slavery advocates and religious reformers bore heavily upon them and kept their purse

144

lean. However, I had no personal needs further than my board, as my clothing was still good in spite of my two years in America.

I found many dear and valued friends during my residence in Cleveland, but none to whom I am bound in lasting gratitude as to Mr. Mayo, who offered me his assistance when he learned that I was in need, my extra expenses having swallowed up the little money that I had brought with me, so that I had not even enough to return to my sisters in New York. As the minister of a small congregation advocating Liberal ideas, he had a hard position in Cleveland, both socially and pecuniarily, yet he offered to share his little with me. I was forced to accept it, and I am now, and have always been, glad that I did so.

No one that has not had the experience can appreciate the happiness that comes with the feeling that a rich man has not cast a fragment of his superfluity towards you (and here let me remark that it is next to impossible to find wealth and generosity go together in friendship), but that the help comes from one who must work for it as well as the recipient. It proves the existence of the mutual appreciation that is known by the name of "friendship." The apple given by a friend is worth ten times more than a whole orchard bestowed in such a way as to make you feel that the gift is but the superfluity of the donor.

Now I was in my element: superintending a very inferior servant girl; providing wholesome simple meals for the invalids; going three mornings a week to an apothecary shop where a friendly man permitted me to assist him in his work, thus acquiring a knowledge of drugs and their preparation; going two mornings a week to my preceptor's office to recite in the usual manner; giving German lessons two afternoons a week; spending one evening a week at meetings in houses of different parishioners for discussions on theological subjects, especially Unitarian and Universalist themes; assisting Mr. Mayo on Sundays at the Sunday school, especially in organizing the same and in substituting for absent teachers; and, after the arrival of the baby girl, taking exclusive charge of the delicate little being, trying to bring it up by hand.

During this summer, I had the pleasure of getting acquainted with Mr. and Mrs. Leander Lippincott (*Grace Greenwood,* a sister of Mrs. Mayo). And later I met a great many renowned ministers and lecturers from the East who either called when passing through Cleveland or exchanged pulpits with Mr. Mayo, being our guests in either case. All these gentlemen were highly interesting, especially when talking on politics, the Free Soil movement and anti-slavery. My knowledge of American civilization was in this way greatly increased and my powers of observation and meditation received full satisfaction.

This quiet yet useful existence was broken by a letter from my father, bringing the news of his having sent my mother and the youngest two sisters to New York for a visit to us, with the intention of following them himself as soon as he could obtain a year's furlough with full salary. All this was meant to see for himself whether I could not be brought back to my senses and persuaded to return to the proper sphere of woman.

Perhaps it may be of interest here to state that my only brother had arrived in New York just before I left for Cleveland and had found a good position as mechanical engineer. And a half-brother of my mother, whom my father had adopted, had arrived after my departure. My father wanted to rescue these two from the fate of being soldiers in Germany, so he expatriated them, sending them to America. But in their new country, the former became a captain in the militia, while later, during the war of the rebellion, the latter became a captain in the regular United States Army.

Shall I attempt to describe the feeling that overpowered me on the receipt of these tidings? If I did, you never could feel it with me, for I could not picture in words the joy I felt at the prospect of beholding again the mother whom I loved beyond all expression, and who was my friend besides; for we really never thought of each other in our relation of mother and child, but as two who were bound together as friends in thought and in feeling.

No, I cannot give you a description of this, especially as it was mingled with the fear that I might not have the means to go to greet her in New York before another ten months were over. Day and night, night and day, she was in my mind; and from the time that I had a right to expect her arrival, I counted the hours from morning until noon, and from noon until night, when the telegraph office would be closed.

At length, on the eighteenth of September, the

despatch came—not to me but to my friend Mr. Mayo—bearing the words,

Tell Marie that she must calmly and quietly receive the news that our good mother sleeps at the bottom of the ocean, which serves as her monument and her grave.

This is the most trying passage that I have to write in this sketch of my life, and you must not think me weak that tears blot the words as I write. My mother fell a victim to seasickness which brought on a violent hemorrhage that exhausted the sources of life. She died three weeks before the vessel reached the port, and my two sisters (the one seventeen, and the other nine years of age) chose rather to have her lowered on the Banks of Newfoundland than bring to us a corpse instead of the living. They were right, and the great ocean seems to me her fitting monument.

This news almost paralyzed me. It was impossible for me to remain in Cleveland, I longed so to be with my sisters in New York. Availing myself of the cheapness of an excursion to the eastern cities, I hastened to them, they being nicely established all in one house headed by my brother-in-law, Mr. A. C. ——

After the first shock of our mother's loss had passed, I called upon my friend, Dr. Elizabeth Blackwell, who, though well established in her newly acquired house, in East Fifteenth Street, could not speak very encouragingly as to practice. For entirely social reasons, people were afraid to employ a woman physician openly, although desirous and ready to consult her privately. Yet even this unsatisfactory practice had prevented her from continuing the little dispensary regularly and it was still closed.

But, during my absence, she had been trying to interest some wealthy friends in the collection of money to enable us after my return in the spring to commence again upon a little larger scale. To effect this, she proposed to hold a Fair during the winter after my return, and we concluded that the first meeting for this purpose should be held during my visit in New York. She succeeded in calling together a few friends at her house, who determined to form a nucleus for a Fair Association for the purpose of raising money for the New York Infirmary.

Dr. Blackwell's experience was so contradictory to Dr. Harriot K. Hunt's statements of the Boston public (in which city a regularly graduated medical woman from Cleveland, Dr. Nancy E. Clark, had also settled) that I decided to avail myself of the fact that my excursion ticket included Boston and to accept Dr. Hunt's invitation for a visit of a few days in order to learn more of the opportunities of that city.

Arriving early one morning, I was conducted through winding streets from Exeter Place to Green Street to Dr. Hunt's house, where I stayed, and where Mrs. Theodore Weld and Miss Sarah Grimké were engaged in editing Dr. Hunt's autobiography, *Glances and Glimpses,* then in the press.

I was shown into a room in the third story, and as I was descending the stairway soon afterward, my

foot caught in the carpet in such a way that I fell
head foremost down the stairs, striking against the
door at the foot of the flight. The noise caused by
this fall brought the inmates of the room to the door
where I lay unconscious. My period of unconscious-
ness was short, and on opening my eyes I saw a
queerly shaped scarlet leg on each side of my head,
and above these a short drapery of the same bright
color but with large flowers printed upon it, while
from a beautiful, gentle and kind face encircled by
soft white curls, came the words, "Are you hurt,
my dear?" It was Mrs. Angelina Weld, in a bloomer
dress of calico, and beside her was Miss Sarah
Grimké, in a Quakerlike costume, trying to disen-
tangle me from the position which I had assumed.

The picture made by the ladies was so amusing
that a burst of mirthful laughter brought me at
once to my senses and to my feet, to the delight of
these two charming ladies who became from that
moment dear and intimate friends of mine.

Dr. Hunt introduced me to many fine people who
consulted her professionally, and also to Dr. Nancy
Clark, then established as a physician in Boston. I
observed that prejudice against women physicians
was by no means as strong as in New York or
Cleveland.

A school established in 1850, for the education and
training of "midwives," had been supported by
Boston's liberal-minded men and women. Some of
the graduates of this school practiced very successfully as midwives. This school developed later
into a medical school for women (New England Female Medical College), and was now giving legal

diplomas of "Doctor of Medicine." The medical school was a small but very respectably lodged concern, with correct and kind men for teachers, and with substantial prospects for getting a larger building and greater advantages for study within a year or two.

However, the greatest event of my three days' sojourn in Boston was my introduction (through Mr. Mayo) to Mr. Theodore Parker, on Sunday evening, I having attended the morning's service in Music Hall. Through Mr. Parker, I met Mr. William Lloyd Garrison and Mr. Wendell Phillips, as well as a number of other prominent men and women. These three men who were pictured so often in Cleveland as three ferocious lions, I found gentle in manners, humanitarian in thought and word and earnest in purpose, possessors of great souls, feeling hearts and sincere patriotism. I was cordially welcomed by them and kept up this relation until the close of their lives, holding even a very honoring relation as professional adviser in their families.

It was a genial circle of friends, at the home of Mr. and Mrs. Parker, who in their easy, informal manner of enjoying each other, impressed me as so utterly different from what I had heard of them, they having been represented by word of mouth as well as in print as the most dangerous and violent revolutionists.

I remember the delicate and graceful figure of Miss Matilda Goddard, the cordial Miss Hannah Stevens, Dr. William F. Channing and Mr. W. L. Garrison, as the center of groups in the spacious parlors, when the talk was of religious and anti-slavery themes, with a frequent easy and cordial laugh at the expense of nobody.

Before returning to Cleveland, I received letters from Mrs. C. Vaughan, a member of Mr. Mayo's congregation, who was shocked to learn of our great bereavement in the death of our mother. She offered me a home for the winter, with the kindest assurance that financial help might be gained by forming German conversational classes for the evenings.

Thus, on my return, I removed from Mrs. Mayo's home, where my assistance had become unnecessary, owing to the death of the little baby, to the hospitable mansion occupied by the Vaughan family and the daughter, Mrs. G. Willey, and her husband.

A few words as to the social and educational standing of this family will be pardonable, especially as they were of so rare an occurrence at the time. Southerners by birth, they were yet opposed to slavery, having set their slaves free by bringing them to Cincinnati. Highly cultivated and talented as well as financially well-to-do, they unconcernedly became true reformers in many ways. The daughter, Mrs. Willey, wrote good Free Soil poetry, then needed by that movement; other members of the family developed their special talents as writers or musicians, while Mrs. Vaughan used her advantages for making propaganda by encouraging Lyceum lectures, which system was then in its infancy. And she invited nearly all prominent speakers to stay at her house while in Cleveland.

I thus saw and heard Dr. Harriot Kezia Hunt; Mr. and Mrs. George Hildreth; Mrs. George Brad-

burn; Grace Greenwood; Rev. Henry Bond; Rev.
Mr. Mumford; Rev. Mr. Chapin; Ralph Waldo Emerson; Dr. W. Elder; Bayard Taylor; James Mur-
dock, the actor; Frederick Douglass; Mr. John
Giles, of the Lyceum lecture system; Rev. Starr
King; prominent professors of the Western Reserve College; and a number of leading *literati* of
those times as well as men distinguished in politics, such as Speaker Colfax, leader of the Free Soil
party, and Secretary Salmon Chase, who were holding political meetings. All these acquaintances were
of incalculable use to me in this educational period.
Although not able to converse with them, I could
observe and learn much that was of greatest importance to my future.

Discussions pro and con on all kinds of subjects
agitated the people, and more than once did I hear
the "Boston Trio"—William Lloyd Garrison, Wendell Phillips and Theodore Parker—denounced as
disturbers of Law and Order.

To Mrs. Vaughan's untiring patience do I owe
my acquiring the English language as well as I was
then capable of doing. I had to write two essays
that winter, one being for an association formed
by the medical students, and one being my thesis.
After having assisted me in correcting the gram-
mar, Mrs. Vaughan made me read over each one
four times, from ten to half-past eleven o'clock, for
fifty evenings, until I got a good English pronunciation of which I was very proud.

My German conservatism was not a little startled
when I found that here also the so-called Woman's
Rights movement (the political enfranchisement of

women) was heartily indorsed. Yet, in all the families whose acquaintance I made from this social center, and who were so different from those in the circles of Mrs. Severance and Mr. Mayo, I soon recognized the same prejudice existing against all women who attempted to step out of the domestic sphere. In spite of their cultivation in literature and music and the fine arts generally, after the completion of school life the women preferred a mere social activity in their own surroundings and a Lady Bountiful attitude among the poor belonging to their respective churches.

I perceived so many contradictions in meeting with these evidently superiorly educated women. For instance, they abhorred the female medical student and would not dare be seen with one of them in the streets, and they considered themselves heroic for including me when inviting any of the Vaughan family to tea or to an evening gathering; yet, in discussing matters of politics, as Free Soilers or sympathizers with anti-slavery, they manifested an independence of speech which showed that they were well acquainted with the subject they discussed. It was so, also, in spiritual and religious matters, in school affairs and in regard to pauperism. The women, young and old, held firmly to their intellectual convictions, and these might be for or against their fathers, brothers or husbands.

It astonished me to see how absolutely quietly and calmly discussions were carried on, without bitterness or excitement, between opponents, and how respectfully men would listen to each other and to

the women in particular, even when directly contradicted in their own views of the case.

It was a great educational opportunity for me,
broadening my whole nature which had been nar-
rowed by the German school training of being *a
subject*, first to the Government and next to Man.

I was often taken by surprise when, on the brink
of forgetting that these manifestations of independence could exist side by side with the most ludicrous prejudice against me and my medical companions, I would be seriously questioned, ''Do you want
to turn women into men?''

And when appearing in a church or meeting, we
always noticed a significant withdrawal of all present so that we medical students could walk or sit
conspicuously by ourselves. This isolation which
bordered on ostracism when exposed to a limited
multitude was very painful to bear, especially as we
were young and at the time of life when the *amour
propre* of the individual would seek obscurity rather
than notoriety.

Elizabeth Blackwell only wished to open ''legally''
to women a field of labor which was successfully cultivated by them ''illegally,'' because we find that
women were numerously employed to relieve pain
and to combat disease.

They appear, it is true, in the capacity of nurses
only, but in this vocation their usefulness increased
to such an extent that the name ''Doctresses'' was
given to them, and their advice and help were sought
by the educated and the ignorant, the rich and the
poor, from far and near.

Legally, their position was not recognized. They

maintained it either through their evident integrity of purpose or through shrewdness, making themselves as useful and as honored as the men physicians, who in reality were often superior to them only because the position of the men was made secure by political laws made by the men and for the men.

Thus when, in the later forties, a woman claimed the right of gaining intellectual power, it appeared as if she stepped out of her sphere. And this claim, so simple and natural, was perverted by a hostile spirit into the claim that she wished "to become a man."

Under the influence of this perverting and contaminating spirit, the sensitive were shocked by her demands; the indolent were vexed; and the wildest apprehensions were excited among both men and women.

I can recall by name even, persons who went to see Miss Blackwell at the college where she studied, really expecting to behold a woman on whom a beard had developed, but who were surprised to find a most womanly woman, delicate in size and figure, timid and reserved in manners, and modest in speech.

Agreeably disappointed in her, proud of her ability, and anxiously wishing her success in all her desires and enterprises, they yet did not dare to invite her to their houses or to request an introduction to her, from fear that they might meet her on the streets and be forced to recognize her in the presence of others.

To associate with or to employ a "doctress" famous merely for common sense, was perfectly respectable and honorable, but to seek the acquaintance of a woman who wished to enter "legally" upon the same work which these doctresses performed was considered of very doubtful respectability.

The consequence was that my three fellow students withdrew entirely into their own abodes and devoted themselves to their professional work. This I could not possibly do. I had to persevere and get acquainted with all phases of American life in order to become what I had always hoped to be, an assistant organizer in the development of the medical education of women.

"The Emancipated Woman!" That was the horror of the day, in social life as well as in the press. And woe to those women who perhaps through lack of physical beauty, or through want of taste in dress, or through a too profound seriousness, did not observe all social graces in detail. They became objects of criticism in private and in public. Exaggerated descriptions and accounts of their every word and act, as well as impertinent and ridiculous delineations, came forth in speech and in print for the amusement of all those who wished to stagnate progress.

Nobody could or would believe that in so few years the admission of the right of women, as "human beings," to do that for which they felt best fitted would lead to the acceptance of the presence of women in all branches of human activity; and not only this, but that these women would be respected and honored, and appointed to positions of responsibility hitherto filled only by men. And, again, that the number of positions calling for them would be greater than the number of women available, thus proving that there is no danger that all women will desert their natural sphere as wives and mothers.

CHAPTER XVII

Interesting adventure leading to acquaintance with Ralph Waldo Emerson—Marie receives the degree of M.D.— The faculty presents her, as a gift, with the note which she had given in payment for her lecture fees—Reflections: direct benefit which the men students derived from co-education; tribute to her college teachers, especially Drs. Delamater and Kirtland. (Twenty-six years of age: 1856.)

This second year of my stay in Cleveland was therefore a most valuable episode of my life, turning all my views topsy-turvy, uprooting me, so to say, from all German conservatism and throwing me into this chaotic medley of contradictions.

However, the one straight aim of preparing myself for the examinations leading to a medical diploma kept me from any alarming detour in my progress of evolution, and the year closed without any other than the usual events in the course of life, as, for instance, the birth of a nephew which arrived in December and which I superintended, my brother-in-law defraying my expenses to and from New York.

But I did have one very interesting adventure. And one daughter, Virginia Vaughan, who had been really the means of my being asked to become the guest of the house, was the leader in this. Mr. Ralph Waldo Emerson had lectured in Cleveland

and he was as usual a guest of Mrs. Vaughan; she had been his pupil when a young lady and at school in Boston and quite an intimacy existed between them. From Cleveland, Mr. Emerson went to Hudson, ten miles away, the real seat of the Western Reserve College, and he was advertised to lecture there at six in the evening.

Virginia, anxious to hear Mr. Emerson again, came to the medical college which closed at four in the afternoon, and proposed our going to Hudson on the half-past four o'clock train to return on the one leaving there at nine. On arriving at the Hudson lecture hall, we found a notice posted on the door informing the public that the lecture would be at seven o'clock.

We went back to the station intending to return to Cleveland and there we found there was no train until the one at nine o'clock. The station was a crude, cold room, having only an insignificant little stove, so Virginia proposed that we find Mr. Emerson who, she knew, was at the house of his cousin, Professor Emerson, a member of the college faculty.

It was a cold, bitter day with plenty of snow everywhere, so we could do nothing better than seek the house of the Professor. There we were made so cordially welcome by Mrs. Emerson that we forgot even our very improper appearance in our common everyday working attire. These kind hosts would not allow us to return in that last train but telegraphed to the family in Cleveland of our whereabouts, insisting that we remain with them over Sunday, there being no trains till Monday morning at eight o'clock.

That evening, after returning from the lecture and while partaking of a cup of hot tea, we noticed a bright rosy light upon the parlor windows. Thinking it was an exhibition of "northern lights," we all started for the door. Alas! it was a great conflagration of magnificent hues of dark red flame. We went to see the spectacle from a little hill between the house and the fire where hundreds of people were already assembled, all of whom were warmed and pleased by the wonderful flames, without any one making any effort to extinguish them or to try to prevent their spreading from the burning cheese storehouse to the adjacent factory. Mr. Ralph Waldo Emerson asked in astonishment of the men standing nearest, "Why don't you try to extinguish the fire?" One replied in a very phlegmatic way, "Because we have no firemen or machines." While another added, "Even if we had, there would be no use for them as we have no water." The little town of Hudson, with its pretty streets and with a college aspiring to become soon a university, was without water. This seemed impossible to believe, yet it was true, as Professor Emerson assured us.

This night will always remain a memorable one, for independently of that glorious illumination of the snow-covered city and landscape which was so fearful and yet so wondrously beautiful, it gave me an opportunity to get acquainted with one of the greatest philosophers of our times. This opportunity was well used during the Sunday morning when all but Mr. Ralph Waldo Emerson and myself went to church, I having no suitable clothes for such attendance. This short acquaintance gave rise to the many kind and pleasant words to people with which Mr. Emerson favored me in later years, and to a very interesting friendship with members of Professor Emerson's family residing in New York and Boston.

During the winter of 1855-1856, my life in Cleveland became doubly interesting because I began to speak English and thus was able to manifest my appreciation of the delightful impressions which I received, directly and indirectly, through the channels outside of my medical studies.

How often was I surprised by the doubts of these more or less radical reformers concerning the success of women as medical practitioners. Only Ralph Waldo Emerson spoke rationally about the innovation of women physicians; yet he doubted that women would enter upon any other profession except that of teaching.

Having spent Christmas in New York with my sisters and the family, who enjoyed the newly arrived baby as only the first one can be enjoyed, I returned to my college life with new zest, and I now had the extra task to perform of writing my thesis for examination.

New Year's Day, 1856, was cold and windy and brought a snowstorm. The lake opposite the house presented a sad and terrible aspect in the presence of an icebound schooner with several dead sailors covered with ice and hanging in its rigging. Attempts to reach the vessel in small boats had failed, and a number of sturdy, sympathizing men were standing on the shore discussing plans for relief that still might be given to some unseen fellow beings on board.

As the day was no holiday, I, of course, had to go to college. But it was a bitter day. I thought my first winter in Cleveland was a severe one, but this was cruelly so and it continued till late in March.

The first ten weeks of the year were spent very industriously by me in preparing to pass my examinations, after my thesis was accepted. The latter was considered exceptionally good, and was the cause of my not failing as a candidate for a diploma, because I received only mediocre marks in all the branches of study, even falling below the passing mark in one branch.

I wish to make a statement of this fact here for many good reasons. One is, that it shows the utter absurdity of giving marks or numbers at all, for independently of my being still very awkward in English expressions, I was, and still am, very slow in thinking out any subject and I have a very poor mechanical memory.

Among my three companions I was very much liked when discussing or reasoning out problems of our studies, often systematizing what seemed to us chaotic on a first reading. They often made me the "quizzer," and I was not a little ashamed to hear with what readiness they gave names and relations of organs, knowing how impossible it would be for me to do the same.

But when it came to practical deductions or applications they always relied upon me. I enjoyed the confidence of those professors with whom I had practical instruction, and I had always out-patients on hand to look after. For this latter, my companions felt they had no time, sitting and committing to memory their lessons, and only one of them had had any practical work in that she had lived in a "water-cure" establishment.

I envied my three friends not a little when I found they graduated with full marks and high honors. However, the desired diploma of "M.D." was also awarded to me. I felt grateful for it, intending to make the most conscientious use of the power thus given to me and which I felt I fully deserved, as I could not help judging my medical knowledge to be as complete as that of any one of the forty-two graduates.

And it is for this reason, also, that I condemn the method of judging of the ability or competence of any student simply from questions and answers. So much knowledge can be acquired by storing the memory with all sorts of details, without making one's self fit to digest what is learned and to assimilate even a part of it. But how necessary is this latter when one is called upon to help all sorts of conditions in people who seek advice for physical, mental or moral ailments. And a physician, in the full sense of the word, must be qualified to help human nature from these three points of view. The mere studying and learning by heart of the symptoms of diseases, and of the origin, preparation and doses of drugs, ought to be the last chapter to be examined upon.

My private studies in which examinations would have given much more satisfactory results, were "biology," "cellular anatomy" and "comparative anatomy," in none of which subjects had we any instruction in the college. And it is my opinion that the medical profession will not, and cannot, make medicine a science as long as these branches (in both their physiological and pathological forms) are not studied profoundly and made a foundation upon which to build methods for averting or controlling disease. So long as physicians are taught to talk of "curing disease," so long will the whole profession wander in the realm of empiricism, if not outright quackery.

It may be excusable that I thus use myself in illustrating what I think is so pernicious, namely, cramming the memory with learning isolated facts and filling the brain to its fullest capacity with the names of authors and their opinions, leaving no room for individual reasoning or research or for the power of making original deductions and applications.

After this apparent digression, I must return to my theme, namely, the last few weeks of my student life in Cleveland. As I have already stated how distrustful the so-called "good society" was concerning female medical students and how ready the so-called "reformers" were to seek them, I must here mention a peculiar aberration which had taken hold of the whole community. I refer to what was then called Mesmerism. The individual thinking and theorizing on this subject assumed with many persons a perfectly preposterous form. The views held were based on no scientific research or study but simply on memorizing what was published (often after the most superficial observation) regarding hysterical or somnambulistic manifestations.

The faith with which statements of so-called "cures" in all sorts of illnesses were received was just as widespread as that which later accepted Clairvoyance, Hypnotism and Christian Science. These, one after the other, followed the Mesmerism and Magnetism waves; but they are all precisely the same thing, under other names, and they are all more or less influenced by what is called Spiritualism. And the countless "miracle" workers, under a host of names, are all of the same class.

The desire for the assistance of superrational influences is one of the greatest obstacles which the human mind has to overcome. It will take centuries of education before the majority of thinking beings will learn that a cell will produce only its like, that modifications of the cell are produced only after a time of slow and, as yet, imperceptible changes, and not suddenly by prayer or personal magnetism.

One of the most perplexing phenomena which I observed was that educated men themselves became victims of these delusions. For instance, I knew a professor of botany who was so completely absorbed in the phenomena of *Spiritualism* and *Magnetism* that he submitted himself to treatment by these uneducated pretenders for an ailment produced by malaria. It is sometimes almost discouraging to see that even education will not prevent faith in the superrational or supernatural.

But the Earth has billions and billions of years to live, and at the rate of mental development as we have observed it, I have no doubt that the human intellect will grow out of its present infantile condition into a maturity of which even the present generations have no conception, although, unconsciously, we all assist in nursing the embryo of intelligence which we call "knowledge" and "science."

One may dream of the greatness of the human mind when all the inhabitants of the earth will be as well-developed mentally as the few out of the billions are to-day. One may imagine that the lowest of the Pygmies in mid-Africa or the stupidest Esquimaux near the North Pole will be able to think, to reason and to enjoy, as much as I do now; and that the then great minds will work and struggle to bring up in the scale such poor ignorant mortals as those of my present level, these then existing by the billions as we have the billions of illiterate existing to-day.

[Walt Whitman had a similar thought, and it is interesting to compare her and his expression of it, remembering the difference between prose and poetry, and the obstruction to expression caused by a foreign tongue which never became easy to her. In "Leaves of Grass," he says:

This day before dawn I ascended a hill and looked
    at the crowded heaven,
And I said to my Spirit, *When we become the enfold-*
    ers of those orbs, and the pleasure and knowl-
    edge of everything in them, shall we be filled
    and satisfied then?
And my Spirit said, *No, we but level that lift to*
    pass and continue beyond.]

In March, 1856, the great event took place. On

Commencement Day, forty-two students, four of whom were women, received the degree of "M.D." The hall in which the exercises took place was crowded, not only with friends of the graduates but with a goodly number of the curious of the city who had come to get a look at the women doctors. A deep silence prevailed after the president had alluded to the female portion of the students, and the dropping of a pin might have been heard when one after the other, according to alphabetical arrangement, they stepped up to the platform, each to receive her roll of parchment. No sign for or against them was made and all went home in a dull, somber mood.

The doors of the college had closed behind us, and the words of advice to "go out and do honor to your chosen profession" with which the whole event had concluded, rang in my ears, though I had not the slightest idea how to realize them.

Shortly after Commencement, the dean of the college (Dr. Delamater) called upon me. A call from this venerable gentleman was a thing so unusual that numberless conjectures as to what this visit might mean flitted through my brain on my way to the parlor. He received me, as usual, paternally, wished me a thousand blessings, and handed back to me the note for one hundred and twenty dollars, payable in two years, which I had given for the lecture fees. He told me that in the meeting of the faculty after graduation day, it was proposed by one of the professors to return the note to me as a gift. To this, those present cheerfully gave a unanimous vote, adding their wishes for my success and appointing Dr. Delamater as their delegate to inform me of the proceedings.

This was a glorious beginning, for which I am more than thankful, and for which I was especially so at that time when I had barely money enough to return to New York, with very small prospects of getting means wherewith to commence practice. The mention of this fact might be thought indiscreet by the faculty in Cleveland were they still so organized as to admit women, which I am sorry to say is no longer the case, though they give as their reason that women at present have their own medical colleges and, consequently, no longer have need of theirs.

Before I quit the subject of the Cleveland College, I must mention a fact which may serve as an argument against the belief that the sexes cannot study together without exerting an injurious effect upon each other. During the last winter of my study, there was such emulation in respect to the graduating honors among the candidates for graduation, comprising thirty-eight male and four female students, that all studied more closely than they had ever done before—the men not wishing to be excelled by the women, nor the women by the men. One of the professors afterwards told me that whereas it was usually a difficult thing to decide upon the best three theses to be read publicly at the Commencement, since all were more or less indifferently written, this year the theses were all so good that it was necessary, to avoid doing absolute injustice, to select thirteen from which parts should be read.

Does not this prove that the stimulus of the one sex upon the other would act favorably rather than otherwise upon the profession? And would not the very best tonic that could be given to the individual be to pique his *amour propre* by the danger of being excelled by one of the opposite sex? Is not this natural, and would not this be the best and the surest reformation of humanity and its social condition, if left free to work out its own development?

On the day following the visit of Dr. Delamater, I received a letter from my brother-in-law in which he told me that his business compelled him to go to Europe for half a year, and that he had, therefore, made arrangements for me to procure money, in case that I should need it to commence my practice. He said that he intended to assist me afterwards, but that as he thought it best for my sister (his wife) to live out of New York during his absence, he was willing to lend me as much money as I required until his return. I accepted his offer with infinite pleasure, for it was another instance of real friendship. He was by no means a rich man but was simply in the employ of a large importing house.

By giving lessons in German, I had earned a little money that served to cover my most necessary expenses. For the last months that I spent in Cleveland, I carried in my purse one solitary cent as a sort of talisman, firmly believing that some day it would turn into gold; but this did not happen, and on the day that I was expecting the receipt of the last eighteen dollars for my lessons, which were designed to bear my expenses to New York, I gave it to a poor woman in the street who begged me for a cent, and it doubtless ere long found its way into a ginshop.

The twenty months that I spent in Cleveland were chiefly devoted to the study of medicine in the English language, and in this I was assisted by most noble-hearted men. Dr. Delamater's office became a pleasant spot and its occupants a necessity to me. On the days that I did not meet them, my spirits fell below zero.

In spite of the pecuniary distress from which I constantly suffered, I was happier in Cleveland than ever before or since. I lived in my element, having a fixed purpose in view and enjoying the warmest tokens of real friendship. I was liked in college, and though the students often found it impossible to repress a hearty laugh at my ridiculous blunders in English, they always showed me respect and fellowship in the highest sense of the terms.

After receiving the degree of "M.D." and leaving the college behind me, it seems quite right to stop for a few moments and cast a retrospective glance at my own situation, objectively. I wonder whether any one can justly claim that one has always followed a well-laid plan in life, or whether conditions and environment do not mold our actions, sustain our firmness and fortify our persistence in following or working towards a positive aim.

I do not think that in youth the individual shapes the *modus operandi* of any undertaking. In spite of having a vague idea, or even a strong desire to carry into effect such an idea, environment as well as outside influences must come to the aid, in order to keep alive and to nourish the hope that his pre-conceived idea or desire can ever be realized. Without such assistance, the young aspirant can easily be diverted and led into spheres of action not intended or desired in the first instance.

After we become older, we may honestly imagine that we followed a regularly planned course in life, when we really lived simply according to whatever chances from time to time molded or influenced our activity.

During the years from 1850 to March, 1856, it now seems to me that no definite plan determined my action, and that all that guided me was the strong desire to make for myself "an independent livelihood" and to assist all persons who felt that same strong desire.

Several times I was tempted to change my field of work so as to obtain this independence. For instance, in Berlin, after leaving the Charité Hospital, offers were made to me by eminent physicians to take charge of private hospitals which were then beginning to be started, especially for surgery. I did not accept these offers, partly because they again placed me in dependence and partly because surgery had been distasteful to me as it was then practiced, without anesthetics, the use of neither ether nor chloroform having become general.

So, as we reason from the concrete to the abstract, I doubt that any one, man or woman, can stand up and declare that one has achieved exactly what one hoped to achieve when entering upon the battlefield of active life. There is no doubt that an intrinsic fitness for a certain kind of activity guides us towards such influences as we need to develop this fitness, but that is all.

It is for this reason, perhaps, that I never married, although educated and trained with the idea that the true sphere of woman is to be a wife and mother. Also, I was very sentimentally inclined towards men, to moonlight walks and to the exchange of friendly letters; but I always grew tired of it all in a very short time and decided that none of these attachments was the right one, proving that my desire for independence was innate. So, happy the man who got released from me and happy was I to remain free.

Again, after arriving in New York, I might just as well have become a manufacturer, as I had begun to be, if I had become familiar with the English language. I was quite happy in that branch of work and was able to assist many a woman in various ways. But the impossibility of acquiring the language in that limited sphere prevented the enlargement of my knowledge and connections necessary in that branch of activity.

Then later came, last but not least, the temptation to go as missionary to the Cherokee Indians. I have not a doubt that in that direction I could have developed my independence and have been extremely useful, had I not been influenced by people in whose judgment I had full confidence—a rare thing in young, impulsive, enthusiastic natures, to accept the advice of others. I was bridled and held in check, not by a clear vision but by influences which overpowered me as the magnet does the iron which it attracts.

Also, do I consider it fair and right and not out of place to speak of the lecturers and teachers connected with the medical department of the Western Reserve College. At the time as well as in the following years, I often heard depreciatory remarks about our professors and their methods of instruction.

There was no doubt that a very few of the students in attendance had a collegiate education superior to that which some of the professors might have had in their younger days, for instance, Dr. John J. Delamater, then over seventy years old, and Dr. J. B. Kirtland, not far from seventy, both of them the kindest of men, true philanthropists and men of a natural genius who had attained a high position among their fellow men.

They had had, perhaps, less advantages in book-learning when young, yet they had the power of inspiring youth to a higher and more thorough study, and their influence in developing the thinking powers of the students was something remarkable. Originality of thought, reasoning and deduction was the example given to us by them. And the form of their teachings was not so much memorizing prescribed methods as the teaching of the students how to observe closely all the phenomena of the case of illness in question and how to study the smallest details, physical, mental and moral, in order to find the primary cause. Such instruction can never be gained from books, although medical literature has now begun to attempt it. Many of the students ridiculed the hints and directions given, while to others they were the inspiration for deeper study even after the degree was obtained.

I know it was so in my case, and works like Kölliker's *Comparative Anatomy,* later Virchow's *Cellular Pathology,* and works on biology, embryology and histology became really the foundation upon which I built my practice, taking little heed of recommendations of how to treat cases or how to administer doses of this or that old or new remedy or system of remedies. I did my own reasoning, I made my own deductions, in as logical a method as possible as the cases revealed themselves to my understanding through physical or psychical symptoms. Originality and spontaneity of mental action are injured by unthinking cramming of mind and memory with booklearning.

It is for these reasons that I love to think, with gratitude and a deep feeling of honor, of the men who then constituted the medical faculty, although two of them were greatly annoyed by the presence of the four women students and did not hesitate to manifest their feelings in word and deed, without being offensive.

Indeed, even this feeling that our presence was objectionable was of use in our training, as it gave us a strong foretaste of the prejudice which we were to meet in our professional lives. And it helped us in many ways to develop the courage which we were to need in meeting the offensive behavior of many physicians and students with whom we were obliged to come in contact when trying to seek fellowship in private practice, or to increase our knowledge, or to gain admittance to public institutions.

CHAPTER XVIII

*Returns to New York to begin practice as an M.D.—
Insuperable difficulties encountered by a woman
physician in finding an office to rent in New York—
Dr. Zakrzewska opens her office in one of Dr. Blackwell's parlors—No admission for women to dispensaries or hospitals—Infirmary remains closed for lack
of money—Dr. Zakrzewska meets Mary L. Booth who
informs the newspapers and social circles of the
medical women—In desperation, she goes to Boston
to visit Mrs. Severance and to seek contributions for
the Infirmary—Meets Mr. Samuel E. Sewall and his
daughter Lucy—Her campaign in Boston is successful—Its extension to Portland, Maine, is unsuccessful—She goes to Philadelphia for the same purpose
but succeeds only in convincing the Female Medical
College there that it must build a hospital for itself—
A second visit to Boston to ask help for the long-
delayed Infirmary Fair—Meets Mrs. Ednah D. Cheney
—Extends campaign to smaller towns around Boston
with no success. (Twenty-six years of age: 1856.)*

WITH regret, I made ready to depart from Cleveland. I dreaded the obstacles which I saw and felt
were before me and which I must conquer. I fully
felt the isolated social position which we four women
medical students had occupied in Cleveland. My
three companions, belonging to the orthodox church
and disapproving of each and every subject discussed in Mr. Mayo's congregation, had absolutely
no outside recreation, "even of the body," and were

shunned even in the boarding house by the inmates there, where we had found an otherwise comfortable home during the first winter, in 1854.

I realized the opposition to women physicians still more after I had learned to speak English. Strange to say, this was far stronger among women than among men in and outside of the profession. My discouragement grew the stronger the nearer the end of my stay in Cleveland approached.

Following Commencement Day, a tremendous snowstorm was the first event which blockaded my next movements; for days no trains could pass the roads; the last quarter of my lessons in German had ended on March 1; my packing made little demand on my time and it was finished. I had no special interests to keep me longer in Cleveland, and I began to consider this calamity of snow a bad omen when Mr. Willey brought home the news that, in a roundabout way and by changing trains four times, I might be able to reach New York in thirty-six hours.

So I started off and I had really a most tedious journey, suffering greatly from the cold before I reached my family, after forty hours in trains, and finding New York just getting free from the snow blockades of the streets.

The welcome at my sisters' was cordial. The one next in age to me had taken a position in a large wholesale millinery establishment, receiving a good salary, while the next younger one superintended the household, and the youngest attended school. We were all hoping that our father would get his furlough for a visit and counsel as to what to do next with the family. Both brothers had gone to the Far West, seeking their own fortunes as brothers usually do.

Although our father sent financial aid to the two younger sisters, eighteen and eleven years old, I had no hope of such assistance from him, and I could not settle down with the family because they resided in Hoboken, New Jersey.

This was too far distant from Dr. Elizabeth Blackwell as well as from the center of the poor among whom it was necessary to seek patients. I felt the necessity of familiarizing myself with general practice in which I had had but very slight training. No clinical instruction was attempted in college, all students depending upon the private practice of their preceptors for this kind of teaching. We women students had received scarcely any such opportunities, as even our kind and beloved Dr. Delamater could not often venture upon such an innovation as to take a female student with him, even when visiting the poorest patients.

My good brother-in-law, who did not have my father's prejudices and his distrust in my eventual success as a practitioner, offered me financial aid, promising to give guaranties to the people from whom I would hire rooms where I might begin practice.

Immediately after my arrival in New York, I began to look out for a suitable office, consulting Dr. Elizabeth Blackwell, with whom I had maintained a constant correspondence, in regard to location.

My fears concerning the opposition to women physicians were fully realized. I found no well-regulated household would rent rooms to me. I investigated everywhere, in all respectable parts of New York wherever signs announced "Parlor to let for a physician" or where I was sent by agents. But as soon as it was learned that it was a woman physician who desired the office, I was denied the opportunity of even looking at the advertised rooms. Thus days and weeks were spent. I even began to explain and to remonstrate with those who sought tenants, but it was all in vain.

Some were afraid to let an office to a female physician lest she might turn out a spiritual medium, clairvoyant, hydropathist, etc. Others, who believed me when I told them that I had a diploma from a regular school and should never practice contrary to its requirements, inquired to what religious denomination I belonged, and whether I had a private fortune or intended to support myself by my practice. While the third class, who asked no questions at all, demanded three dollars a day for a back parlor alone, without the privilege of putting a sign on the house or the door.

Now all this may be very exasperating when it is absolutely necessary that one should have a place upon which to put a sign to let the world know that she is ready to try her skill upon suffering humanity; but it has such a strongly ludicrous side that I could not be provoked in spite of all the fatigue and disappointment of wandering over the city when, with aching limbs, I commenced the search afresh each morning, with the same prospect of success.

Finally, in a moderate-sized house, I was admitted by an introductory letter from an agent. The lady was kind and pleasant, entered into conversation with me and informed me that a cousin of hers had drawn her attention to the fact that women studied medicine in Cleveland. On further talk, she spoke of one who was especially liked by her cousin through the interest which Ralph Waldo Emerson took in her. And thus I found that this lady was a cousin of Mrs. Emerson, of Hudson, Ohio.

Of course, my heart was delighted to find a cultured woman not only interested in me and my profession but who was also willing to have me become a member of her household, if—her husband agreed to such an arrangement. Alas! in a few days came a letter in which she regretted that her husband could not reconcile himself to a woman doctor. He feared all sorts of annoyances should he take such a step as to have a woman doctor go in and out of his house. At any rate, he could not bear the thought of having the sign of a woman physician on his house.

Such was the horror that beset every one, that woman would disgrace decency and undertake abhorred practice. The name of "Madame Restelle" was on every one's tongue as typifying the "female physician." She was then the leading abortionist, of whom a prominent lawyer said, when Dr. Blackwell and I called upon him to see if something could not be done to stop her in her vile career, "She is a social necessity, and she will be protected by rich and influential personages." However, I may here remark that after many years of agitation, her infamous business succeeded in placing her and some of her disciples in prison, and, eventually, she killed herself by drowning in the spacious bathtub of the extravagantly luxurious house on Fifth Avenue, where she resided under her real name.

Thus time passed, and I could find no abode. My lack of success was similar to that of Dr. Blackwell who had finally been obliged to rent a house, and she now proposed that I should join her at her home, she letting me have the back parlor for office purposes. Thus I was able to arrange for office work as well as for general practice. Arrangements were concluded and, on April 17, I established myself with her, yet independent of her, in business.

Still, small as was Dr. Blackwell's practice, this association was of great benefit to me. Her household consisted of her relatives and was headed by an older sister and her mother, a fine, cultivated lady. Antoinette Brown Blackwell and her husband joined us just before their oldest daughter was expected, and there also came Lucy Stone and her husband, Henry Blackwell. In fact we were a delightful family, suffering more or less from social ostracism but happy in spirit, and feeling far above the ordinary run of mankind in the belief of our superiority in thought and aim.

I love to remember the friendship which developed between Dr. Elizabeth Blackwell and myself when, wearied and disappointed in waiting for patients who seldom appeared, we renewed our courage by getting temporarily away from the field of struggle. On Sundays, we took long, long walks in Staten Island, in Jersey Heights, yes, even as far as Hackensack, watching the budding trees, the inspiring scenery and the glorious sunsets, and renewing our faith in our calling as physicians. And we discussed all kinds of plans as to how to become of use to our fellow men and to ourselves.

[These must have been memorable walks, for Dr. Blackwell refers to them again and again in later life in her letters from England to Dr. Zakrzewska, recalling "the picture which is hung up in memory, the dark-haired young physician with whom I used to walk on Weehawken Heights."]

Alas! money was wanting. To resume even the little dispensary work of two years previous was impossible, for the reëstablishment of that called for a sum of five hundred dollars and this we could not raise. Meanwhile, we tried to get opportunities to improve our practical knowledge by endeavoring to get admission into dispensaries or hospitals. Everywhere we met objections, and everywhere we found denial.

Many high-stationed professors and physicians to whom Dr. Blackwell had applied were willing, but the general practitioners objected, just as remains the situation at present in most instances. The fear that women doctors would diminish their practice was the real cause of their objection; although the denials were usually expressed as the moral conviction that women could not take any serious responsibility, or, if they did, that they would unsex themselves. However, a German physician, Dr. Aigner, and a Scotch physician, Dr. McCready, occasionally allowed me to accompany them to their respective hospital and dispensary.

Meanwhile, I had regularly attended the Fair meetings which were held every Thursday, wonder-

ing how persons could afford to meet to so little purpose. There was scarcely any life in these gatherings, and when I saw ladies come week after week
to resume the knitting of a baby's stocking (which
was always laid aside again in an hour or two, without any marked progress), I began to doubt whether
the sale of these articles would ever bring ten thousand cents instead of the ten thousand dollars which
it was proposed at the first meeting to raise in order
to buy a house. I used to say on Wednesday, "To-
morrow we have our Fair meeting. I wonder
whether there will be, as usual, two and a half persons present or three and three-quarters."

After weeks of this idle waiting, for the few patients who came through acquaintances did not fill
much of my time, I began to feel desperate, especially as social life also was so utterly closed against
us, and this latter was such a necessity to my temperament. I then proposed to go canvassing with
circulars giving information of our previous experiment, to try to collect money for the establishment
of a dispensary.

The idea occurred to me to go from house to house
and ask for a dime at each, which, if given, would
amount to ten dollars a day; and, with the money
thus collected daily for half a year, to establish a
nucleus hospital which, as a fixed fact, should stimulate its friends to further assistance.

I took my notebook and wrote out the whole plan,
and also calculated the expenses of such a miniature
hospital as I proposed, including furniture, beds,
household utensils, everything, in short, that was
necessary in such an institution. With this book

which I still have in my possession, I went one evening into Dr. Blackwell's parlor and, seating myself, told her that I could not work any longer for the Fair in the way that the ladies were doing; and then read my plan to her, which I advocated long and earnestly.

She finally agreed with me that it would be better speedily to establish a small hospital than to wait for the large sum that had been proposed, though she did not approve of the scheme of the dime collection, fearing that I would not only meet with great annoyances but would also injure my health in the effort. At that time, after some discussion, I agreed with her. Now I think that this plan would have been better than that which I afterwards followed. On the same evening I proposed, and we agreed, that on a year from that day (the 1st of May, 1857), the New York Infirmary should be opened.

I went to rest with a light heart, but rose sorrowfully in the morning. "In one year from to-day, the Infirmary must be opened," said I to myself, "and the funds towards it are two pairs of half-knit babies' stockings." The days passed in thinking what was the next best scheme to raise money for its foundation, when an accidental visit from Mary L. Booth to Dr. Blackwell turned the tide in another direction. Miss Booth was serving her apprenticeship as a journalist through the kindness of the editor of the New York *Times*.' Her sister who was a patient of Dr. Blackwell had interested both Mary and him in the idea of women doctors, so Mary came to interview us concerning our practical progress.

This interview led to the disclosure of our wishes and plans regarding the dispensary, and Miss Booth, taking up the idea, made our wishes known in the *Times,* very guardedly, of course, but decidedly. The effect of this little notice was remarkable, and it gave both Dr. Blackwell and myself new hope and also the courage to ask for similar remarks in other papers.

At the same time, my social circle became a little widened through this acquaintance with Miss Booth which I developed when I found that she also was a beginner in her career and had obstacles to overcome; as, for instance, hiding her sex by signing only her initials to whatever she wrote, or not signing at all.

Thus a few new friends were obtained for our cause, and a few of Dr. Blackwell's patients who belonged to the sect of Quakers, and who had sustained the former dispensary, came forward promising small subscriptions towards a new effort. Yet no sum was large enough to warrant the expenditure of five hundred dollars, the amount absolutely needed to open this charity for the poor and the chance for us to gain practical experience.

About this time, Dr. Harriot K. Hunt, of Boston, sent a patient of hers to Dr. Blackwell. This patient was accompanied by Dr. W. H. Channing, who was not in practice but who attended this patient with Dr. Blackwell. Becoming acquainted with Dr. Channing, I disclosed to him our financial, professional and social position, enlarging upon the difficulty of obtaining that practical experience in clinics which is so absolutely necessary to the young physician.

Then as I told him of the plan of establishing a dispensary which could have a small number of indoor patients, in fact, the nucleus of a hospital for which Dr. Blackwell had already obtained a charter from the Legislature, his enthusiasm created not only hope but courage.

He spoke so ardently of Boston as being liberal and "the hothouse of all reforms" that I proposed visiting that noble city in the interest of our plans and asked him for introductions, as I knew only Dr. Harriot K. Hunt and Mrs. Severance, the latter recently removed to Boston from Cleveland. He gave me a list of names of Boston ladies—Miss Lucy Goddard, Miss Mary Jane Parkman, Miss Abby May and Mrs. E. D. Cheney.

When I look over my diary and see that the time of my receiving my degree and leaving Cleveland was in March and that this proposition to go to Boston was only three months later, it seems a fact impossible to believe. For the restlessness caused by the want of opportunity to further our desires seemed to turn days into weeks and weeks into months. I find in one of my notes the words, "It seems an impossibility to find friends for our cause; nobody seems to feel the need of hospital or dispensary for the practical training of women physicians. Even our gentlemen friends in the profession say women must find this training for themselves among the poor."

I may here remark, perhaps, a fact which amused me greatly. So far, I had had but very little opportunity to write prescriptions, but whenever I gave any I added my initials, M. E. Z., as signature, thus proving my responsibility. Every time such a prescription was received by an American apothecary, a messenger called to inquire the meaning of those mystical signs. And when I explained that it was my name which was too long to write in full, I was told that signatures to prescriptions were not customary or needed. However, I continued to sign mine, for I felt from the very outset that I must establish the position of being responsible for all I did, so that in case of trouble from either patient or apothecary I could protect myself. So I never followed the then prevailing custom of giving prescriptions without indicating for whom they were intended and by whom they were issued. Perhaps I may add that my practice by the end of the year had brought me one hundred and twenty dollars.

The earnestness with which Dr. Blackwell advocated not only the necessity of having women as physicians but also their thorough education and training for practice was convincing to a few friends, who promised to assist with subscriptions as soon as the idea had taken shape and had materialized itself in a building in which the experiment could be tried.

Nobody has fathomed the depth of Dr. Elizabeth Blackwell's soul as I have had the opportunity to do. On our delightful long walks she was the speaker, and her reasoning was so sound, her determination so firm, her love for humanity so true, that she seemed to me a prophet of no ordinary insight and foresight. Even now, when doubts arise in me whether women will develop fully all the chances provided for their higher scientific education, I recall her words and quiet my doubts, remembering that what one woman has done, thousands can do and will do. To me she was, and is, not preëminently the physician but the philanthropic philosopher, the standard bearer of a higher womanhood.

To such a nature, it is given to inspire others with an idea or an ideal but not the faculty of execution or organization. I was able to supply these latter qualities, and, encouraged by the description of Boston's liberal element, I proposed to Dr. Blackwell to search for a house which would suit our purposes and to get an estimate of the rent and the expense of furnishing it, so as to have a definite sum for which to beg, since simple statements were not sufficient.

[Dr. Blackwell refers to such complementary relations in a letter to Dr. Zakrzewska, written in later years, in which she alludes to the days here described and says:

"I work chiefly in Principles, and you in putting them into practical use; and one is essential to the other in this complex life of ours."

Again she refers to these days, "as we sat in Fifteenth Street planning those everlasting bazaars," and she writes:

"You are a natural doctor, and your best work will always be in the full exercise of direct medical work. . . . You know I am different from you in not being a natural doctor; so, naturally, I do not confine myself to practice.

"I am never without some patients but my thought, and active interest, is chiefly given to some of those moral ends—for which ends I took up the study of medicine."]

The house was found in Bleecker Street close by the poor quarters, at an annual rental of one thousand, three hundred dollars, and an estimate was made of another five hundred dollars for furnishing, as well as an outlay of one hundred dollars for fuel. My proposition was now to go to Boston and try to get half of the rent pledged for a three years' lease, Dr. Blackwell to raise the other half of the three years' rent from friends in New York, and then to hold a Sale or Fair to raise the remaining six hundred dollars.

On the next day, the regular Fair meeting was held at Dr. Blackwell's. The new plan was brought forward, and, although it was as yet nothing but a plan, it acted like a warm, soft rain upon a field after a long drought. The knitting and sewing (for which I have a private horror under all conditions) were laid aside, to my great relief. And the project was talked of with so much enthusiasm that I already saw myself in imagination making my evening visits to the patients in the New York Infirmary; while all the members present (and there were unusually many—I think, six or seven) discussed the question the next day among their circles of friends whether Henry Ward Beecher or a physician of high standing should make the opening speech in the institution.

This excitement increased the interest exceedingly, and the succeeding meetings were quite enthusiastic. The babies' stockings were never again resumed (don't think that because I detested those stockings so much I am cruel enough to wish the little creatures to go barefoot), but plans were made for raising money in New York and for getting articles for sale on a larger scale.

Thus it happened that I went to Boston for the second time in the beginning of July, visiting Mrs. C. M. Severance and using my introductions to begin a regular, systematized campaign "to beg for an institution for American women." For myself I could never have begged; I would sooner have drowned myself. Now I determined to beg money from Americans to establish an institution for their own benefit. Dr. Blackwell agreed to this plan, as there was nothing risked in it, I taking the whole responsibility.

In spite of finding the women of Boston quite ready to listen to me, it was not an easy task to get a three years' promise of six hundred and fifty dollars. The first question put to me was always, "Can you not raise this small sum in rich New York?" The explanation had to be repeated over and over that only a very few women in social life dared to connect themselves openly with "such radical reformers" as we appeared to them. To turn upon "the sphere of woman" and declare openly that she can take the whole responsibility of managing a public institution, as well as the care as a physician of sick women and children, seemed so monstrous to most men and women that in New York money was intrusted to us only with incredulity.

The second and more important question was as to "why we needed and wanted a dispensary and a hospital for women physicians." Nobody at this present time would or could believe that this need then had to most people a preposterous sound.

And here I may tell you an episode which occurred to me in Philadelphia, to which city I went after returning from Boston with my six hundred and fifty dollars pledged. In Philadelphia, the first medical college for women (the Female Medical College of Pennsylvania), had been established in 1850, and it was housed in extremely modest quarters in a rear building on Arch Street. I was introduced through Dr. Ann Preston, one of the first graduates of this college and now one of its professors. And I spoke to the friends of this enterprise at a gathering of both men and women, explaining the need of a practical professional training after a merely theoretical course of instruction. I tried to make plain the greater difficulties which beset the introduction of the young women students to the private patients of their preceptors even though these patients were ever so poor, and I illustrated the situation by quoting Dr. Ann Preston's conscientious refusal to practice under such circumstances, she simply teaching physiology in the college. I also spoke of others going to Europe to seek this clinical instruction from foreign physicians and maternity hospitals.

After having exhausted the subject, as well as myself, one of the ladies present said—it was in the

parlors of Lucretia Mott— "Then thee thinks
that a hospital must be connected with the college?"
I replied, "Yes." "Then thee thinks that practical
training cannot be got by the young physician among
the poor?" I said, "No." "We thank thee for
thy coming to tell us so, and we promise thee that
we shall exert ourselves at once to get a hospital of
our own."

Thus ended my efforts in that noble city. But the
Philadelphia Woman's Hospital was established
there within the five years following my visit.

In Portland, Maine, where I went by the advice
of Mr. Samuel E. Sewall and his aunt, Miss ——, I
also met with no success for the Infirmary. Here,
in spite of my being the guest of some of their relatives, none dared to expose themselves to the ridicule of asking acquaintances to see or hear a woman
doctor. To illustrate again something of the feeling regarding a woman doctor, I must tell an incident which in after years caused us great amusement.

Dr. Harriot K. Hunt had introduced me, in Boston, to Mr. Joseph Sewall, and we had been invited
to meet Mr. Samuel E. Sewall, Miss Lucy E. Sewall
and Miss ——, their aunt. While sitting in the parlor waiting for the dinner hour, Lucy Sewall went
upstairs and, as she told me in later years, examined
my cloak, bonnet and gloves in order to find out
whether they were neat and respectable, she feeling
a great uncertainty as to whether a regularly graduated and practicing woman physician could attend
to the minor details of proper habiliments. Dr.
Hunt was accepted by them as a curiosity but she

had never been a regular student in a college. However, all this company became our truest friends, as the history of the New England Hospital for Women and Children testifies.

The season being July, it was not favorable for doing any more than securing signatures, guaranteeing for the New York Infirmary for Indigent Women and Children six hundred and fifty dollars, for half the rent annually for three years. But friendly invitations to revisit Boston caused me to return in early October.

The encouragement which I brought back to New York from the Boston friends rendered it easy for Dr. Blackwell to secure among her friends the other half of the rent. However, we also needed money to furnish and to prepare the house as a hospital and dispensary. But we hoped to obtain this additional money from the Fair which had been so long in preparation, and it was in connection with this that I again appeared in Boston.

It was then that I made the most valuable acquaintance of Mrs. E. D. Cheney who has ever since been a true and devoted friend of the medical education of women.

This visit was rich in experience as I was introduced by my acquaintances made in July to a great number of the leading women in the anti-slavery cause. From these I learned how the anti-slavery bazaars were managed, and I obtained a promise to provide a table at our New York fair in December, as well as the names of several ladies who would superintend it, so that accommodations for their sojourn in New York might be made. Another table was promised by Dr. Blackwell's English friends to whom she had appealed by letters.

I also visited a number of the smaller towns around Boston for the same purpose but without success. A list of the Boston people in whose houses I spoke, creating enthusiasm, and who subscribed towards the half of the Infirmary rent as well as towards the table for the Fair, is still in my possession and I will here copy the names:

Miss Lucy Goddard	Mrs. Sarah S. Russell
Miss Abby May	Mrs. W. L. Garrison
Miss Mary Jane Parkman	Mrs. E. D. Cheney
	Miss Sarah Clarke
Mrs. George Hildreth	Mrs. James Freeman Clarke
Mrs. George Hilliard	
Miss Anna Lowell	Mr. George W. Bond
Mrs. Mary G. Shaw	Mr. Samuel E. Sewall

besides a goodly number of others not so prominent in benevolent and advanced work for women.

CHAPTER XIX

Boston's help for the Infirmary stimulates New York, sometimes to unconscious humor—Meeting with Fanny Kemble—Dr. Zakrzewska obtains entrée into the variety of social "circles" then existing—The Cary sisters—Women of the Press—The educational circle—The esthetic group—The so-called Free Lovers—The artistic circle—Mrs. Z.'s social circle—The philanthropic circle—The Fourierites—The demonstrating Spiritualists—Woman's Rights meetings—Dr. Zakrzewska and Horace Greeley opposing speakers in discussion on "Divorce"—Dr. Emily urges Dr. Blackwell to give up New York for London, opposition there being lessened by Florence Nightingale's work—The Fair finally materializes and is successful—Dr. Emily Blackwell returns from Europe, making the third physician working upon the Infirmary plans. (Twenty-seven years of age: 1856.)

MEANWHILE, the letters from Dr. Emily Blackwell, who was completing her medical studies in England, urged Dr. Blackwell to give up her life in America and come to England as a more promising field for developing the introduction of medical women into practice.

But Dr. Blackwell held fast to the fact that in America the first Woman's Medical College (Philadelphia) had been in existence for several years, and she felt that it would be unwise to desert this beginning.

The struggles of this little college were so great

because all aids to foster its growth were so hard to acquire; and also because many a student withdrew from the school after a few months of attendance upon learning what great obstacles were to be overcome in acquiring medical knowledge and how great was the social prejudice against female medical students. Hence, only the brave, the courageous, the determined, and the financially equipped women could remain and weather the stormy days of their student life.

Thus it was felt best that the realization of the New York Infirmary should be carried on; and Dr. Emily promised to interest her English friends to contribute to the English table. Dr. Blackwell's friends and well-wishers began with great zeal to arrange sewing circles, while new friends were acquired who were willing to assist in the charity even if not inclined to the "reformers," as we were called.

An old lady, Mrs. T——, residing on Fifth Avenue, was one of the newly acquired friends. She also wished to assist us by introducing us into her circle and she invited me to her reception days which were held from eleven to one—the fashionable hours at that time.

The difficulty was not in my name, for it was very fashionable at that time to introduce exiles and their friends into society, but what should be my title? She said that I was too young to be called "Madame"; and "Miss" would not sound well with my unpronounceable name while "Doctor"—oh! no! she could not call me that; and "Doctress" was not reputable. So, what?

Then, what would I talk about? "Hospitals," of course. Yes, of course—and then she added, tolerantly, "Well, if you must talk on hospitals, do not mention women doctors but say for the purpose of 'training nurses,' which is now so fashionable in England through Miss Nightingale's training at Kaiserswerth, Germany."

Another lady invited me to dine with her. And she remarked, "I shall be all alone and we can talk your plans over without being disturbed or ridiculed by my husband and sons. You see," she added, "my daughters are married and we hold by our fortune a position which would equal that of a duchess in your country, so we must be very careful not to offend good taste by inviting reformers without a thorough knowledge of their plans." When I replied that my ancestry was about as good as her money as we dated our name back to 911, she was quite relieved and asked permission to tell this fact to her friends in order to explain her interest in me.

Then there was the little incident which I never can forget, so ludicrous did it appear to me, when Dr. Blackwell and I called upon Fanny Kemble, and she most tragically exclaimed, "*Women* DOCTORS! NEVER!"

During the summer months, Dr. Blackwell gained a number of new acquaintances who, being inclined towards the elevation of woman's education, were sent to us by Dr. Harriot K. Hunt, of Boston. Among these were Miss Elizabeth Peabody and Miss Anne Whitney (the latter then known simply as a poet, now also as a sculptor) who interested themselves deeply in our projects. And through them we became acquainted with Mrs. Angelina Grimké Weld and her sister, Miss Sarah Grimké, and Mrs. Spring, all these being our neighbors across the Hudson, residing at Eagleswood. Other valuable aid came through Mrs. Lucy Stone and Mrs. Antoinette Brown Blackwell who, sharing the home with us, formed strong links with all the liberally inclined members of the anti-slavery movement. My friend, Mary L. Booth, became of great assistance to me, and I joined an association of women, called the *Alpha,* of which she was secretary.

There was a quiet revolution going on in all strata of social life. The present generation can form only an approximate idea of the spirit of the time in those years. New England transcendentalism had influenced all intelligent people throughout the country. It was a real *Sturm und Drang* period which pervaded men and women alike. Abolitionism was at its height. Everywhere, the *pros* and *cons* of the means to abolish slavery was the topic of conversations and discussions. And transcendentalism was interpreted into all kinds of *isms* because nobody could define its meaning. Thus it happened that there arose a great many circles and cliques in which one or more theories were nurtured.

One of the pleasantest of these circles was that formed by the sisters, Alice and Phœbe Cary, who kept open house every Sunday evening from eight to eleven o'clock These were not the fashionable, senseless receptions of the present day, but real social gatherings where everybody came regularly and often took up the conversation where it was left unfinished the week before, or brought the new events of the week for discussion. All was informal; no sitting down, the little parlor often holding fifty or sixty guests, many representing the press or politics; no refreshments except a pitcher of cold water and glasses in the hall. Eminent men were always the center at these gatherings—the names of Greeley, Colfax, Ripley, Garrison, and a host of similar leaders were never wanting.

This description answers very well for all the other circles. The charm of all these gatherings consisted in the fact that they were not receptions but places where everybody came regularly when disengaged otherwise, or while in New York if not resident. No refreshments were served but a liberal supply of ice water, with plenty of glasses, stood in a little room or in the hall, while conversation or discussion or music or even dancing formed the attraction.

One circle was the promoter of women in the press, and this was headed by Mrs. Elizabeth Oakes Smith. She held open house on Thursday evenings, and here all the then-known press women, musicians and artists met in the most liberal spirit.

In the educational field were Mrs. Kirtland and Miss Haynes, who each had the best school for young ladies but to whose houses invitations were needed.

The esthetic group, representing those who aspired to the cultivation of the fine arts, and including exiles of renown, gathered at evening receptions under the leadership of Mrs. X. In her elegant parlors every one who was introduced by those already accepted was welcomed and entertained with music,

conversation and card playing. Mr. and Mrs.
George Hildreth could be found there week after
week, as well as the then most-renowned musicians
and actors.

Another very prominent circle was that of the
Free Lovers, then so called. Mrs. Grosvenor was
called by Mr. Alcott, whom I first met at her evenings, the "high priestess of free love." This circle
was most frequented by all persons who represented any *ism*. Mr. Alcott held his conversations
often in this house. Messrs. Ripley, Greeley, Albert Brisbane; the pianist, Gottschalk; the advocate
of Spiritualism, Andrew Jackson Davis; the com-
munist, Stephen Pearl Andrews; representatives of
legislatures and of Congress; as well as literary
women and artists—all could here find people who
were intellectually congenial to them in this field of
speculation.

A purely artistic circle gathered at Miss Freeman's studio apartments. She being then the most
prominent illustrator of books, drew around her
delightful aspirants in art and music. In her parlor, I met Miss Charlotte Cushman, who kindly patronized me and my internes and students after the
New York Infirmary was established, by sending
us tickets to her performances.

An important social circle gathered around Mrs.
Z., the leader of taste and fashion, who entertained
in her elegant and spacious parlors. Here also
whist playing was cultivated under the leadership
of Mr. George Hildreth, who patiently taught me
whenever I could join his table.

The philanthropic circle was the smallest. Its

leaders were Mr. Charles Brace of "Five Points" fame, Mr. Peter Cooper, Miss Elizabeth P. Peabody, and the Sedgwick family, of which Miss Catherine Sedgwick was the most prominent member. I attended meetings of this circle through Dr. Elizabeth Blackwell.

Another important and active influence was exerted by the admirers of the socialist Fourier. A movement was initiated similar to the Brook Farm movement, in Boston. Mr. Marcus Spring had erected a phalanstery, in Eagleswood, New Jersey, where ideal housekeeping, education, the cultivation of literature and high-grade amusement were the objects pursued. To this phase of social life, I was introduced through Mrs. Theodore Weld, Miss Sarah Grimké, Miss Elizabeth P. Peabody and Mrs. Horace Mann. Menial labor was abhorred, in contradistinction to Brook Farm ideas; the culture of mind and of body was preëminent, and Mr. Theodore Weld was the High Priest.

A strange center was that of the demonstrating Spiritualists, who were held together by Mrs. Cleveland and her sister, Mrs. Horace Greeley. Here, as it happened, abolitionists appeared most prominently, and general invitations to the house were extended only during the "Convention Week" in May. The Fox Sisters have been said to perform wonderful feats on such occasions. I never witnessed any, as each time that I happened to be present disturbing elements were said to prevent the materialization of the spirits. Soon after this, the Fox Sisters joined the Roman Catholic Church and were said to have confessed that all their performances were well-arranged deceptions.

Thus I became acquainted with the leading minds who agitated the public, and who helped to advance our plans for the establishment of a hospital where women physicians could prove their capacity and skill by attending sick women and children.

Unfortunately, Dr. Blackwell was not in general harmony with these different phases of social development; on the contrary, she often felt repelled by the theories advanced by them. And I was not only interested and instructed in the various ways of freedom of thought and speech, but also greatly amused by the frequent extravaganzas and oddities of persons and occurrences, especially at the Anti-Slavery meetings and, later, at the so-called Woman's Rights conventions.

For instance, on one occasion Mrs. Ernestine L. Rose was speaking, when a mob of men was determined to quiet her by making unseemly noises. A handsome, delicate little woman, she stood silent on the platform listening to the roaring of these men. All at once they became quiet, impressed by her statuelike dignity, and one of the disturbers called out, "Go on, old steamboat!" to which she calmly replied, "As soon as you have done." She then spoke for a whole hour without further interruption.

Similar interruptions can be related by Lucy Stone and Antoinette Brown Blackwell. Both of these ladies at that time formed part of Dr. Elizabeth Blackwell's family, in New York, which was presided over by the most genial, kind and efficient old lady, Mrs. Blackwell, the mother.

A great misfortune for us was that the components of these circles, while not exactly poor, were certainly not rich. All the assistance which they could give us was in good will and good wishes. Yet these were of great help after all, for they opened channels which led us to the well-to-do. These latter were influenced by motives of philanthropy and also by the general awakening of the spirit which began to demand nobler fields of action than the providing of mere physical comforts. They also opened the way for us to friends such as Mr. George W. Curtis, Rev. O. B. Frothingham (then in Newark), Rev. Henry Ward Beecher, Drs. McCready, Kissam and Porter, Rev. Mr. Bellows, Rev. Mr. Chapin, Dr. Tuthill (one of the editors of the New York *Times*) and his wife and sister; Mrs. R. G. Shaw (mother of Col. Robert Shaw), Mrs. Marcus Spring, the Misses Sedgwick, Mrs. Howland and many others, who came to our assistance and turned the social scale somewhat in our favor.

I might here record an experience which I had as a member of what we would now call a "Woman's Club," and which was named the "Alpha." This association was composed of women who were striving for the advancement of women. Its leader and president was Mrs. Lyons, Miss Mary L. Booth was secretary, and Miss Sarah Tuthill was treasurer. Its meetings were held alternately at the houses of Mrs. Lyons and Miss Booth. It also held social gatherings several times during the year, and to these gentlemen were invited and asked to take part in the discussions. Among these latter were Horace Greeley and George Ripley, but there were also all persons well known in literary or professional life.

At one of these latter meetings the divorce question was made the subject for discussion, and Mr. Horace Greeley was appointed to take the negative side and I the affirmative. As I was with and in the spirit of the times in discussing the subject, it was decided by the judges that I had the better of the argument.

Mr. Greeley was so excited and provoked that he said, "Then, Madam, I understand that a man has the right to say to his wife on Sunday morning when he finds that a button is missing on his shirt, 'Wife, I demand that we get divorced!'"

All were rather confounded by his argument and looked dubiously at me. Fortunately, my wits were previously rather excited, and so I replied:

"Mr. Greeley, the sooner such a man seeks a divorce from his wife, the better for her, because if he considers such a trifle as he mentions a cause for divorce, he is not married in the sense he ought to be."

This incident he related soon afterward in the *Tribune,* with the addition of pointing out the danger to which the "thinking" of women will lead. And he markedly ignored me whenever by chance we met afterward.

All these experiences were of great interest and advantage to me personally, and I developed all these opportunities for forwarding my plans and gaining friends, little by little, for the idea of employing women physicians. But the main object at that time was to gain friends for the proposed Fair in December.

As I now look back on that time when a little pin-cushion or mat was presented for this enterprise and think how joyful we were, as we saw in every little gift the desired dollar, or even fifty cents, and then compare that state of affairs with the present, when we calmly announce that ten thousand dollars must be raised by a Fair, I cannot hope to describe the happy emotion which I then felt over the gift of fifty cents.

It is not the size of the gift or the amount of money which it represents which swells our breast with thankfulness and happiness. It is, after all, the sympathy which the gift conveys which makes its value, and this value is greatest when such sympathy is most needed.

Oh! the golden time of Youth and Hope! How little we improve the chances in our later years to assist the young in their aspirations! And thus do we deprive both them and ourselves of that which means true happiness, namely, sympathetic relations between on the one hand, those who keep the world and its interests moving by their aspirations; and, on the other hand, those who have retired, often with disappointment, because of the little they could effect individually.

It is youth and the superior wisdom of the young, no matter whether they have it in reality or only in their imagination, which leads humanity onward toward the millennium. Humanity is, and must remain, young; and no olden times are worthy of being held up as an example.

Meanwhile, letters from Dr. Emily Blackwell, who was continuing her studies in England, came cheeringly with promises of help towards the Fair. But she also continued to urge the abandonment of the work in the United States and its transference to London, where a desire to promote the education of medical women had begun to manifest itself after Miss Florence Nightingale had so successfully shown the necessity of educating nurses in their profession.

One of the great advantages in such transference to England urged upon Dr. Blackwell was that we would not there have to live down or fight the nefarious and criminal practice which was being carried on chiefly in New York City, but also more or less in smaller places, and which by its advertising in the newspapers had created such a strong prejudice against "Doctresses," as its practitioners were styled.

We were obliged to place the intention of training nurses in the foreground when appealing for sympathy or assistance in our work, in order to get any kind of hearing among the philanthropists, or in sending articles to the newspapers.

Finally, in November, we saw the result of our efforts becoming substantiated in boxes, in baskets, in trunks and in the closets, so that we now were ready to decide upon a locality where we might offer our treasures to the benevolent of New York City.

Dr. Blackwell called a meeting in her parlors of all the ladies who had interested themselves during the summer, and we discussed halls, as well as vestries, which might prove attractive to the public, and a committee was appointed to visit the different places and to seek interviews with those in control of them.

I was, of course, one of the members of the committee, and we decided to go to the places in groups of two or three and to report the result at the end of a week. In less than three days, however, the chairman called a meeting of the committee because of the experiences of the three groups who had spent two days from morning till evening visiting the agents of the different desirable, and even undesirable, locations. Everywhere they had received the same answer, namely, "We don't want to have anything to do with women doctors or irresponsible ladies wishing to hold a Fair in our place."

Not the proposition to pay in advance nor the promise that we should not advertise the fact that it was intended to furnish a hospital for female physicians, as they were then called, could soften the hearts of these men, who simply closed all discussion by saying, "It is not our custom to deal with ladies." Even the kind words of Dr. Bellows could not induce the men of his church to allow us the use of their vestry. What was to be done?

A general meeting was again called, and the husband of one of the committee, Mrs. Haydock, suggested that we hire a large loft in a building, in the business quarters, of which he had control. This was an unfinished room with a bare floor of unplaned boards with numerous knot holes and protruding nails. It had no fixtures for lighting and no ornaments overhead but rough beams and rafters. Another lady of the committee proposed to send her parlor chandeliers to be connected with the gas pipes; while a friend of Dr. Blackwell made a drawing showing how to cover bare, rough walls with evergreens and wreaths. Others loaned rugs for the floor and draperies for the walls, and we used evergreens to conceal the bareness above.

The necessity to have a place at all caused us to accept these propositions and, in spite of three long rough flights of stairs, we advertised our Fair largely and also the motive for holding it, praising its arrangements and enlarging upon its novelty as well as upon its choice goods. We charged ten cents admission and we drew a good attendance for four days, realizing six hundred dollars net profit. And what an immense sum this seemed to us all!

CHAPTER XX

WE at once entered into negotiation for the house we had in view and obtained the refusal of it for the 1st of March, 1857. We also ordered the twenty-four iron bedsteads needed, for the sum of one hundred dollars, and all the ladies went to work begging and preparing house linen, so that when the year closed we held a most joyful New Year's Day, and received so many congratulations that we actually thought ourselves in the command of thousands of dollars.

The house was an old-fashioned mansion of the Dutch style, at the corner of Bleecker and Crosby Streets, just at the outer end of what was called the "Five Points," fully respectable on the Bleecker Street side, and full of patients and misery on the other side and at the rear. And we spent the few weeks which elapsed before we could begin to arrange it in getting the good will of editors, ministers and business men, in order that we might procure the means for carrying on a charity for which we had nothing but an empty purse.

Dr. Blackwell's influence among the Quakers, many of them rich, and Miss Mary L. Booth's indefatigable notices in the newspapers, opened to us the ways of procuring the necessary materials for the dispensary, which occupied the lower front room. It contained a consulting desk, an examination table behind a large screen, shelves for medicines and a table for preparing the ingredients of prescriptions. The front entrance hall was comfortably arranged with settees for the patients to wait their turn. Donations from several wholesale druggists were received, and second-hand furniture suitable for our purposes was cheaply acquired.

A door was put in to separate the back hall from the front hall, and in this back hall was placed a large stove which heated the stairways, there being no furnace in the house. This back hall also served as a dining room for the officers, while the large kitchen opening into it was ample for all culinary purposes and also allowed space for the servants' dining table.

The second floor was arranged for two wards, each containing six beds; while the third floor was made into a maternity department, the little hall room serving as a sitting room for the physicians. Open grate coal fires provided the only heat throughout the house.

The fourth, or attic, floor contained four rooms— two large ones and two small ones, with a square hall in the center. The two large rooms served as sleeping rooms, one for four students and the other for three servants. One of the small rooms served a similar purpose for the resident physician and one student, while the other was the much needed store and trunk room. As the attic was rather low studded, the doors were all kept open, and the skylight of the center hall was kept lifted except during a storm.

These apartments were furnished with such material as benevolence provided. It was the most curious mixture of elegant old furniture and cheap stands and chairs, without any comfort or system, each of us doing the best we could with our belongings as the house was almost entirely devoid of closet room.

Into this primitive, first true "Woman's Hospital" in the world, I moved in March, superintending all its arrangements, with the kind assistance of a few ladies appointed by the now organized board of directors. We ventured to hire one servant to clean, wash and do general work, as I was the only inmate until the house was regularly and formally opened on May 1, 1857.

Dr. Blackwell was aided in procuring speakers by Dr. Emily who had returned from Europe a few weeks before this memorable event. Henry Ward Beecher, Dr. William Elder from Philadelphia and Dr. Kissam, a prominent New York physician who was in favor of our experiment, carried out the program and solemnized the undertaking, while the audience, seated among the snowy white little beds, felt proud of having accomplished so much.

But even here my proposition to have one of the

Drs. Blackwell also speak and explain our intentions was refused by our patrons, because it was feared that she might speak "like a Woman's Rights woman." So we remained in the background, in the most elated spirits yet modest in appearance.

A sign on the front door told the purpose of the house, and very soon our old patrons of the Tompkins Square Dispensary found their way to the now comparatively speaking, quite stylish place. And before a month had passed, we had our beds filled with patients and a daily attendance of thirty and more dispensary patients. Drs. Elizabeth and Emily Blackwell and myself each attended the dispensary two mornings in the week, from nine to twelve, while four students from the Philadelphia college came to live in the hospital in the capacity of internes, apothecaries and pupils of nursing.

The students spent thus their summer months between their lecture terms in Philadelphia, grateful to have at last an opportunity to see actual practice. Of course, they had to pay for this opportunity, three dollars a week for board, as the establishment could not afford to feed them.

We also had two nurses, one for the general wards and one for the maternity department. They were both unskilled and considered the training as more than sufficient equivalent for their services, receiving simply an allowance of two dollars per week for their necessary clothing. Thus we kept true to our promise to begin at once a system for training nurses, although the time specified for that purpose was only six months. However, one woman remained with us for several years, and in the course of time she became invaluable as head nurse.

As for myself, I occupied a peculiar position. I was resident physician, superintendent, housekeeper and instructor to the students of whom none was graduated, so that I had the full responsibility of all their activities, both inside and outside the little hospital. In order to give an idea of the situation, I want to relate from my notes the record of one day of my work.

At 5:30 A. M., I started in an omnibus for the wholesale market, purchasing provisions for a week, and at 8:00, I was back to breakfast. This consisted, for all inmates except patients, of tea, bread and butter, Indian meal mush and syrup, every morning except Sundays when coffee and breakfast bacon were added.

After breakfast, I made my visit to the patients in the house with two of the students, while the other two students attended upon Dr. Blackwell in the dispensary. Then a confinement case arrived and I attended to her, giving orders to students and nurses. After this, I descended into the kitchen department, as the provisions had arrived, and with the assistance of the cook I arranged all these so as to preserve the materials, and I settled the diet for all as far as possible.

I then took another omnibus ride to the wholesale druggist, begging and buying needed articles for the dispensary and the hospital, arriving home at 1:00 P. M. for dinner. This consisted every day of a good soup, the soup meat, potatoes, one kind of well-prepared vegetable, with fruit for dessert. On

Sundays, we had a roast or a steak, while in the
winter we occasionally had poultry when this was
sent in as a donation and when the amount was more
than was needed for the patients.

After dinner, I usually went out to see my private
patients, because receiving no compensation I depended upon my earnings for personal needs. On
this day, however, I was detained by the confinement case mentioned and could not go out till 5:00
P. M., returning at 7:00 P. M. for tea. This always
consisted of bread and butter, tea and sauce or
cheese or fresh gingerbread. After again making
the rounds of the patients in the house, it was 9:00
o'clock.

Then the students assembled with me in the little
hall room, I cutting out towels or pillow cases or
other needed articles for the house or the patients,
while the students folded or even basted the articles
for the sewing machine as they recited their various
lessons for the day. After their recital, I gave them
verbal instruction in midwifery. We finished the
work of the day by 11:30, as I never allowed any
one to be out of bed after midnight unless detained
by a patient.

This day is a fair illustration of our life. If I
had not food to provide, it was something else; if
not drugs, it was drygoods; and if neither, I attended the dispensary at least two forenoons, and
if either of the Drs. Blackwell was prevented by
private business from attending her regular forenoon, I attended in her place.

The strain upon us all, added to the very meager
diet, was immense, and it became a necessity to

provide relaxations. So I arranged that during the summer, once a month, we all went on a picnic during an afternoon in the hills across the Hudson; and in the winter, once a month, we went to a good theater which was near by, and where we often saw Joseph Jefferson, Laura Keene, Karl Formes or Brignoli. These entertainments were highly refreshing, and, what was very important, they were cheap; theater prices were then very moderate and simple picnics were furnished at low rates.

Oh! how delightful were those days, in their youthful enthusiasm and filled with hopes. They were full of hard work, both day and night, for our outdoor poor practice increased almost faster than the dispensary morning clinics, but a few leisure hours once in a while were enjoyed as we had never before in our lives enjoyed the most desirable events or festivities.

Also, we were patronized by those families who, in favor of our medical work as reformers, often invited us to their receptions where we enjoyed intellectual diversion. Among others already mentioned were the Sunday evenings at the house of the sisters, Alice and Phœbe Cary, where distinguished men and women filled the homelike parlors and partook of plenty of ice water as refreshment.

Another house open to us was that of Mrs. Oakes Smith, where art and literature were represented. Another was that of the leading lady of fashion, Mrs. Cole, where whist and music formed the entertaining pleasures. Here I felt especially at home with Mr. George Hildreth as whist partner, his being almost deaf giving me a fine opportunity to be diverted without exertion when too tired even to talk.

To be seen and noticed in these circles was an advantage to medical women and to our little hospital, for, in spite of our very simple diet and the plain living of the patients, we were always in debt; and we had to make great efforts to raise money, holding even a little Sale again before Christmas. This Sale was held in our own wards, the patients being removed for a whole week, but we raised the two thousand, six hundred dollars which was the cost of our first year's experiment, not including the rent which was pledged, as already told.

It was a great oversight and much to be regretted, that we considered this hospital experiment and ourselves of so little importance in themselves that no printed report had been preserved until the year 1868, that is, eleven years from the time we opened the Infirmary.

I have also only very imperfect private notes, but I find that the expense, all in all, including the board of the students, was a little over two thousand, six hundred dollars, from May 1, 1857, to May 1, 1858; and that the average morning dispensary attendance was thirty; while the in-door patients were about one hundred during the year. But we had a very large out-door practice, one of the four students alone, Dr. Mary E. Breed, attending fourteen cases of childbed in one month; while I was often sent for in the night to assist them with advice when their knowledge was not sufficient.

The practical gain to these young women was so great that they were not only devoted, hardworking and conscientious in their professional duties, but they were more than willing to bear great physical discomfort, as well as the ridicule which they encountered when they attempted to demand the recognition and the respect due to their calling. Everywhere among the better situated people, they met with discouraging remarks and questions, giving evidence that the opinion was that the practice of medicine by women would, in the course of time, be impossible, even if the present few were received as exceptions, or as the novelties of a fad. And the greatest tact was called for in accommodating ourselves and our work to the need of even the poorest people.

I may here describe one picture which memory recalls. Dr. Breed had been attending a difficult case of childbirth, in a negro quarter, and she called on me for consultation and assistance.

I entered a room which seemed filled with people of all sizes, and with faces shading from pitch black through all colors to what seemed pure Caucasian. This latter was the woman in the corner, near the table on which stood the lamp, and she was just being delivered of a mulatto baby by the doctor.

The rest of the swarm were both male and female, of whom the woman in the corner claimed eight or more. We did not concern ourselves with the relationship of the remainder, as they all seemed perfectly healthy and did not require our attention. It seems to me that there must have been about twenty-four persons in that room, to judge from the number of beds and the air.

We medical women all went home together at about one o'clock in the morning. It is strange to say but we had no fear about going to these squalid places, and there really was no need of fear either.

The greatest politeness and attention was given to our students when they were once accepted and, as in this case, the young doctor had to be nurse and comforter during the whole day, as well as doctor at the moment of crisis.

She felt quite safe during her stay and was provided with fresh milk—which she drank from the tin can of the store in which it was bought; and she ate the pie from the paper in which it was wrapped. She felt strong and at ease, and happy to have the opportunity to exercise her best influence during the twenty hours of her stay—which may or may not have sowed some seed for the better.

At any rate, gratefulness was gained in more than one way, for this kind of people being more or less under the control of the police and of missionaries at large, did much to spread a good reputation for us and for our work. In this way, women physicians became known and sought by just the class in whom they were interested and among whom they desired to work.

The need for the friendliness of the police towards us I can illustrate here also. A woman died in the hospital after childbirth. We had informed the many relations whom the poor and forsaken usually possess of the seriousness of the case. There was always one woman of the kinship at the bedside of the patient for about sixty hours before the death, which took place in the forenoon.

It was not an hour after this sad occurrence before all the cousins who had relieved each other at the bedside appeared, with their male cousins or husbands in working attire and with pickaxes and shovels, before our street door, demanding admission and shouting that the female physicians who resided within were killing women in childbirth with cold water.

Of course, an immense crowd collected, filling the block between us and Broadway, hooting and yelling and trying to push in the doors, both on the street and in the yard; so that we were beleaguered in such a way that no communication with the outside was possible. We could not call to the people who were looking out of the windows in the neighboring houses, our voices being drowned by the noise of the mob.

At this juncture the policeman who had charge of Bleecker Street and the one from Broadway came running up to the scene. On learning the complaint of the men, they commanded silence and ordered the crowd to disperse, telling them that they knew the doctors in that hospital treated the patients in the best possible way, and that no doctor could keep everybody from dying some time.

CHAPTER XXI

Social success—Growth of private practice—Professional recognition—Consulting staff of leading medical men for Infirmary—Occasional opening of some dispensary clinics to women students who there introduce a needed reform—Incident of Dr. J. Marion Sims, and why a woman was not appointed assistant surgeon in the New York Woman's Hospital of which he was chief—Second mobbing of the Infirmary following death of a patient—Definite beginning of training of nurses—Trying experience of two fires in neighborhood—Dr. Zakrzewska's health begins to show effects of overstrain—Inquiring visitors from all parts of the United States and even from England. (Twenty-nine years of age: 1857-1859.)

DURING the winter of 1857-1858, our entrance into the social circles already mentioned was an immense help to the spreading of the idea of women physicians through our meeting what was then called the "higher kind of Bohemians," among whom were preëminently women artists, aspiring journalists and dramatic students. Although we medical women were not cordially accepted, as only a few of them dared to make our acquaintance, our repeated weekly appearances (as one or more of us made it a point to attend these receptions, no matter how tired we were) familiarized these small publics with the thought that women doctors are as good as anybody.

The fashion then was to attend these "socials" regularly; and *social* they became. They were not stiff and meaningless as is the present fashion, where one goes once or twice during the whole season, shakes hands with the hosts, says some nothings, meets friends and foes and says more nothings, shakes many hands without knowing why, and takes some refreshment in thimble cups, which is no refreshment so scanty is it in quantity and so poor in quality, mere elegant nothings only pretty to look upon. No; in those years, receptions meant intellectual recognition, social grace, conversation, and enjoyment in whatever suited the different tastes, whether a song, or some music, or a quiet game of whist in a retired corner; and no "refreshment" to make a show of pretense, but simply plenty of good ice water.

Among these good people, of whom many have since become of eminence in literature and in art, we gradually developed professionally a small clientele who, if not paying in lucre, paid with grateful remembrance in speaking of us, spreading the idea of us and occasionally writing little articles concerning the New York Infirmary for the leading papers and journals.

I much regret not to be in possession of any of these writings for, as I remember them now, they seem to me so juvenile, so absolutely simple in their tenor, that it might appeal to our sense of humor to read them in the present altered position of women physicians.

For instance, the public was assured that none of us wore short hair like men, but dressed gracefully within the fashion; that we appeared neat in costume, nothing extraordinary indicating our calling, etc., etc. The only disagreeable thing which they found in us was that we objected to being called "Doctress," but insisted upon the neutral appellation of "Doctor of Medicine." This led even to lengthy discussions as to "whether the English language would conform to such a title for a woman."

However, this publicity helped "the Cause" and, strange to say, men were the first who took to the innovation of employing a woman physician by advising their daughters and wives to avail themselves of our services.

Thus, at the end of the year 1857, I had quite a comfortable private practice established. And I took great pains to assure those to whose families I ministered that, year by year, an increase of better women doctors would be the consequence of widening their practical experience and giving them equality of opportunity with the men physicians.

Here my notes read very sanguine, as some of the men highest in professional standing were exceedingly friendly, both professionally and privately; and it is with deep gratitude that I mention the names of Drs. Kissam, Willard Parker, McCready, Aigner and Buck, who gave us their most cordial assistance.

Dr. Kissam, a prominent obstetrician, was on our consulting staff and he became quite friendly to our students, though still believing that Dr. Blackwell and I were exceptions to all womankind. Dr. McCready, attending physician at Bellevue Hospital, was another one who had put aside prejudice. The influence of these men procured for our students attendance at some of the larger dispensaries. In one, the Eastern Dispensary, Dr. Aigner, one of the Austrian exiles and a man of high education, took a sincere interest in the whole movement.

When our students expressed their surprise that no books of patients were kept in these large and rich institutions, no records of cases or prescriptions retained, in fact, that no methodical system was followed, these men inquired into our doings and came and looked through our system, by means of which every patient could be traced—the name, residence, diagnosis, treatment and subsequent course. This was a revelation to them; as it was further when I told them that I never allowed in out-door practice any student to give a prescription without signing her name to it. Thus, in case of any question being raised as to mistake in the prescription or mistake by the druggist (who was by no means in those years always a professional person in that line, but often a mere business man who opened an apothecary store), this signature would always tell where to place the responsibility for the writing of the prescription.

At that time I did not realize, as I do now, that these men, like all those whose position is fully established both professionally and financially, could afford to step outside the pale of professional custom and take up what was not recognized in the strict sense of common daily life.

It is the insecure, struggling physician who is hostile to the woman innovator, actually fearing for

his bread and butter much more than for any al-
leged inferiority of intellect or of professional skill
in the woman, although these latter have always
been used as the war cry against women doctors.

The Boston *Medical and Surgical Journal*, Feb.
16, 1853, expresses this point of view in an editorial
on female physicians, apropos of Dr. Hunt's receiving an honorary degree of M.D. from the Female
Medical College of Pennsylvania. It says:

It is not a matter to be laughed down as readily
as was at first anticipated. The serious inroads
made by female physicians in obstetrical business,
one of the essential branches of income to a majority of well-established practitioners, makes it natural enough to inquire what course it is best to pursue.

Among the young men at that time, Dr. J. Marion
Sims played such a peculiar rôle and one which is
so characteristic that I must relate it here. Dr.
Sims had come from the South to New York in 1853,
poor and unknown. He had perfected an important
operation which was based on a German theory,
but for which no material to practice on could be
found either in Europe or America, until he was
able to utilize the negro slave women. Dr. Sims
quotes "the great Würtzer, of Germany"; and he
told me by word of mouth that he had operated one
hundred and eleven times before he had the first
success. This first success followed the performance
of the thirtieth operation upon one of the six or
seven slave women upon whom he had unlimited
freedom for experimentation.

As it happened, Dr. Sims was introduced into the same social circle in which we were acquainted, and learning from certain members that they were enthusiastically interested in women physicians, he advanced in a year's time in such a friendly manner that he had hard work to live down his friendly advances when he later learned from his professional brethren, as well as from a wider public, that women physicians were by no means popular and could in no way forward his plans. However, he remained outwardly polite to the Drs. Blackwell and myself, inviting us to his operations in the then small beginning of the Woman's Hospital, but excusing himself from further assistance to medical women as a hindrance to the philanthropic enterprise of enlarging the above-mentioned institution.

Dr. Sims stood on common ground with the women physicians in that he also found the medical profession unfriendly, and realized that his only hope of establishing himself was to open a hospital for himself. He says in his autobiography, which was published under the title of *The Story of My Life,* "I said to myself, 'I am a lost man unless I can get somebody to create a place in which I can show the world what I am capable of doing.' This was the inception of the idea of a woman's hospital. . . . If the profession had received me kindly in New York and had acted honorably and gentlemanly and generously towards me, I would not have thought of building a woman's hospital. . . . When I left Alabama for New York, I had no idea of the sort in the world. I came simply for a purpose the most unselfish in the world—that of prolonging my life."

While no more fortunate than the women physicians in enlisting the coöperation of the medical profession, Dr. Sims had greater success with some prominent and wealthy women, who eventually established the hospital for him. The work of Dr. Blackwell and the movement in favor of women physicians had evidently made an impression upon these women also, because they adopted a by-law providing that "the assistant surgeon should be a woman"; and Dr. Blackwell and her sister, Dr. Emily, both well-qualified by their added clinical training in Europe, were the logical candidates for this position.

Dr. Sims cynically refers to this by-law as follows: "One clause of the by-laws provided that the assistant surgeon should be a woman. I appointed Mrs. Browne, a widowed sister of my friend, Henri L. Stuart, who had been so efficient in organizing the hospital. She was matron and general superintendent."

Six months later, he told the board of lady managers that he must have an assistant. He then offered this position, successively, to two young men who had just been graduated and who declined it. His third choice was made because the man had married a young Southern friend of his youth!

Returning to the friendly physicians mentioned above, they dared to introduce our students into their dispensary clinics, and they gave clinical instruction to us at the Infirmary, thus helping on gratuitously the few women who were struggling faithfully to fit themselves for their responsible calling. It was the more estimable in these men

that their audience was a small one whenever they
came to our hospital during the winter evenings,
the largest number never exceeding six. And they
were always ready to come in consultation, even if
they were requested to attend the same case re-
peatedly.

My heart is still full of joy when I think how
kind and helpful these men were in protecting us in
this way; and even, also, against brutal assault, as,
for instance, in a case of appendicitis to which Dr.
Kissam had been every other day in consultation
and which ended in death. His advice had been the
application of cold water compresses, which were
in vogue at that time.

On the morning following the day on which the
patient died, a number of men appeared before the
Infirmary, demanding entrance and creating within
ten minutes a large mob to whom they were talking
loudly, declaring that this was an institution of
some cranky women who killed people with cold
water. I had found means for sending a messenger
from the back door to Dr. Kissam, and it was
through his presence that no harm was done to the
institution. He addressed the mob and advised the
disturbed people to have a coroner sent for to make
an examination in the presence of twelve of themselves as a jury. It was a sight to behold—these
poor distraught men in overalls, with dirty hands,
disheveled hair and grim faces, standing by during
the autopsy, and at its close, declaring their satisfaction that death had been an unavoidable consequence of the disease.

New Year's Day, 1858, was one of the brightest

and pleasantest winter days we ever enjoyed. A friend to women physicians had placed money in my hands for gifts to our faithful servants; and another friend sold to me at half price a whole piece of thibet, so that I was able to present each one of my hardworking women with a dress, as well as with some sweetmeats, all of which were duly appreciated.

Perhaps nobody, nowadays, can understand the willingness and devotion of the women who assisted me in carrying on this primitive little hospital: who were willing to work hard, in and out of hours; who fared extremely plainly and lodged almost to uncomfortableness; yet who felt that a good work was being accomplished for all womankind. And this was true of all—students, nurses and domestic help.

The eight months of experiment had stimulated us all with great hope for the future, and we now began to make more positive plans for the education and training of nurses. The first two who presented themselves for this training were superior women, one a German, the other an American, but neither was willing to give a longer time than four months, during which they received no compensation except their keeping and one weekly lesson from me on the different branches of nursing.

After these left, it was again a German woman who presented herself, and who, after four months' training, remained as head nurse for several years. The second pupil nurse was sometimes of American, sometimes of Irish, descent and nothing remarkable.

This whole year had nothing special to note except that the press began to take a little more favorable notice of our doings and was ready to speak in favor of a Fair which again was arranged for at the end of the year; and this publicity spread the idea of women's competency to take care of sick people.

We had constant applications from students to share in the experience of practice which we offered, and who were willing to live outside in order to attend the dispensary; while the number of patients in daily attendance at this latter increased so rapidly that we had to establish the rule of locking the door against admission after a certain hour.

Among the applicants were all sorts of extremists —such as women in very short Bloomer costume, with hair cut also very short, to whom the patients objected most strenuously; others were training as practitioners in a water-cure establishment, and wished to avail themselves of our out-door practice in order to introduce their theories and methods of healing. In fact, we were overrun with advisers and helpers whom we had to refuse. Popular prejudices could be overcome only in the most careful and conservative manner; and even our most ardent friends and supporters shared to a certain degree in the feeling of uncertainty as to the success of our experiment.

Personally, I received during this year great comfort in the acquaintances and lifelong friendships gained. And the recollection of these friends calls forth such a deep feeling of gratitude for their devotion in our work of love, and for their trust in me, and of admiration for their high purpose to

serve humanity, that I consider it worth while to
have lived if for no other reason than to realize
through them the goodness of womankind.

So the year closed upon us as one which had
brought great satisfaction in all we expected to
gain, professionally and as bearers of a new idea.
Youth was with us all, and our hopes of success
knew no limit. We were the happiest, even if ma-
terially the poorest, of a group of women which
included friends engaged in different lines of work,
such as journalism, art and music. Of these, none
identified herself so closely with us as Mary L.
Booth, later editor of *Harper's Bazar,* who spent
every Sunday with us, and who often shared my
room and bed when she was out at night as reporter
of the New York *Times* too late to return to her
home in Williamsburg.

Oh! happy days! Springtime of life! It was the
"May" which never returns to the human being, and
the beauty of which we realize only long after it has
passed. Memories of these glorious days keep with
us and reconcile us to the many sad, dark, anxious
and trying hours through which we all have to pass
in one form or another. These latter make us wiser,
perhaps, but certainly not happier, even though we
have struggled successfully through the years and
feel that we should be contented with what we have
accomplished.

Still, there was a dark side to my experience during that year. The sick headaches, to which I had
been subject off and on since childhood, came upon
me quite often and very unexpectedly, evidently due
to the overstraining of all my forces, physical and

mental, and I was quite often obliged to relinquish some very important duties.

Before leaving this year's record, I must add a few remarks concerning our work, that is, mine and that of the ten or twelve students who had been connected with the Infirmary now for twenty months.

The prejudice against women physicians was by no means confined to that stratum of society where education and wealth nurtured the young. We found it just as strong, through habit and custom, among the working people and among the very poorest of the poor. Their coming to our dispensary was not *a priori* appreciation of the woman physician, but was the result of faith in the *extraordinary*, just as now faith-curers with other claims are sought and consulted in illness.

Our work was that of real missionaries. Even among the well-to-do and intelligent, little or nothing was known of hygiene. If "a goneness in the stomach" was felt, whisky, brandy or a strong tonic was resorted to for relief. Diet, rest and the sensible use of water were never considered.

So among the poor we found everywhere bad air, filth and utter disregard of food. And sponges, as well as soap, were carried in the satchels of our young medical women along with the necessary implements of the physician. And the former were given to the patients' friends, after showing them the use of water and soap in fever cases as well as in ordinary illness. It was an innovation in the minds of the people, the teaching that sick people must be bathed and kept clean, and that fresh air was not killing.

The good results obtained by the addition of these sanitary auxiliaries whose use was permitted only through our persuasion, created almost a superstitious faith in us and resulted in sending to us patients from a distance of ten and twelve miles from Bleecker Street. This made increased demands on our physical and nervous powers, for we made it a point not to refuse any person if it were at all possible to see her.

Thus we placed foundation stones here and there all over Manhattan Island upon which to build our superstructure of medical practice by women. In this respect, as in all solid production in nature and in civilization, a sound foundation must be created first. No reform, no culture can be successful if we limit ourselves to the higher intellects. We must under all conditions be careful not to speak over the heads of the mentally mediocre crowd.

The soil in which the seed is sown must be examined, then prepared, and then cultivated in the most prudent and careful manner—only then can we expect to have the seed take root and grow.

The gaining of confidence is not obtained by showing your own superiority; nay, it is by hiding this latter and allowing the persons whom you want to benefit to think well of themselves, yet continuing to lead them, indirectly, to the idea that there is a possibility of their bettering themselves. Only by such a proceeding is it possible to bring about confidence; then an attachment follows and, finally, a dependence upon your higher wisdom which will always end in admiration and gratitude. Whenever this is not the case, it shows failure in our having been wise, or kind, or comprehending of the situation; in short, it is the fault of the would-be benefactor.

We had two strange accidents in the neighborhood during that year. Our backyard and outbuildings faced the rear of a livery stable containing more than forty horses. This stable took fire one afternoon about five o'clock. I was just coming home, and I felt so sure of the solidity of our own buildings that I was able to control the excitement of all our inmates who, in bed and out of bed, were perfectly quiet and remained in their rooms in spite of the smoke and noise and all the confusion which a large fire causes.

A few months later at four o'clock in the morning, I was just retiring to my room after having attended a patient below when I heard the cry of "Fire!" And looking out of my window, I saw that a man had upset a fluid lamp, filling the whole room with flames, while he with his night shirt on fire was seeking to escape through the door which he could not find, thus burning to death before my eyes. It was an appalling spectacle, and before I could really comprehend the situation, firemen appeared and worked hard, for the conflagration soon included several buildings.

Again, I could control my patients and the other inmates, although our students and servants dressed hastily and were ready to obey commands in case of need. Fortunately for us, the wind blew the flames in the opposite direction from our house, and I trusted in this fact. Had I had the experience of the Chicago and Boston conflagrations, I would not have trusted to the wind nor perhaps have been able to control a family of nearly forty heads. Such is the blessing of youthful inexperience! But the strain of anxiety on these two occasions was tremendous, and I was laid up each time for a couple of days with a severe sick headache.

Visitors interested in women physicians came from all parts of the United States as well as from England, but especially from Boston. I was often at the same time amused and pained when disappointment was expressed over the smallness of our hospital, and we had to take great pains to explain our out-door department work.

From the very beginning, I had instituted record books in which the name, age, residence, occupation, diagnosis and treatment of every individual case were written—of those who were in the hospital, those who came to the dispensary clinics, and those who were attended at their homes.

These books revealed to the visitors our activity, and they were admired also by our professional brethren. No such records then existed in their dispensaries but were introduced after our example, primitive as it was in those years. However, having such records saved us a great deal of annoyance in many ways, as we offered them for inspection to all whom they concerned; and they protected us against any accusation of carelessness, ignorance or malpractice of any kind.

It was the same with the prescriptions given when the medicines were not provided by us. I insisted that every one who wrote a prescription should sign her name, if not also the name of the patient. As my name was so long, I have always signed *M. E. Z.*

CHAPTER XXII

Dr. Blackwell goes to England for vacation—Dr. Zakrzew-
ska's health suffers under increased strain—Goes to
Boston for vacation—Is there urged to become pro-
fessor of obstetrics in the New England Female Medi-
cal College, and to establish a hospital for this college
—Accepts offer and removes to Boston. (Twenty-nine
years of age: 1859.)

NEW YEAR'S DAY, 1859, was a very cold one, bleak
winds prevailing after a snowstorm. A number of
invitations were extended to us by friends, who did
not simply array their houses for callers bringing
their congratulations in Dutch fashion and receiving
the customary refreshments. I decided to accept
the hospitality of Mrs. and Mr. Booth in Williamsburg, the home of our friend and companion, Mary
L. Booth, while the rest of the household was treated
to a dinner of roast goose which kind patrons had
provided. We never could have thought of such
luxuries ourselves, nor on Thanksgiving Day nor
Christmas, either. However, we never suffered for
the want of them—they always appeared in due time
on these holidays.

This furnishes proof that it is a pleasure to be
kind and that there are more good people in the
world than we may realize. If only one half of
humanity could be brought into absolute contact individually with the other half which is neglected,

degraded and discouraged, there is no doubt that we would witness the same equalization in the large cities as that which prevails in the country towns and villages. Not that there is no difference of subsistence in these latter, but the absolute poverty is not to be found in them as we find it in the former.

Dr. Elizabeth Blackwell now went to England for a vacation and to visit old friends. Her absence caused an increase in work and responsibility, as Dr. Emily and myself had to divide the work which she had done in the dispensary. This increase was just the little more which I could not bear, and the sick headaches returned so often and with such violence that I had to relinquish a good deal of supervision to my head nurse, and finally I was obliged to keep to my bed for a whole week.

When they were visiting the Infirmary, the Boston friends of woman's medical education, of whom I have spoken, had kindly asked me to visit them. So I concluded to take a short vacation in February, placing my senior students in charge of the medical work, under the supervision of Dr. Emily Blackwell.

My visit to Boston, towards the last of February, was exceedingly interesting. I found that Mr. Samuel E. Sewall, as well as his associate directors of the *New England Female Medical College,* had been anxious to add a clinical department to their purely theoretical school.

And outside friends, who had become interested in me personally as well as in my plans to aid the education of medical women by training them in practical work, also were anxious that I should change my place of residence from New York to Boston and accept the position of organizer of this clinical department.

The impression which I received when first visiting Boston in 1856 was deepened. And it was exceedingly favorable as to the earnestness of all the women with whom I came in contact, and as to their desire to elevate the education of womankind in general and in medicine especially. I felt that a larger field for my efforts might be opened there in connection with a medical school rather than in New York where the two Drs. Blackwell controlled the direction of efforts towards what seemed to them wisest and best.

Besides, the financial condition of the Infirmary was improving so steadily that the services which I had been rendering gratuitously could now be hired; while the medical applicants were of an unusual talent and more and more willing to make arrangements for a longer period of service with increased responsibilities, although they still had to pay their expenses.

Also, my private practice had increased to such an extent that I was free from debt, having repaid all loans advanced to me during my studies save the two hundred dollars which the Cleveland society had expended towards my first year. This, I could not now repay as the society had dissolved. But I kept this amount to loan to poor students, without note or interest. Some repaid the loan of fifty dollars or one hundred dollars from time to time; others, not able perhaps to do so, are still holding it, and I am unable to say positively who they are as I did not record the names. I am only sure that these amounts, and some more, are in their hands. The first one to whom I loaned the whole two hundred dollars was Dr. Susan Dimock, when she was going to Europe to study, she repaying it before she made that fatal trip abroad in 1875.

All these considerations influenced me when Boston's liberal friends of women, or of "the Cause," as it was styled, offered me the position of organizer and head of the clinical department which they were ready to establish. And the directors of the medical college offered me the chair of obstetrics in that school, which being my specialty had great attraction for me.

After hesitating for a long time as to what course to pursue, I went to Boston in the spring to define in a public address my views and position in respect to the study of medicine. I found so great a desire prevailing for the elevation of the medical college for women to the standard of the male medical colleges and such enthusiasm in respect to the proposed hospital, that I felt a great desire to make the new hospital department as useful to the public and to the students as the New York Infirmary had become.

The chance of being able to carry out my own plans of work instead of being simply assistant to the Drs. Blackwell was a final temptation, and after inquiries and consultations with Dr. Emily I decided in May to accept the offered position and to remove at once to Boston. My decision was aided by two facts: the first, that Dr. Blackwell's absence had proved that the Infirmary could be sustained by two doctors, not only without loss but with a continuance of its steady increase, this latter being the consequence of the good already done to the community through its ministrations. And the second was that my health was becoming uncertain under the strain of the work which, by virtue of necessity as well as of habit, would remain my share in New York.

Having fulfilled my promise of contribution to the Infirmary of two years' gratuitous services and having put everything in order and divided the duties which I had been discharging, I left the Infirmary on June 1, 1859, taking a short vacation in New York but arriving in Boston on the sixth, as I found to my great disappointment that no short vacation would bring back the strength which I had wasted in my zeal to advance "the Cause" more rapidly than the law of evolution permits.

Thus ended my New York career. I left feeling that I could be spared, although the breaking up of several true friendships saddened the departure. Of all the friends, Mary L. Booth was the dearest to me. It is not through blood kinship that we feel the strongest; nay, we may even feel no affinity at all towards the sisters and brothers we so love, while the few kindred spirits we meet fill our souls with life and inspiration.

The few friends to whom I was thus sincerely attached remained such for life, and the professional affinities stand to-day in the same relation to me as when we were young, while a few non-professional New York friends find time and opportunity to meet me occasionally to exchange reminiscences of the golden days of our youth.

About this date, there were already a goodly number of women upon whom the degree of M.D. had been legally conferred, but the minds of those who understood the conditions which prevailed were far from being satisfied with results.

Recognition in the profession and opportunities for a good education for others who wished to cultivate this field of labor were our aims. And so we labored on, the Drs. Blackwell and myself in New York and Dr. Ann Preston in Philadelphia—the latter for the "college," and all the former for the "hospital" education of female students.

Meanwhile, a number of spurious institutions proclaiming the same aim had sprung up like weeds which threatened to choke the wheat in the field. After the interest of a few high-minded male physicians had been secured, the battle with and against these institutions had to be fought—and it is still to be fought.

The best of these secondary institutions existed in Boston, and it was thither that I was going with the hopefulness which befits the missionary spirit.

[As has been elsewhere stated, most of the preceding chapters were written by Dr. Zakrzewska in a letter to her friend, Miss Mary L. Booth, in New York. And she closes this letter with the paragraphs which follow.]

. . . I could not refrain from writing fully of this part of my life which has been the object of all my undertakings, and for which I have borne trials and overcome difficulties which would have crushed nine out of ten in my position. I do not expect that this will be the end of my usefulness; but I do expect that I shall not have to write to you any more of my doings. It was simply in order that you, my friend, should understand me fully, and because you have so often expressed a wish to know my life before we met, that I finished this letter. Now you have me externally and internally, past and present. And, although there have been many influences besides which have made their impressions on my peculiar development, yet they are not of a nature to be spoken of as facts, as, for instance, your friendship for me.

On looking back upon my past life, I may say that I am like a fine ship that, launched upon high seas, is tossed about by the winds and waves and steered against contrary currents until finally stranded upon the shore. There, from the materials a small boat is built, just strong enough to reach the port into which the ship had expected to enter with proudly swelling sails. But this ambition is entirely gone and I care now very little whether or not people recognize what is in me, so long as the object for which I have lived becomes a reality.

And now, my good friend, I must add one wish before I send these last few pages to you, namely, that I may be enabled some day to go with you to Berlin to show you the scenes in which my childhood and youth were passed, and to teach you on the spot the difference between Europe and America. All other inducements to return have vanished. Nearly all the men who aided in promoting my wishes have passed away, and the only stimulus that now remains to make me want to revisit the home of my youth, is the wish to wander about there with you and perhaps with two or three other of my American friends. Until this can be accomplished, I hope to continue my present work in the New England Female Medical College which, though by no means yet what we wish it to be, is deserving of every effort to raise it to the position that it ought to take among the medical institutions of America.

CHAPTER XXIII

*Details of the College building—Dr. Zakrzewska meets
many men and women leaders in advanced thought
in Boston—Differences between Boston and New York
with regard to the question of "woman's sphere"—
History of the New England Female Medical College
—She finds the educational standards of the College
low, and she meets opposition in her attempts to elevate them—She establishes the hospital (Clinical Department) along lines similar to those she had
developed in the New York Infirmary—Several leading men in the profession acknowledge her qualifications but refuse to act as consultants for the hospital,
or to countenance the College—Letters from Dr. John
Ware—Hardships of the Out-Practice. (Thirty years
of age: 1859-1860.)*

THE New England Female Medical College had its
home in Springfield Street, in the building erected
for the Boston Lying-In Hospital and later occupied
by the Home for Aged Men. Here the lectures were
held, the officers had their rooms and the directors,
their meetings; and yet, not half of the building was
occupied. So I had there my office and bedroom, furnished by the lady managers of the college.

I assigned the basement rooms to the dispensary,
while the rest of the lower rooms served for domestic purposes inclusive of servants' rooms. The
middle story was taken for the indoor clinical department, or hospital; while the upper floor, or
attic, was arranged for students' chambers, and for

243

these we received rent and pay for board from those actively serving in the hospital department.

This whole affair, however, had to be organized and superintended, and as I felt unequal to added medical responsibilities I devoted myself during the whole summer (1859) to arranging this department and getting it in working order, taking every now and then a whole week's vacation at the seashore or in the country.

New friends in the form of a board of lady managers were added to the college because increased funds were needed to carry on the new department, the most noted name on this board being that of Harriet Beecher Stowe. And the ladies and gentlemen who favored my plans when I came, three years earlier, pleading for the New York Infirmary, now bravely advanced and provided the means for this new enterprise.

Through all of my former acquaintances I at once found warm friends and protectors here in our beloved city of Boston. I may mention the names of Theodore Parker, Wendell Phillips, William Lloyd Garrison, Samuel E. Sewall, F. W. G. May, Francis Jackson, Rev. William E. Channing, Dr. W. F. Channing, Dr. Samuel Cabot, Dr. E. H. Clark, Mrs. Sarah S. Russell, Miss Abby G. May, Miss Lucy Goddard, Rev. and Mrs. James F. Clarke, Mr. and Mrs. Bond, Miss Mary J. Parkman, Mrs. R. G. Shaw, Mrs. Ednah D. Cheney, Mrs. F. Fenno Tudor, Miss Susan Carey—and there were a host of others, both men and women.

I wish I could mention all of the noble minds, pioneers of a new era in the broadening of thought.

No specialism was represented, except perhaps that of Abolitionism and the Advancement of Women. Free scope of the intellect was admitted, and every one who promoted culture of mind and body was welcomed. Scores of able women sought instruction, demanding to know what was objectionable in woman's aspirations.

These and other activities were evidences of the smoldering volcano which burst forth into active conflagration in the outbreak of the Civil War, in 1861, and which gave birth to a new type of Woman—as Minerva was said to have issued forth from the head of Zeus fully armed with weapons of force and intellect.

The names of Lucy Goddard, Abby May, Ednah D. Cheney, Sarah Shaw Russell and Anna Lowell should be engraved on plates of gold for remembrance by those who will come after, for they took a stand which made history in life, and especially in the life of women.

For, let it be understood, the impression of the great liberality of Boston society, which I had cherished and fostered as a belief, was not as well-founded as I thought, and upon closer acquaintance I was soon convinced that here also it required a great deal of courage to advocate a new era in woman's sphere.

Although I found much less tendency to ridicule, to treat with contempt, or to prophesy failure than we had met in New York, yet the fear of losing social caste was strong here also. Declarations that the study of medicine would unsex girls or break down health and beauty prevailed throughout the community, and newspaper remarks were discouraging rather than otherwise.

In short, I had to go over the same ground as in New York, explaining the possibility of a woman physician's being able to do precisely the same work as the average man physician. The only difference I found in the two cities was that in spite of doubt and prejudice against woman "leaving her sphere," as it was called, intelligent men and women in Boston were ready to listen to and to discuss all possible chances.

The fact that this small medical college for women had now lived for nearly ten years induced the liberal-minded to go a step farther and to begin to employ women, especially in midwifery cases.

One of the graduates of this school was still practicing in Boston as midwife on July 1, 1889, she having by that time attended five thousand confinement cases. Although she was never sought by the well-paying portion of the Boston community, she held a very reputable position among her patients and among such of the profession as had business relations with her. Her name, Mrs. Hassenfuss, has been mentioned to me quite often by the best of men physicians. Therefore, honor to whom it belongs. This good, sensible woman, the mother of eleven children, has done her share in overcoming prejudice against women physicians.

Several other ladies who had graduated from this school tried to practice in Boston although as they told me with very little financial result. They were obliged during the first years after establishing themselves to seek practical experience among the poor, either as assistant to a friendly man physician or on their own responsibility. In either case, they appeared to the people's minds more like well-trained nurses than physicians who assume an authority which creates confidence. Their position was by no means an enviable one, and only the self-assurance produced by the American education could hold them up socially.

Here it should be said that the graduates of this school labored under disadvantages produced by obscurities in the minds of those who controlled it.

Ever since the men physicians began to organize themselves into a compact body or guild, their endeavor has been not to educate the women whom they everywhere found called to be the natural obstetricians, but to drive them entirely out of such practice and to monopolize it for themselves. This struggle continues everywhere, all over the world. And it is a struggle which will continue until both men and women are educated equally well, so that the individual patient may exercise her choice of the "trained doctor" of either sex.

A public agitation begun in Boston in the summer of 1847 culminated in 1848 in a revulsion of feeling among the laity against this attempt of the male physicians to monopolize the practice of obstetrics, and in favor of the restoration of at least a part of such practice to the hands of women. And this revolt was countenanced by a large number of the leading citizens of Boston as well as of the rest of New England.

As a result of this agitation, the *Boston Female Medical School* was opened on November 1, 1848, with twelve pupils. And to aid this School, the *Female Medical Education Society* was organized on November 23, 1848, with six members. This membership increased to a thousand or more during the following year, its larger part consisting of men of prominence in all walks of life. And in the following year, 1850, this society was incorporated "for the purpose of providing for the education of Midwives, Nurses, and Female Physicians."

In the earliest printed report of the Boston Female Medical School (1851), most stress is laid upon the course of study for *Midwives,* which is as follows:

Candidates for Diplomas as Practitioners in Midwifery, must be at least twenty years of age, and must present testimonials of good moral character; they must have studied at least one year, including the Lecture terms; must have attended two full courses of Lectures, one of which must have been in this institution: and must pass a satisfactory examination before the Board of Examiners, in Anatomy and Physiology, in Obstetrics and the diseases peculiar to Women.

Nurses are referred to in the statement that:

Courses of Lectures and Instruction will be given to Nurses in reference to their important and responsible vocation of attending the sick.

And *Female Physicians* are considered in the paragraph:

The candidates for full Medical Diplomas must

have pursued a course of Education equivalent to that required in other medical institutions; and at least two terms of their instruction must have been in this School.

While all groups are urged to seek to prepare themselves, "Persons intending to become members of the School will do well to study, in advance, some elementary work on Anatomy and Physiology—Cutter, Jarvis, etc.," closing with the naïve statement whose wisdom cannot be gainsaid, "And any other preparatory knowledge will be useful."

Thus we see that the Boston Female Medical School aimed as high as any of the male medical schools of the day. Really, its aim was higher, in that from the beginning it planned to have a Hospital and to make "practical" instruction in obstetrics and the diseases of women an integral part of its course. In advocating this latter procedure, it claims superiority for itself, making the statement that "the Harvard Medical School furnishes no facilities in the way of 'practice' in a Maternity Hospital—the most important part of an obstetric education."

But, presumably, this school found itself practically confined to the education of midwives and nurses—groups whose qualifications were apparently not regulated by strict legal enactment. Because, in 1856, an act of legislature was passed changing the name of the Female Medical Education Society to that of the *New England Female Medical College,* and giving this latter body power to "appoint Professors, who shall constitute a Medical Faculty; and to confer the usual degree of Doctor of Medicine," provision for these latter legal necessities having evidently been overlooked in the earlier incorporation of 1850.

The New England Female Medical College says nothing in its reports about midwives, but speaks only of medical students, of nurses, of female physicians, and of its purpose to have "a part of the Faculty consist of female Professors." But it lists its medical alumnæ from 1854.

Thus becoming acquainted during the summer with the new field for my activity, I found still an added difficulty among the few women who possessed a medical diploma, namely, that not being accustomed to work with one another on a common plane, they rather feared any one whose standpoint differed from their own and who brought new views of the subject in question.

"What is, or was, sufficient for me ought to be sufficient for all who come after me," was the common human principle on which they based their indifference towards improving or enlarging their stock of knowledge. Medicine was then taught, even in the best of colleges, not as a scientific vocation but as a practical business.

For instance, after having been connected with the New England Female Medical College for a year, I ventured to express my surprise that no microscope was in the college, and to say that I wished for one because much that it was necessary to explain could only be done with such an instrument.

My petition for one was refused. And Mr. Sewall informed me that one of the gentlemen who was a leader in the college, after having listened to my written petition, said, "That is another one of those new-fangled European notions which she tries to introduce. It is my opinion that we need a doctor in our medical department who knows when a patient has fever, or what ails her, without a microscope. We need practical persons in our American life." This man is long dead, yet I feel sorry that he could not have lived longer in order to see that we teach the new-fangled notion of the use of a microscope even in our public schools.

It can easily be understood that my position, both as professor of midwifery and as head of the clinical department, was not very agreeable, with such opponents among the directors of the school and having to meet the indifference of the established women doctors of Boston; and also, I am deeply sorry to say, receiving only limited support from the men physicians with whom I was associated in the college.

Although in favor of the school, the students were regarded by these physicians more in the light of trained nurses who were to become their handmaids in practice. This fact revealed itself to me when, feeling the need of consultants, I tried to reorganize the hospital staff. I found that none of the prominent Boston physicians was willing to give me his name, and the excuse was that the standard of the school was below par. On the other hand, the physicians connected with the school thought they were teaching all that a woman doctor ought to know.

Here I want to anticipate a little by telling of my

first examination of students for the degree of M.D. This was to be carried on by the professors of the school, in the presence of a committee of three from the directors, but only one of the latter appeared. Several of the candidates who presented themselves for their examination were possessed of such elementary education that they had no other recommendation to the examiners than that they had attended two courses of medical lectures of twenty weeks each, and had studied with a preceptor to make up three years of reading medicine, but whom I had never seen in our clinical department.

I objected, of course, to these students as unfit for a position of the gravest responsibility. While all the rest reluctantly took my side, they added, "Nobody in Boston would employ a woman doctor in serious cases, anyhow!" However, I prevailed, and I did not have to place my name on the diploma of women who, excellent as nurses, were unfit to take the position of physicians.

By October 1, 1859, I considered myself strong enough to begin regular daily work. The housekeeping cares which I had hitherto assumed were divided with a competent woman. Financial difficulties, however, were not so easily overcome, and we had to charge a board payment of three dollars a week to such students as wished to avail themselves of residence within the building.

This arrangement added a good deal of care to me as superintendent, for, in spite of exercising the greatest impartiality between the resident students and those from outside, a feeling naturally grew up among the students that favoritism was practiced.

What really happened was that, as a consequence of constant presence, the internes appeared better equipped to render assistance than the externes. A few of these latter, however, gave me credit by word and deed that, if anything, I favored the externes rather than the internes and these few became real and true friends in later years, often calling upon me or writing for advice, as well as giving me their sincere friendship.

To be appreciated as just, conscientious and unselfish has always been my ambition—other honors, or wealth, I have never sought nor received. Even at this moment, when age has come to me and health has failed, my small income from my savings gives me greater satisfaction than if I had accumulated a large competency. Though I should still like to have this latter in order that I might help many a struggling woman to whom I have to refuse aid because I am poor myself.

Among the resident students, were Lucy E. Sewall, my private pupil and devoted friend and co-worker during her life; Anita E. Tyng, a woman of talent, at present living in California; Mary H. Thompson, who became famous by establishing the *Woman's Hospital* in Chicago, reëstablishing the same after it was burned during the great conflagration; Helen Morton, my associate in practice after her return from Paris in 1867, and still residing in Boston; Lucy Abbott, who became resident physician at the New York Infirmary; and others who became of more or less importance in after years.

Again our household assumed more of the condition of a family circle like that of the New York

Infirmary, having a similar intimacy. This was due to the fact that, although women physicians were more tolerated in Boston society, they had not yet conquered all doubt or prejudice among the women of Boston, while the profession at large would not recognize any of them at all.

However, I made the attempt to call upon a few prominent men. For instance, I saw Dr. Henry E. Clark, who had visited the Hospital Charité in Berlin when I held the position of *Accoucheuse en chef* in the Maternity Department of that institution. And I had the opportunity of being very helpful to him in all he wished to gain as a young doctor seeking experience in a foreign land. He received me with kind politeness, but told me frankly that he could not sanction the study of medicine by women. He yielded so far as to pronounce me "an exception" to my sex, and he promised to assist me in private practice should I require consultation. Also, in the course of the winter, he sent me several patients, and he spoke with recommendation to those who inquired of him about me and my former position in Berlin.

Another one, Dr. John Ware, accepted me as an exceptional woman, and fatherly and kind as he was, he laughed heartily when I told him that the exceptions would multiply by the hundred.

[Dr. Ware writes, under date of February 11, 1860:

My DEAR MADAM:
I ought before now to have acknowledged your kindness in sending me a copy of your Lecture. I

have read it with much satisfaction, and wish most
heartily that every one of my professional brethren
entertained views as just and elevated of the nature
of their calling, and were as conscientious in regard
to its responsibilities as you would have all be who
assume them.

I take the liberty of sending in return a few pub-
lications of my own, relating in part to the same
topic. You will find on the 24th page of one of the
Lectures—that on "Success in the Medical Profession"—a brief expression of my opinions on the
subject of Female practitioners, which, altho' you
may not agree with them, I hope you will find no
reason otherwise to disapprove.

I am, with sincere respect and regards,

Yrs.

JOHN WARE

To Marie E. Zakrzewska, M.D.

Again, referring to the earlier chapters of this
autobiography, he writes, on December 13, 1860:

MY DEAR MISS ZAKRZEWSKA:

I received yesterday a volume which I supposed,
certainly I hoped, came from you. I read it at once,
and with the deepest interest. I have a right, therefore, whether it came from you or not, to thank you
for it. Neither can I let the opportunity escape of
expressing the admiration and sympathy with which
I followed you in the long struggle you endured, and
which you maintained with so much of that energy,
courage, perseverance and fortitude, which we are
apt to call manly—as if they were our peculiar possession—and yet without any infringement of that
womanly delicacy, which we certainly cannot claim.

You know perhaps my doubts about the medical education of women. It is not because I do not think well enough of women that I entertain these doubts, but rather, I suspect because I think too well of them, to be willing they should go through with a medical education, or endure a medical practice. I have put it to myself whether I could be willing that one of my daughters should go through the discipline and lead the life that I have done myself. The idea is intolerable. That you have accomplished what you have with success and honor does not satisfy my doubts—how few of either sex could do the same.

I may be mistaken, for it is very hard to be sure that we are not influenced by early impressions and the prejudices of society, and I am quite willing to find myself in the wrong, for I have the most earnest desire that every possible avenue should be opened for the admission of women, not only to places for labour, but of honor and profit. I sympathize not only with every attempt to enforce "Woman's Right to Labour"—but to think, speak, act and enjoy.

With sincere regard, I am your friend,

JOHN WARE

To Marie E. Zakrzewska, M.D.]

Drs. Henry I. Bowditch and Samuel Cabot regretted to refuse all aid so long as I was connected with such an inferior school as they considered the New England Female Medical College to be.

Dr. Cotting, of Roxbury, was the most cordial; he expressed himself as favorable to having women physicians as auxiliaries to the professional men. He sent me more patients than any one, and they were rich as well as poor. The latter were the most desirable, as our dispensary practice was small, lacking material for the benefit of the students.

This was the great difference between New York and Boston. Within three months after opening the New York Infirmary dispensary, we were obliged to close the doors for admission after a certain hour, so full became our reception hall; while in Boston we kept open all the forenoon without getting all the patients we wanted, and we even attended to them the whole day.

This may have been due to the fact that the college and hospital were located in what was then a demi-fashionable quarter of the city, the South End, where not many poor lived; and distance was not then annihilated by street cars, of which none existed. But it was also due to a greater prosperity among the poor of Boston, this creating a prejudice against free dispensaries in general, and women physicians in special.

To all these reasons was due the very hard work which we had to do, because if a family in the distant poor quarters inclined to favor us with their patronage, we had to rejoice. And the disadvantage of such events because of walks of two or three miles in the midst of winter nights was overcome by the enthusiasm of having gained another foothold among the poorest of the poor. Thus we had our clientele not only, though chiefly, at the North End of the city but also in the suburbs, where not even omnibus travel was possible, there being none to South Boston, Dorchester, Roxbury, Jamaica Plain and other outlying districts.

What would life be without the enthusiasm of the

young! And how much or how little would be accomplished in the evolution of reforms and progress, if the young were not ready and happy to live up to the fullest inspiration of this enthusiasm! Reasonable or unreasonable, let us not stint or discourage any enthusiastic young person in the ways and means of living up to its fullest extent! Youth will always meet with more or less success in realizing its ambition, and even if premature death should be the consequence of such efforts, it does pay to have favored and encouraged the activity of such aspirations.

The happiness which is enjoyed by enthusiastic workers is impossible to describe in words, for, though ever so little be gained from the opposition, or by perseverance, this gain gives moments of joy which cannot be outweighed by many a disappointment or by any amount of fatigue. Oh! the single hour of happiness which victory brings! Even in humble aspirations, it is worth living for. It is not the quantity of anything which satisfies a noble heart—it is the quality, and the feeling of conscious satisfaction that the best of which the person was capable has been done.

CHAPTER XXIV

Formal opening of the College term—Professor Zakrzew-
ska delivers the Introductory Lecture—Father dis-
approves of her removal to Boston—This increases the
shock of news of his death. (Thirty years of age:
1859.)

THE term of 1859-1860 of the college opened well.
A goodly number of students had registered, among
them the fine women already mentioned who assisted
much in giving a high tone to our work, and I felt
greatly supported by their earnestness and zeal.
[According to the college announcement, this term
opened on November 21, 1859, with the "Introductory Lecture by Professor Zakrzewska." A few extracts from this formal address will help still further in developing the portrait of the speaker.]

The study of medicine is so great and comprehensive a field that within its horizon we find included
the whole moral world. It comprises mankind in
all its conditions, in all its changes of opinions and
in all its modes of society. It has been subject to the
highest wisdom in existence, to the greatest folly
and mysticism which superstition could produce and,
in our days, to the most profound learning and scientific speculation. And though I am now addressing
a miscellaneous audience of which only a few are
physicians or students of medicine, every one is in
some way connected with the profession, be it only

as a patient. Every one receives this liability as an inheritance from nature and, therefore, ought to be interested in a science which occupies itself with mankind.

The only motives that this profession permits to its votaries are the clear and decided conviction of an inborn taste and talent for the practice of medicine and an earnest desire for, and love of, scientific investigations concerning the human being—its construction, its condition of health and disease, and all its relations with the surrounding world.

It is a positive fact, acknowledged among all nations and at all times, that there is in the mass a growth of the human mind from generation to generation similar to that in the different periods of individual existence. And to these varying stages of mental growth we must ascribe the different forms through which the practice of medicine has passed.

Disease is as old as mankind. The first sore finger made the first patient, and the first physician was the one who bound it up or who inquired how it was doing. Pain awakens the instinct to relieve, one following the other, and this must have existed from the creation of mankind.

The practice of medicine dates back, therefore, to the morning of life; the shadows of a hoary antiquity gather around its cradle. The annals of history do not reach back of it, but only open the portals of fable in whose shadowy domain it is supposed to dwell. Æsculapius was the grandson of Zeus, whose father was Time himself.

Gradually we see it emerging from this hazy atmosphere in the form of a mysterious science, assisted and appropriated by the mysticism of the oracles and astrologers, until it found its devotees in the priesthood who pursued the practice upon the body in connection with their duties as priests for the soul.

It is only since medicine has ceased to stand isolated from the other sciences that the erroneous belief that disease was produced by supernatural agency has waned. Nothing has more retarded the progress of medicine in becoming really scientific than its separation from general learning; and nothing could favor empiricism and superstition more than the promotion of this separation.

That this separation produced an apparently inextricable confusion was very natural, just as it was natural that medical sects should have been formed of which the one renounced this, the other that, and the third something else—each individual sect being distinguished by its one-sidedness. The only sect— if we may thus term the regular physicians—which at no time could be accused of one-sidedness in its proclamations was that based upon the principles of Hippocrates and the Alexandrian School—these advising practical, experimenting science, a course of reasoning which Lord Bacon in his works has approved with such justice. And how necessary it was to follow this recommendation continually and in every particular is best illustrated by showing how one branch of medical practice could fall almost into oblivion by neglect to pursue it as an *experimental* science.

For instance, in the history of Obstetrics, we find that very little was done to promote its elevation from the times of Hippocrates and Celsus until within the last one hundred and twenty years, when Pareus, Mauriceau, De la Motte, Deventer, and Justina Siegesmundin and others began to investigate it and to raise it to its proper place as a science.

Until this time, the obstetric art was so entirely neglected that it was considered beneath the dignity of an honorable man. Low and uneducated persons appropriated this practice to themselves, even in cases of the greatest emergency. The degradation of this branch alone proves the need of the introduction of new ideas formed by constant observation in science at large; it also proves that we cannot abandon speculations and experiments on the natural laws which pervade all organizations; and that it is a matter of great necessity that every student of medicine should be provided with ample opportunities for so doing. And how successful and beneficent, although difficult, such reforms are, I shall illustrate by speaking again of the resurrection of obstetrical science.

New life had to be introduced into it before new light could be thrown upon this field; and this new life was finally introduced when the persons just named entered upon the study. They found that midwifery as it was then practiced must be reorganized. Observations on nature needed to be made and these were to be followed by scientific analysis, and the results introduced into practice.

A new era for the studious was opened, and many young and brilliant minds now found their attention directed towards this branch of learning which before they had considered as a subject beneath their dignity. Very soon after the first attempt for improvement, an ardent enthusiasm was created in the subject, since in it a field for new investigations, and consequently for new honors, became apparent to the eyes of the ambitious or the learned. In a very short time, the practice of obstetrics was regulated in such a manner that not only had the horror towards the persons engaged in it entirely disappeared, but the terrible operations often practiced had also become lessened to an insignificant number, these latter belonging to the class of unavoidables.

Every country produced authorities. England boasted her John Burns and Hunter, while France raised up her Baudeloque, her Madame Lachapelle, Madame Boivin and many others. But no country gave to the profession such thoroughly scientific investigators as did Germany, and of these a *woman* took the lead. Justina Siegesmundin was the pioneer of this great reform, and her work, written upon the subject in 1741, came upon Europe like a thunderbolt. In every country, minds which had been preoccupied with a thousand other things, forgetting the most important, were awakened to an activity which would but a short time before have been deemed impossible. In Germany, therefore, the subject of obstetrics is still considered as of momentous importance, the foundation almost of all other practice . . . and the statistics prove that in this branch of practice less loss of life occurs there than in any other country, though its proportion of difficult cases is the greatest of any.

Reformations similar to this will be constantly demanded in all the different branches of medical science. . . . Every day brings results of new researches which are throwing fresh light upon subjects not yet understood.

And this is the position which a physician must assume to-day, and for which those who are entering upon this field of study should fit themselves. To be an honorable acquisition to the profession, a consoler to those who require assistance in overcoming disease, a public instructor in the art of preserving health, a reformer from the artificial to the natural—these are the aspirations which must animate every one who dares attempt to step forward to the platform of the benefactors of mankind.

This is the aim which the beginner must have in her mind, and if she falls short of attaining it, she must be able to say that it was neither through indolence nor indifference, but through absolute powerlessness. If you doubt this to be the position which the student should take, then look around and ask yourself what you want of your physician.

If you are educated, you want your physician to be still more so; if you possess perception of conditions and circumstances, you demand this of your physician still more. You want of him that he shall not only perceive and penetrate into the secret relations and conditions of the body physically and psychically, but that he shall also explain to you those phenomena which are incomprehensible to you in spite of your great perceptive faculties.

You further demand of your physician that he shall know everything belonging to medical science. If you understand physiology well, you demand that your physician shall explain in a moment every fact that is dark to you, while a lifetime may not be sufficient to prove a hypothesis. If you are at home in chemistry, you will certainly be greatly surprised if your physician makes a mistake in some combinations, and you will be ready to say that he is stupid. If you have great skill in nursing, you will expect your physician to teach you how to improve; if you are kind and agreeable and amiable, you demand the same qualities in him; if you are irritable, fretful and capricious so that you have been designated by your neighborhood as a fury, you want at least that your physician should comprehend your subtle nature. And in addition to all this, your physician must be sociable, entertaining, wise in every word, overflowing with great thoughts, and uttering new truths whenever you invite him to your table.

All this is really demanded of the physician, but how far it may be justifiable, I leave it to the thinking ones to decide. But of this we may be sure— the physician of the present day occupies a higher station than ever before and greater qualifications for the study of medicine are increasingly demanded.

I mentioned in the beginning that the motives for the study of medicine must be the right ones; now I have to add that these alone will not suffice to make a good physician such as we want to-day. These motives must be accompanied by certain qualifications. The latter are twofold, and may be divided into those belonging to the intellect, and those belonging to our personal and affectional nature.

It is of infinite importance that the intellect should have been previously developed by a course of study which shall train the student in logic and reasoning and familiarize him with natural as well as with moral and mental philosophy. Observation and experiment are the two great auxiliaries to medical study. Those who possess the first as a natural gift and who have judgment enough to apply it whenever they have an opportunity will take the lead; but those in whom both must be developed will always limp behind unless they study most industriously and perseveringly.

Foremost among the second group of qualifications stands the matter of age. The student ought to be mature enough to think and to reason, but not advanced beyond the time when the mind is naturally predisposed to acquiring knowledge. Physical health and prepossessing appearance are of the next importance; while cultivated manners and agreeable behavior, as well as talent in adapting himself or herself to all conditions, all circumstances and all persons, are by no means the last to be considered.

In addition there are some qualifications yet to be mentioned which form a part of our affectional nature and without which no practitioner can succeed. Of these, the most essential is sympathy—not sentimentalizing sympathy, but the sympathy which never betrays weakness or timidity and which is firm and persevering, controlling every action that it may not become rashness. Modesty and reticence, sobriety and unselfishness are other virtues much desired in the practitioner. And I add here a word of warning against temptations into which physicians are constantly led because I know how often pecuniary gain or social position can be obtained by being untrue to one's best self. I have also had occasion to see the consequences in those who have yielded to the temptation to abandon their principles.

No greater misery can perhaps be imagined than contempt for one's self; no greater punishment can be endured than the consciousness of having acted meanly and despicably. A man who when alone in his chamber is forced to blush for himself carries hell within him—the loss of a clear conscience is the source of much despair. Conscientiousness, so important for every man of whatever station in life, is still more important in a physician. To be scrupulously honest, to satisfy his own conscience even at the cost of material profit, is absolutely essential for him.

It is human life—that most divine element in creation and irreplaceable when once lost, for which the practitioner is responsible; and no regrets, no penitence, no despair will be accepted by those who mourn or will reconcile them to their bereavement. The loss of a beloved wife and mother perhaps brings another life to the grave, or it may fix the unhappy fate of a dozen human beings of whom she was the guardian angel, and who now are left alone.

Pause and think for a moment, and try to appreciate the weight of misery which in lonely hours such a picture reveals to the mind of one who in a critical moment was made responsible for life and death, and who must confess that such victims fell a sacrifice to the ambition which prevented him from owning his inability for the work intrusted to his hands.

I must leave the subject here and allow you to decide if I have pictured clearly enough what we want in a physician of to-day. If I have succeeded, you will certainly join with me in giving voice to your convictions that not only the very best method for instruction should be provided, but that every facility should be offered to the student to make him or her acquainted with the past history of medicine. Only those who are familiar with all that occurred before they stepped on the platform as public instructors or practitioners will thoroughly comprehend their duty. Great deeds stimulate to greater ones, and so much has already been done in the profession that in order to understand his or her own position the newcomer needs to have knowledge not only of to-day and yesterday but of all times.

[The foregoing definition of the medical profession paints a picture far removed from that of Dr. Johnson, as quoted in one place by the speaker— "The profession of physic is a melancholy attendance on misery, a mean submission to peevishness and a continued interruption of pleasure.''']

The men professors, of whom there were four, and the other woman professor (teaching physiology) were in apparent harmony with my plans. These were to devote my teaching—which was threefold, namely, obstetrics, diseases of women and diseases of children—to only one of these subjects at a time instead of giving two lessons a week on each.

This seemed to work very well; but as it left only four weeks for treating the diseases of children, while obstetrical teaching ran through the winter, the students of less intelligence began to be dissatisfied and my college troubles had already begun before the winter session had ended.

Meanwhile, I was not happy in my relations with my father, whose letters disapproved of my having left New York, where he felt that I was under the supervision of the Drs. Blackwell with whom all responsibilities for the hospital enterprise rested. He now became really distressing to me because his conviction was that whether I succeeded or not I was disgracing the family, and German womanhood in general, by accepting a position which caused my name to come prominently before the public.

I finally felt that I must write a strong and decided letter to him, requesting him either to stop writing to me altogether or else to preserve silence as to his judgment of me and my actions. This letter arrived in Berlin at a time when he was ill in bed and he died a few days later.

I received the news of his death in November from his wife, he having married again. But I never knew whether he read my letter or not. The shock was very great and it upset my nerves, not only as the loss of so near a relative naturally would but also from the fact that I had written a letter which I had for several years hesitated to write, not wishing to place myself in a hostile position to a father who, after all, had been kind and had done the best he knew how to do for his children.

This news also added another care and responsibility, as my father left two younger sisters unprovided for. Being a salaried civil officer in the government, he had no opportunity to accumulate money, and both these sisters were above the age when government pensions are allowed to children. Although my sisters who were married and lived in New York and Washington gladly joined in this financial care yet their own family interests could not be sacrificed.

Thus ended the year 1859, and Christmas time was a rather *triste* one, especially as that cheerful festival was not then celebrated in New England, and schools and colleges continued in session as usual.

In looking back upon it, it seems to me that that year was one of the most delightful as well as the most tragic, and one of the most peaceful yet most conflicting, in emotion, in judgment and in making decisions.

Often have I meditated how differently would we act if we clearly saw events a little before they occurred. And how utterly tales of fiction fail when they describe how rightly instinctive wisdom decides at a moment when emotions and intelligence oppose each other, always leading the hero to do the right thing. The calm reasoning of the author knows what aim he has in view and what will be the end. In real life it is quite a different affair, and no one can judge the result when in a condition of conflict between heart and head.

CHAPTER XXV

*As part of her struggle to elevate the College standards,
she insists the students must be trained practically as
well as theoretically—Confirmation of her views by
experience of Dr. J. Marion Sims—Persistence in her
convictions and refusal to pass students whose work
is below her standards make many enemies for her—
Private practice increases—She applies for admission
to the Massachusetts Medical Society—Is refused because she is a woman—Militant ostracism of women
by the Philadelphia County Medical Society—Sketch
of the Female Medical College of Pennsylvania—Ap-
palled by the death rate among babies, Dr. Zakrzewska
establishes a temporary asylum for infants—Continuing unable to elevate the standards of the College,
she decides to resign—Her resignation is accepted,
with the request that she relinquish her last year's
salary—The occurrence causes a split in the College,
many of the men professors and trustees also resigning—The hospital is discontinued, and its furniture
is bought by friends of Dr. Zakrzewska. (Thirty-
two years of age: 1860-1862.)*

IF the Christmastide were prosaic, the New Year's
Day (1860) was not the less so. Business went on
everywhere just the same, only that every one
shouted to each other without any kind of feeling,
"Happy New Year!"

As the year progressed, lectures and dispensary
work, as well as the hospital department, went on;
private practice increased, adding to my income,
which was small. As professor, I received three

hundred dollars, and as superintendent of the clinical department, an additional three hundred dollars. Each of the gentlemen professors also received three hundred dollars while the lady professor of physiology had the benefit of an endowment of that chair and received five hundred dollars. From this it must be admitted that it was not money that induced these people to work hard every day, five times weekly, to instruct the students, but a real interest in the cause of educating professional women.

Had the originator of the school (Samuel Gregory), an ambitious man, originally a missionary, been a man of higher education and broader views, the school might have been taken up by the men standing highest in the profession. The prevailing sentiment among these men seemed to be that if women wanted to become physicians, the trial should be made by giving them the same advantages as were offered to men students.

But in a monograph which had been published by this originator to promote his plans, under the title of *Man-Midwifery,* he not only challenged the prevailing method of practice but abused even the best of physicians by intimating the grossest indelicacy, yes, even criminality, in their relations with their patients. This was the reason why no physician in Boston would openly acknowledge me as long as I remained in connection with the New England Female Medical College.

Besides this handicap, the non-professional portion of the trustees exercised a very fatal policy in trying to increase the number of students regard-

less of their preparatory education, so that there
existed a great contrast among the students. Some
had the best of education, while others fell far below a proper standard in their preparatory studies,
to say nothing of the age of some of them. Thus,
we had a number of students over forty—one was
fifty-six years old.

I admired the courage and persistency of these
middle-aged women in studying their lessons, often
mechanically without understanding their depth, yet
I could not conscientiously consider them fit subjects to enter upon the practice of a profession which
requires so much knowledge in various scientific directions as well as a broad education, so as to enable
one to comprehend the effects of all kinds of environment upon the individual patient.

How absolutely necessary it is to cultivate in the
student not only the scientist but also the philan-
thropist, the humanitarian, yes, even the philosopher, in order that one shall be fair and just in all
situations when consulted by persons morally, mentally or physically afflicted.

I constantly taught that the treatment of patients
cannot be learned from books but must be studied
practically. This was a principle which only a few
of the students would admit. The idea which I emphasized, that any other view of treating patients
belongs in the realm of quackery, was considered
by these ignorant students as an insult when I tried
to explain it to them.

But it must be remembered that at this date such
was the prevailing custom in even the best medical
schools for, as I have already explained, students

were expected to procure their practical training at
the hands of their private preceptors.

That this training was liable to be a will-o'-the-
wisp even with male students who had no difficulty
in finding preceptors has been well shown by the
personal experiences related by Dr. J. Marion Sims
in his autobiography called *The Story of My Life*.
Nowhere have I seen the consistent results of such
a method of medical education as everywhere prevailed even at this time, so clearly described as in
this book which was published in 1884.

Dr. Sims had a preceptor and he was graduated
from the Jefferson Medical College, in Philadelphia,
in March, 1835. He states that his preceptor was a
very great surgeon who was often unfitted for his
professional work by the habit of drinking. He also
states that he was very glad when he was able to
leave the office of this preceptor and attend medical
lectures.

About two or three weeks after Dr. Sims opened
his own office he was called to his first patient, "a
baby about eighteen months old who had what we
would call the summer complaint or chronic diar-
rhea." He continues his story, saying, "I examined
the child minutely from head to foot. I looked at
its gums and, as I always carried a lancet with me
and had surgical propensities, as soon as I saw some
swelling of the gums I at once took out my lancet
and cut the gums down to the teeth . . . but when
it came to making up a prescription I had no more
idea what ailed the child or what to do for it than
if I had never studied medicine."

Telling the mother to send to his office for medicine, he continues, "I hurried back to my office and took out one of my seven volumes of Eberle, which comprised my library . . . and turned quickly to the subject of Cholera Infantum and read it through, over and over again. . . . I knew no more what to prescribe for the sick babe than if I had not read it all. But it was my only resource. I had nobody to consult but Eberle. . . . He had a peculiar way of filling his book with prescriptions, which was a very good thing for a young doctor. . . . At the beginning of his article of twenty or thirty pages there was a prescription. . . . So I compounded it as quickly as I knew how and had everything in readiness for the arrival of Jennie."

Speaking of his next visit, he continues: "As the medicine had done no good, it was necessary to change it." He once more returned to his office and "turned to Eberle again and to a new leaf. I gave the baby a prescription from the next chapter. Suffice it to say that I changed leaves and prescriptions as often as once or twice a day. The baby continued to grow weaker and weaker." And in a short time it died, although Dr. Sims says, "I never dreamed that it could die!"

About two weeks later, he was called to his second patient, another baby which was ailing similarly to the first one. He writes, "I was nonplussed. I had no authority to consult but Eberle; so I took up Eberle again, and this time I read him backward. I thought I would reverse the treatment I had instituted with the Mayer baby. So, instead of beginning at the first of the chapter, I began at the last of the chapter, and turned backward, and turned the leaves the same way, and reversed the prescriptions. The baby got no better from the very first. And soon this baby died.''

Dr. Sims was so disheartened, he decided to leave that town, and he did so. But it is just to him to add that he further wrote, ''Being obliged to continue in the profession that I had started in, I was determined to make up my deficiency by hard work; and this was not to come from reading books, but from observation and from diligent attention to the sick.''

Thus it happened at the New England Female Medical College that, feeling as strongly as I did as to the necessity for clinical training, I made but few friends among my listeners, and I felt out of place except with those few who had had superior educational training. This difference in education naturally divided the students, and the feeling of favoritism grew stronger with the majority, while my interest in this majority naturally grew weaker. The clinical department was frequented only by the few, as no rule of compulsion demanded of the students a regular attendance.

My position became tedious in its teaching duties and unendurable in its relation to the students, yet I had nothing to complain of which could be corrected without changing the whole policy of the school and eliminating the most active directors, in fact, starting a college on college foundations.

My male co-workers, men of education and experience, fully agreed with me and told me that indorsing my election, they had hoped I would prevail upon the founders to elevate the standard of the school.

I, a foreigner who, as such, was not greeted with a cordial welcome by two thirds of the directors! And the Know-Nothing spirit prevailing strongly during those years in all strata of the community!

Besides, I did not feel called upon to condemn and to reform the part of their enterprise which had been justly praised in speech and in print, and which had been sustained for years by the efforts of regular physicians in the capacity of professors and private preceptors.

So, when my first college year closed, in March, 1860, and I flatly refused to agree to the bestowal of the degree of M.D. upon several women who presented themselves, I had laid the foundation of a hatred which rendered my work extremely trying and hard, and which to a certain extent prevented the growth of our out-door dispensary practice.

However, my private practice steadily increased, and in it I had the good will, as well as the assistance when in need, of the most prominent physicians in Boston. Among these were Drs. S. Cotting, Walter Channing, H. I. Bowditch, E. H. Clark and S. Cabot.

These men advised me to attempt to gain admission into the Massachusetts Medical Society, of which they were prominent members. After preparing for the necessary examination, I presented my claim but was refused because I was a woman, their charter allowing only male candidates for the examination.

This refusal on the ground of sex decided these men not to break the rules of the Massachusetts

Medical Society by consulting with me or by assisting me when advising patients to seek my attendance.

To be sure, their friendliness had not been withal an admission of the principle that women ought to be, or could be, physicians. On the contrary, I was informed in private conversation by some of these men that I was considered an "exception" to my sex; that such exceptions had existed in ancient times and were honored, and that during all the centuries such exceptions had continued to occur. Only one famous old physician, Dr. James Jackson, told me frankly and politely and in the kindest manner that it would be impossible for him to recognize as a lady any woman who was outside "her sphere."

A similar ostracism was practiced by the Philadelphia County Medical Society against the other medical college for women, the Female Medical College of Pennsylvania, which had been opened in 1850, two years after the New England Female Medical College began under the name of the Boston Female Medical School. But the Philadelphia college had taken the precaution from the beginning to obtain the same legal authority as the male medical colleges for conferring the medical degree.

Nevertheless, it led a precarious existence and had to be closed for the session of 1861-1862, and Dr. Ann Preston feared that the institution to which she had given so much time and strength was doomed to succumb to the weight of opposition and the absolute refusal of the male physicians to meet the women physicians in consultation. However, a few of the ablest men disregarded the rules of their society and stood by the women who had just then succeeded in opening their little hospital for women and children.

It was not until 1867 that the Philadelphia College could be considered as on a firm basis, but within ten years from that time it produced the first woman ovariotomist in America, Dr. Emeline H. Cleveland, who was resident physician of the Woman's Hospital after her return from study in Europe, principally in the Maternité in Paris.

Thus for me the year of 1860 ended. The college course which began in October had not varied in kind from that of the previous year, though I could note increased personal success in practice as well as in social connections.

The year of 1861 began for me in no way differently from the first in Boston. The dispensary practice increased in numbers of patients and also in greater variety and interest.

There was an especially large increase in the practice among children and infants, which gave me an insight into the neglect which the latter had to endure when boarded out among ignorant, and often indifferent, families, where the small sum received for the maintenance of these little unfortunate beings was of more consequence than their health and existence.

The frequency with which we were required to sign death certificates of infants whom we had seen but a day or two before, and who were then in an almost dying condition, was out of all relation with the number who applied in the early stages of what was then called "cholera infantum."

This led me to inquire how far the law protected such little beings, and how far institutions gave relief either to poor mothers by boarding their offspring, or to foundlings. This brought me in contact with one of the greatest philanthropists to these little creatures, namely, Miss Matilda Goddard, who had at that time provided good homes for about eight hundred infants, keeping a record as well as an oversight of them all. No public provision existed save a few places in connection with a Roman Catholic institution.

I therefore proposed to a few friends of mine the establishment of a temporary asylum for infants, and an apartment for this purpose was secured at the corner of Washington and Oak streets. Small as was this beginning, we having about eight babies, it drew the attention of a large number of philanthropists to the need of looking after these poor beings. And then the Massachusetts Infant Asylum, as well as other provisions for these dependents upon the Commonwealth, were called into existence. The result was the saving of many a valuable life and the directing of the attention of the benevolent to the absolute need of watchfulness over those helpless beings who are at the mercy of strangers during the first days or years of their lives.

The work at the college continued to be unsatisfactory to me, and the year 1862, which was to become of such great importance to womankind in general and to me in special, opened in the usual prosaic custom then prevailing, namely, with every day filled with routine work.

However, I felt very excited, as well as very uncertain how to shape my plans and prospects, for I had decided to leave the college and its little hospital at the close of the term in March. I had communicated my intention to the directors of the college at the close of the year of my engagement, in June, 1861.

One of the most interested of the directors was Mr. Samuel E. Sewall. He asked me what my reasons were for giving up the position, and I replied in a letter to him of which I here make a copy:

About two years have passed since I became connected with the New England Female Medical College. Twice I have signed the diplomas of the graduating class, both times with reluctance and under protest.

My work as teacher in the college and as physician in the medical department has not been performed with that ease which is the result of a mutual understanding of all engaged in the same purpose, nor has it given me satisfaction.

Not one of my expectations for a thorough medical education for women has been realized; indeed, I could not even do what has been in my power heretofore, namely, discountenance as physicians those women who do not deserve that name. On the contrary, I am obliged by the resolve of the majority to put my name to diplomas which justify the holders in presenting themselves to the community as fitted to practice.

If it were the intention of the trustees to supply the country with underbred, ill-educated women under the name of physicians in order to force the regular schools of medicine to open their doors for the few fitted to study, so as to bring an end to an institution from which are poured forth indiscriminately "Doctors of Medicine," I think the New England Female Medical College is on the right track.

Allow me to say a few words about the school in justification of this. To a critical observer, it will soon become apparent that the majority of the class of students could be made to be only good nurses; whilst some might become respectable midwives; and a very few, physicians. Yet we have to give the diploma of "Doctor of Medicine" to all, after they have passed the legal time in study.

After the first year of my work here had expired, I hoped to effect a change by remonstrating in the faculty meeting against the admission of all sorts of women, old and young, with and without common sense, and the distribution of diplomas to them all.

But I found very little support, and I was told that it would be hard to disappoint some women who had perseveringly labored for a diploma. According to my ideas, which agree, I know, with the ideas of the profession generally, perseverance alone does not entitle persons to receive a diploma. Even should a disappointment prove to be a deathblow to the student, it is better that one should die rather than receive permission to kill many.

It will be perceived by you that these circumstances are not such as to make success possible, and consequently they cannot make me contented in my position. I therefore ask you to accept my resignation as soon as the time expires for which I agreed to remain.

Knowing well how difficult it is to find a suitable

professor for a college for women, I thought it well
to inform you of my intention a full year in advance.
Yet should you find a desirable person to fill my place
before that time, I wish you to remember that I shall
be thankful to be released from duties which are
burdensome and unsatisfactory in result.

I hope that you will not consider this an impulsive
or rash step, and in order to convince you of the
deliberation with which I have made this decision,
and my firm determination not to alter it, I hope
that you will allow me an opportunity to state to you
personally, more fully, my views of the condition of
the school under your patronage.

Respectfully,

Marie E. Zakrzewska

Mr. Sewall gave me this opportunity, especially
because as a lawyer he wished to explain to me that
this letter could not be presented to the directors
and trustees of the college, as it suggested many
points which would necessarily lead to legal investigations and which would involve us all in a notoriety
absolutely fatal to the whole cause.

Yet I felt that no malicious intent was in me to
injure the school or any one. I simply expressed
my opinion and the opinion of professional men outside the college, who would not countenance the
school nor assist me personally so long as my connection with it lasted.

But in consequence of Mr. Sewall's opinion, I
resigned at the end of the college term without giving any other reason than that I felt not contented in
my position.

This led to many meetings of the trustees as a

number of them were anxious to retain my services, especially as the hospital department depended so largely upon my superintendence. On the other hand, a number, under the leadership of the secretary, Samuel Gregory (who had already pronounced against such innovations as microscope, thermometer, test tubes, etc., as proof of incapacity to recognize the ailments of patients), tried to convince the others that "foreigners" are not fit for American institutions, as they invariably are pedants and too rude to treat the free American woman with that courtesy to which she is accustomed.

Mr. Gregory brought proof of this declaration by calling before the meetings several of the women students who were opposed to me because I had frankly told them that they might in time become good nurses.

He also tried to convince the directors, who were in great financial straits, that the school had existed for ten years without such an expensive experiment as a hospital department, and that, by my leaving, this would be discontinued as a matter of course.

Thus my resignation was finally accepted, with the request that I relinquish my last year's salary of three hundred dollars, as the treasury was empty. I therefore became a benefactor to the college for that sum, though the treasurer did not acknowledge it in his report.

Besides this, an agreement was entered into between the college directors and my friends (who now more than ever wished to establish a hospital for women, managed by women physicians, and for the training of women as physicians and nurses) that all the furniture and fittings of the hospital department of the New England Female Medical College should become the property of these friends of mine for the sum of one hundred and fifty dollars.

[The Annual Reports of the New England Female Medical College during Dr. Zakrzewska's connection with it, from September, 1860, to September, 1862, show total expenses for the Clinical Department of $5,362.97, and total receipts for the same department of $5,024.13, making a total deficit of $338.84. But it must be remembered that Dr. Zakrzewska's connection with the department ended six months before the date of the last report.

Dr. Zakrzewska's forced "donation" of her salary for her third and last year, of three hundred dollars, brought the deficit down to $38.84; and the receipt of one hundred and fifty dollars from her friends as purchase price of the furniture left a net profit in the hands of the college of $111.16.

The last Annual Report contains not only the interesting omission of acknowledgment of Dr. Zakrzewska's donation of her three hundred dollars salary, but also the interesting acknowledgment of "donations" of one hundred dollars each from the two men professors who retired from the faculty at the same time.]

The whole occurrence brought about a split in the college and the most intelligent men, among whom was the Hon. S. E. Sewall and some of the men professors, also resigned. This was the beginning of the end of the college which, in 1874, was merged into the Boston University Medical College by an act of legislation which preserved to women as full rights as students as if they were in a college by themselves.

Thus it came about that Boston had a medical school for both sexes, though this then became a homeopathic school.

Dr. James R. Chadwick, in an article ("The Study and Practice of Medicine by Women"), in the *International Review,* October, 1879, states that

"in 1874, while the proposition to transfer the New England Female Medical College to Harvard University was under consideration by that corporation, the trustees suddenly merged the college in the School of Medicine of Boston University, which is under the exclusive control of homeopaths."

And he adds the following comment:

While this act may have involved no betrayal of trust in a legal sense on the part of the trustees, it certainly was an indefensible breach of trust toward those who had contributed funds to enable women to obtain a medical education in accordance with the tenets of the regular school.

During the three years of my life in Boston, from June, 1859, to 1862, it was necessary to educate the laity to consider a woman doctor a necessity in family life; to teach it that a woman can have the endurance and fortitude of body and mind to meet the demands of the profession, night or day, winter or summer, rain or shine. Also, to get the profession accustomed to the thought that women will study and practice medicine honorably and systematically. The attainment of these ends was the real satisfaction of these first years.

Fortunately, the eyes of the laity were fully upon us and criticism was not wanting. With watchful eagerness to grasp at the least mistake or failure, this kind public kept us at the work.

PART II

(1862—1902)

CHAPTER XXVI

A third American beginning—Founding of the New England Hospital for Women and Children—Incorporation for threefold object, to aid women as physicians, nurses and patients—Dr. Zakrzewska is resident, attending and dispensary physician, and in charge of the out-practice—Later, with the aid of paying guests, she is able to establish her home separate from the Hospital—The charitable policy of the Hospital. (1862-1863.)

THE quest approaches its goal. But the seeker knew it not, for she writes:

In 1862, after disconnecting myself from the New England Female Medical College in Boston, I stood alone once more, now for the third time, and still at the beginning of my life's work, as it appeared to me. I was no longer needed in New York, yet nothing could I show as the result of my eight years' labor.

Standing there alone as she felt herself, her soul filled only with the vision and her movements directed only towards following the gleam, she was all unknowingly already bound to Boston by constraining bands, the weaving of which she had shared with Clotho who spins, and with Lachesis who allots. And around her was gathering the atmosphere towards which her spirit had been yearning, an atmosphere made by kindred souls who needed her for their life's satisfaction as she needed them for hers.

Many men and women had upheld the New England Female Medical College because they felt called to assist in the evolution of medicine as a field for *human* endeavor rather than one forbidden to all but male workers. When Marie E. Zakrzewska appeared, some of these men and women realized that they had mistaken the light of the torchbearers for the chariot radiance, and when she concluded to leave the college they decided to go with her and to uphold the determination which she expressed when she said:

"I decided to work again on the old plan, namely, to establish the education of female students on sound principles, that is, to educate them in hospitals."

She continues:

Whoever is acquainted with the miraculous progress of medical science made in Europe, and especially in Germany, will know how far behind medical education in America had remained. This was chiefly owing to the want of well-organized hospitals. Clinical training and practical study can be had only at the bedside and in the deadhouse. No pathological or physiological discovery can be made in a college, behind the *cathedra*—it can only be proclaimed from this place.

Therefore the lecture room for the study of medicine had become secondary to the hospital all over the continent of Europe, and our best-educated young men and women were all longing to go to that Eldorado of medical research and knowledge.

It was the lack of this method in all medical

schools here which we felt when starting the New York Infirmary, especially as the few existing hospitals remained—and still remain for the most part —closed to women students. It was our perception of this true method for educating a physician that determined us to establish a hospital prior to a college. We women decided to start from a sound and correct foundation, and to this principle we owe the great success so far attained, although it may appear small to those who now enter upon the work.

Here let me remark that we willingly allow the newcomers to make their criticisms of the present conditions; we admit the truth when it is spoken, but we expect the newcomers to work as hard and to strive as untiringly and perseveringly as we pioneers have done, to improve and to complete what has been undertaken.

A few friends—Mr. George William Bond, Mrs. Ednah D. Cheney, and Miss Lucy Goddard—true, firm friends of the education of women, stood beside me, with no other ready means than some remnants of hospital furniture, valued at one hundred and fifty dollars, which remained from our experiment in connection with the New England Female Medical College. On June 22, 1862, we hired, on our own responsibility, a sunny, airy house with a large yard, located at No. 60, Pleasant Street, corner of Porter Street, at a rent of six hundred dollars, and here we commenced operations.

And thus was born the *New England Hospital for Women and Children,* which began its work on July 1, 1862, a few men physicians being willing to aid us by giving us their names as consultants.

Other friends of women's education soon joined us and became directors. Among these Samuel E.

Sewall, the old friend of the college, and F. W. G. May, the ever-hopeful treasurer of a then empty purse, gave us their indefatigable aid and unremitting interest.[8]

Thus in the midst of the Civil War we started our work. And many a soldier's family thanked us for so doing, for just then the darkest days of the struggle gave us special opportunity to advise and comfort.

A Provisional Committee managed the new institution. Four of the committee became responsible for the rent, and each of the ladies pledged herself to obtain her proportion of the expenses from month to month. As an example of the faith and courage of these supporters of Dr. Zakrzewska, it is related that Mr. Bond met Mr. Abraham A. Call and told him that a house on Pleasant Street had been rented for a hospital but there was not a penny to pay the rent, whereupon Mr. Call handed him a contribution of five dollars for that purpose and later became a director of the Hospital, his daughter, Dr. Emma L. Call,[21] becoming in time one of its leading physicians.

Meantime, Dr. Zakrzewska repeated the superhuman work which she had already done at the New York Infirmary and again at the Clinical Department of the New England Female Medical College—organizing the details of the Hospital and Dispensary, serving as resident and attending physician and responding to all calls in both out-patient and private practice.[9]

The new institution began at once to grow and on March of the following year (1863), it was incorporated, Miss Lucy Goddard and Mrs. Ednah D. Cheney joining her as legal sponsors for the undertaking.

The name, the New England Hospital for Women and Children, was chosen because Boston was considered as the center of this cluster of States which seemed to have so generally the sentiments and relations of a family group within the larger Union. But common usage has always been to shorten the longer, detailed title and to call the institution simply the New England Hospital, and by this latter title it has become known all over the world.

The objects of the Hospital, as stated in the first by-laws, were declared to be three:

1. To provide for women medical aid by competent physicians of their own sex.
2. To assist educated women in the practical study of medicine.
3. To train nurses for the care of the sick.

During the first transitional year, 1862-1863, Dr. Zakrzewska's duties were again increased by the resignation of Dr. Breed as resident physician, and this added care continued till September, 1863, when Dr. Lucy E. Sewall returned from study in Europe and became the new resident physician. As this year progressed the need for an attending surgeon was felt and, as there appeared to be no sufficiently qualified woman available, Dr. Horatio R. Storer was appointed.

This latter is the only instance in which a male physician has been appointed on the attending staff of the New England Hospital. And this cutting of the Gordian knot, which was made necessary by the lack of opportunity for surgical training for women, is characteristic of Dr. Zakrzewska's attitude of mind. While her greatest interest was directed toward developing women she was profoundly interested in all forms of human activity, and she believed a balanced life required everywhere the presence of both men and women. The New England Hospital was forced to be limited to women physicians because all other hospitals denied them entrance. Even when they were, later, grudgingly admitted to some of these latter, it was only to the lower positions, and opportunities for advancement were never, and are not to this day, equalized.

When the appointment of a resident physician no longer made it necessary for her to live in the Hospital, though retaining her office there, she rented a house in Roxbury and once more had the joy of possessing a home of her own, sharing this with two of her sisters. These were the youngest, who had been sent to her after her father's death, and another whom she was educating for self-support as a teacher.

However, as her financial condition was very precarious, she was obliged to admit to her household as paying guests some friends and patients. She thus found herself the head of quite an establishment, and over this she presided with that executive ability and that atmosphere of elder-sisterliness which we have already seen her manifest in her first New York home.

The most notable members of this family circle were undoubtedly Miss Julia A. Sprague, who became her faithful friend and home companion for life, and Mr. and Mrs. Karl Heinzen. It is easy to understand how such a personality as that of Karl Heinzen [10] would appeal to her, especially as his name had been a household word in her home in Berlin. She writes:

From early childhood I had heard of Karl Heinzen as the pioneer of republicanism in Germany, whose writings my father read in secret. He was very poor and he published a paper which was unpopular, as it advocated not only the abolition of slavery but also "woman's rights." Our friendship was, therefore, based not simply on affinity by nature but also on principle; and we pledged ourselves to devote our strength and our means to furthering the realization of our convictions.

This friendship lasted as long as Karl Heinzen lived (he died in November, 1880) and its influence on both of these independent thinkers was profound and far-reaching.

In addition to her other work she increased the Hospital funds by lecturing to the public; some of her private patients furnished greatly needed assistance by holding a Fair in Roxbury; and an especial service was rendered by Miss Sprague who gave three months of her time to serve as matron of the Hospital.

An item of interest is the contribution given by the trustees of the Boston Lying-In Hospital who had at that time no hospital of their own. During the years of 1861 and 1862 this body gave to the New England Female Medical College donations of twenty dollars and fifty-one dollars, respectively, these donations being contributions for the care of obstetric patients in the Clinical Department under Dr. Zakrzewska's management. During this first year of the existence of the New England Hospital (now become the only lying-in hospital in the city) the donation was made to this hospital, and it reached the sum of two hundred dollars.

Striking evidence of the growth of her work and of the faith of her supporters is shown in the formation, already in this first year of the life of the New England Hospital, of a Building Committee and the beginning of a Permanent Fund, the birth of this latter being marked by a donation of three thousand dollars from Mrs. George G. Lee and by one of one thousand dollars from a friend of Samuel E. Sewall.

The charitable policy of the Hospital was one which presented great practical difficulties of administration, difficulties which have always fallen to the lot of every one who has attempted any philanthropic work. The point of view adopted by Dr. Zakrzewska and her director associates is admirably shown in the first annual report (1863) and its appendices. It is especially to be noted here because of attacks which were later made upon it, as we shall presently see.

CHAPTER XXVII

Extracts from letters to her first Boston student, Dr. Lucy E. Sewall, now studying in Europe—Lectures to public on "Hospitals: their history, designs and needs." (1863.)

THE daughter of Samuel E. Sewall became an enthusiastic admirer of Dr. Zakrzewska during one of the visits which the latter made to Boston in the interest of the New York Infirmary, and a close friendship between them resulted. An amusing incident of their first meeting has been related in an earlier chapter.

This friendship led to Lucy E. Sewall's decision to study medicine and she entered the New England Female Medical College as soon as Dr. Zakrzewska became connected with it, in 1859. She remained a student there during the entire three years that Dr. Zakrzewska continued on the faculty, being assistant student in the Clinical Department, and being graduated in March, 1862. Following the advice of Dr. Zakrzewska, she then went to Europe for clinical study and for the practical training which was denied her in her own country.

From the correspondence which ensued many interesting sidelights are thrown on Dr. Zakrzewska's personality and activities during these days. Thus, she writes:

October 16, 1862.

DEAR LUCY:

I suppose you want long letters and in order to meet this want I will write as often as I find time, so as to fill the sheet as I go along. After that forlorn day yesterday, I am established again as usual this morning at the table writing.

Now let me tell you that I consider you one of the greatest intriguants possible. You thought, I suppose, that you could catch two flies in one beating by providing me with inkstand and pens. Of course, I have to write if I have the materials; while the things will not get used up in so doing, and will even be ornamental next year after you have returned and we have an office together! But wait till you do come home, and then see whether your speculation turns out as you calculated.

I gave the match box and tumbler to Mr. and Mrs. Heinzen who were greatly pleased with the little memento. Now this is all for one morning, only let me assure you that you sha'n't leave me again behind you; or if you desire to do so, you shall not see me when you start.

October 21.

I have had two letters now from Dr. Morton, the one I told you about and one other, dated September 24, in which she spoke of her safe arrival and of her terrible homesickness. She calls Paris a cold city. She likes England very much and wants to hear from you, all about yourself and your experiences. . . . Minna writes pleasantly about her life and wants to hear from you, too. I suppose I will have to send her your letter when you send me one that I can send about.

. . . Dr. Cabot called here the other day. He was very pleasant and accepted all as very good—arrangements as well as physicians and students. I asked him about consultation in forceps cases. He said it was not necessary to call him for such cases, as forceps when skillfully applied were without danger to either mother or child. You see, he rightly supposes we use the forceps "skillfully."

The student, Miss Cook, has left for the Philadelphia college. I really don't know what else to write to you unless I tell you some of my domestic affairs, namely, that I got, all in all, eight barrels of pears and seven of apples; and I have any quantity of tomatoes pickled and barberry jelly made. . . . On the 12th of November, we shall have the Dress Party, which will be given by Miss Nichols in honor of Miss Sprague's birthday.

Boston, Pleasant Street,
Saturday, November 29, at 9 P. M.

I am in Miss G.'s (the matron of the hospital) room, which is my present abode during the nights. I have just arrived from the depot where I left Mrs. —— (one of her home patients) and Mrs. Heinzen, who are going to New York. The first goes to see her son who is going to the war, and the latter accompanies her for safety's sake. They both return day after to-morrow.

Before starting for Roxbury, I read your letter to the whole company there. They all send love to you and say that it is Holiday when your letters arrive. . . . We read all your letters, even those to your father, and I assure you they are all much too short.

. . . Why don't you tell me more about Miss B.'s

nephew, or have you decided on a compromise? You
remember that I don't want you to marry a German,
and your uncle forbids an Englishman; so you must
try to find one who combines all the good points of
German, English and American.

. . . I was very much amused at your descriptions of the English doctors. I hope they will be
of use to you. What you say about Dr. —— and
Dr. —— is, I am afraid, correct, for they have at
times a special faculty for being haughty and making themselves as disagreeable as anybody can do.
I should like to hear more about it because, from
Mrs. ——'s expressions, I inferred the same. I
am very sorry that she has left London. I know
her; she spent an evening with me at the Infirmary
and my acquaintance with her was interrupted by
another matter which took my attention.

. . . What kind of a bonnet did you buy? And
why did you not complete the last page of your
letter by giving a description of it?

. . . There is no need to tell me not to forget to
miss you. I am sure I never missed any person
more than I do you. I almost had it in my heart
to wish that you may not succeed in London and
that you then make a visit to Paris during the rest
of the winter, and then go along the River Seine and
come home in June. I feel almost wicked to make
you homesick yet certainly I do feel provoked when
you say that you are not so; for I am homesick for
you.

It is very strange how you have grown yourself
into my heart. I never before have felt such strong
attachment for a woman, that is, so "tenderly"
strong. I have always appreciated and loved women
more intellectually. But you are my child. And I

am going to have the first grandbaby all to myself as my well-deserved property.

You see, I am not so very selfish. I want you to enjoy all happiness that exists for us poor mortals— which is by no means in the single life.

Roxbury, Attic Room, Southeast Corner,
Sunday Night, 10:30.

I hope this is dated explanatorily enough to need no comments. But where under this wet heavens are you? We have plenty of water from above, have you still the same below you? I would almost envy you were I not so cosily covered.

Henceforth, I fear we will have to pity you on Sundays in that pious England. I can appreciate your loneliness, for I often have a taste of it here on Sabbath evenings. For in spite of all the liberality of our inmates, we have to be stupid Sunday nights to please them, and I am always thankful when the day is over.

Mr. Heinzen said to-day that I am a great talker, and he is not so very wrong, for it distresses me to see a whole company sitting together doing nothing, saying nothing, and thinking nothing, because it is Sunday and they can't go to church, in order to hear nothing—but words and phrases.

I often think I will make these latter myself, using innocent subjects for the sake of conversation. The presence of people disturbs me and prevents my thinking deeply, so I talk out what comes along. Have you ever found me so very talkative—unless I am with people who don't interest me very much above a certain degree, say one above zero?

I hope this letter and the one I wrote to Miss Morton will not be called belonging to this class.

Still, I am writing to-night chiefly to let out some steam. Some people will not do this and therefore often burst when least desirable.

. . . My finger which became infected during the treatment of that little Mrs. —— is now progressing so that I do not fear future trouble. It has been the most curious development of pathological changes that you can imagine. I am sorry that you could not watch nature in a small trouble and see her action in repairing damages.

Be careful of yourself for you know that at the time when my finger became infected, it was apparently perfectly sound, yet there must have been some point of entrance for the infection which followed. I am glad that it proved to be so slight.

I have not been to see your father as I was so very busy, but I shall go there to-morrow unless the storm continues too severely.

Roxbury, December 28, 1862.

Merry Christmas and Happy New Year! I shall not tell you any more that I miss you at any time, for I don't, not a bit. On the contrary, I am glad that you are gone.

I just read this paragraph to our parlor assembly and they wanted to tear it up. Now, don't you think that is quite a despotical sign of our regiment here? I am sure I don't want to write anything else, for you shall not get too vain about yourself.

We, that is, myself and Mrs. —— and Miss Sprague, as well as Mr. and Mrs. Heinzen, feel quite proud of our little doctor in England, only we feel as if that little M.D. should write a little oftener.

. . . Mrs. W—— has a splendid little girl of nine and one-half pounds. She had a very hard time, thirty-six hours' labor, and I finally delivered her with forceps, Miss Tyng officiating as assistant. Mother and child are doing well and send love to you.

Christmas was a very pleasant day and evening with us. We had the parlors trimmed beautifully with laurel and holly, and when I came home in the evening, I covered the chandeliers with wreaths.

Then we placed white cloths on the front parlor center table and on another small one, and set plates on them with German gingerbread and apples and nuts.

Returning from supper, we found large baskets and bundles which Santa Claus had brought to the room and left for me to distribute.

So after each one had appropriated a plate, I called out the names, and lots of handsome little things came out of the brown and white papers, by and by covering the tables completely, so that the room looked like a charming little fair, and we had ever so much fun, and many funny things, and I only wish that you had been here, too.

Now, tell me how you are getting on in London, how your health is, how much you are learning and how you spent Christmas.

I have been nonsensically busy, so much so that I am completely worn out, and to-day I proposed that I go to London to bring you back for the purpose of getting rested. Everything goes the same old, old way. Miss —— is with me but she stays in the same old place and, although I like her very much, yet there is no mutual sympathy between us.

Lucy, never marry a man with whom you do not agree on all points! I feel it more and more, the older I grow, that love grows stronger only towards those with whom we sympathize; and that we become more and more a burden to each other if we do not

agree well. And although we may avoid quarreling
yet coldness is sometimes harder to bear than an
absolute quarrel. I feel all this with Miss ——, and
yet she is far more agreeable to me than a good
many other of my acquaintances. I really feel an
attachment for her, perhaps for the very reason
that I feel we will not be obliged to be always together.

Miss —— charged me with a great deal of love for
you, and you may help yourself to as much as you
want. . . . On the 20th, I am giving a lecture for our
Hospital, at Chickering Hall, on the subject of "Hospitals." I shall let you know how it comes off. . . .
Write soon and put yourself into the letter, and I
will send you back by the next mail.

Roxbury, January 25, 1863.

It is Sunday morning, and I am tired and worn
out. I felt miserable all last week, so miserable that
I had to give up my work and my lessons for the
last three days and rest. Yesterday afternoon we
all went to the minstrels, and I am the only one
who got used up by it.

I have had a great deal of practice this winter,
more than is good for me, yet I did not make so
much money. People are all poor, everything being now so dear.

Nevertheless, I am satisfied with my affairs if I
can only keep strong under the strain. My sister
Anna is again quite sick, and Rosalie will therefore
come to live with me in April. Minna had everything arranged to go to Paris in April or May, but
now that gold gets higher every day, she thinks she
must give it up for another year. Would it not be
nice if she could arrive in Paris when you do?

I wish gold would come down again so that could come about.

Now, a few words as to the talk in England about a medical college for women. Elizabeth Blackwell wrote to me about this as follows: "She may get a great deal of valuable knowledge there, but I can judge far better than she can of the value of their speeches. What they mean by a 'college' is a school for a better class of midwives. To the broad, true ground of admitting women to an equality in the profession, they are stubbornly opposed; and they hold the power of exclusion entirely in their own hands. The law in England makes medicine and surgery a close corporation, very different from the freedom here."

Miss Garrett seems to verify all this, and more. I know, myself, that the same talk and the same help would be extended to you should you go to Berlin. But all that means a different thing from native women taking the same work, as a general thing. There are *some* liberal men, to be sure, but they are so much in the minority that their voices cannot even be heard.

The work for us is in America, and nowhere else. I therefore feel extremely glad to find that some of the most prominent men in New York have taken up the matter; they have published a circular asking the public to give fifty thousand dollars which is to be invested, and the interest of which is to go for scholarships in one of the great New York medical schools, for the use of such women as are able to meet all the demands for a preparatory education.

This is the best plan after all, both here and abroad, and the best you can do is to learn all you can so as to come home well prepared to enter the ranks as a practitioner. Every well-educated woman works more for the cause of her fellow beings by doing well herself rather than by meddling and trying constantly to help others. For the next few years, I shall make this my working principle and after that, I shall see what is best to be done next.

. . . You are very much mistaken if you think Vienna or Berlin better than the Paris Maternité for real knowledge. For instance, in Berlin, no student, not even a male, is permitted to perform "version" or do anything in the way of an operation. In Paris, every midwife gets her case of "version."

In Vienna, only the male students get "versions." And both there and in Berlin the men take the places close to the beds and the women have to stand on the outskirts; while in Paris no man stands in the woman's way.

. . . I felt very sorry that you were so homesick during the holidays. I really missed you more than I ever missed anybody before. I hope you will be at home next Christmas.

. . . I sent Miss —— on Christmas Eve a little ivory bookmark, beautifully cut, Swiss work; it can be used also as a paper cutter though it is very weak.

. . . I am not seeing Miss —— since she came home. I think my friendship, or rather hers, is over, since she cannot convert me.

Roxbury, February 20, 1863.

It seems to me an eternity since I wrote to you last, and the cause of it is that I was very sick and unnaturally busy. I delivered my lecture on January 20th. and the Hospital got some fifty dollars profit.

I had been extraordinarily busy and had the house full of patients in Roxbury. Besides, I was short of help at the Hospital which worried me very much. The consequence was that I got really sick, gave up practice entirely for a week, and when I did not get better, I packed my bundle and went to New York on a "spree." Now, is it not curious that what we wanted to do for so long, namely, to take a journey together, was realized with Miss ——. She volunteered to take care of me, and consequently went with me and we had a real good time, at least as far as I could have it, being really sick and blue.

Since then I am a little better, but not very well, and so busy that I have had to disappoint Aunt Hannah three evenings, after I had appointed the day to take tea with her and to spend a lively hour. Yet I could not help it.

So much for myself! Next thing is the Hospital. Dr. Breed has resigned her position, and I am therefore without a resident physician. Miss Tyng takes charge in my absence, while Miss Abbott stands second. She is resident student and also aids in the nursing. Miss Tyng is splendid in all mechanical work, and together they are very helpful to me.

As to a resident physician, I am authorized, and appointed a committee, to ask "you" whether you will be willing to fill this post after your return. In case you accept, we shall go on as at present, and wait for you. Write me, therefore, at once what you think about it.

My great desire is that we shall have an office together. Now, I do not like Pleasant Street at all, although it would not make any difference to you where you begin practice. Perhaps we can find a more suitable house for next fall. Ours is too small anyhow. However, this must be left to the future. So far, we are doing very well at the Hospital. And yesterday, Dr. H. R. Storer called upon me and invited me to call upon him, as he is anxious to extend colleague-ship to me. He was a student of Simpson, in Edinburgh, and a classmate of Priestley, and he studied with Dr. B. Brown. By the way, you must get certificates from all these men that you studied with them, or that you visited their respective hospitals. If it is nothing more than a simple recommendation, it will help you amazingly over here, and also do good to the general cause of women studying abroad. Therefore, try to get something written.

I shall go to see Dr. Storer next week and show him some of your letters. I am sure you will find a good reception here, as I am preparing the way for you somewhat among the physicians. I also read some extracts from your letters in my lectures, reading especially loudly the one where Dr. Brown introduced you as "Dr. Sewall from America."

. . . I will send you a Philadelphia catalogue next week, but I would advise you not to encourage any students coming here at present. Dr. Blackwell is trying very hard to make arrangements for women to enter the New York University of Medicine. If she succeeds, it would be much better for any woman to go there rather than to Philadelphia.

[The Female Medical College of Pennsylvania was still struggling for existence against the bitter opposition of the men, and especially of the Philadelphia Medical Society. It had at this time just reopened after being obliged to close for the session of 1861-1862.]

Rather, let the English women fight their way in England. Don't get too much interested in the establishment of a woman's college in London. Dr. Blackwell is correct in her statement as to the position women would occupy there in case they study separately from the men.

. . . I have not yet seen either your father or the books as I can hardly find time for anything except my practice.

Roxbury, May 7, 1863.

. . . I received your first letter from Paris on Saturday, May 2d. I am very glad to hear of your success and hope you will profit by it. We are going on beautifully here with our Hospital if only we had more money.

. . . We had five days of incessant storm, and now it pours down like a deluge. Spring has been very forward this season. Our cherries were in bloom and we sat on the hill on April 13th. What did you do on your birthday? We celebrated it by being out of doors all the morning and wishing for you. . . . I went to New York again for about four days. . . . My health is tolerably good again, I think better than last spring. . . . Miss Sprague is now in Minna's place, and she heads the Roxbury house beautifully. I like her very much in this position, she takes such an interest in the whole affair. Rosalie is with me now and acts quite nicely as nurse.

I don't mean to have many patients this summer; everything is so dear, and besides it is a great burden. I would rather live by myself and pay more for the comfort of having a free home than to make a little profit.

. . . In the Hospital we are so busy that the back parlor is turned into a ward for four beds.

. . . We have a fine Dispensary now—about one thousand patients this year and an interesting Hospital. Next week we shall have one great operation, and probably a second one.

Don't be alarmed about my health. I am as well as usual, and I think a little better than last spring. There are a good many things that worry and trouble me besides my work, things which I cannot control, and which have a good deal to do with my running down in health. At present I feel quiet and happy. . . . I got a fresh supply of young chickens this morning. . . . What buttons did you buy? I want to send you the money very much.

Elsewhere Dr. Zakrzewska, in speaking of her lecture mentioned in one of the preceding letters, says that the founding of the New England Hospital had given rise to so many inquiries as to the need for hospitals that she was requested to give a lecture on the "History, designs and needs of hospitals" in general and of special hospitals in particular. She also corrects the figures for receipts, later returns showing a net profit of one hundred dollars, although the admission fee was only twenty-five cents. She continues:

It is surprising how at that time hospitals were considered as places for merely the poor and the wretched, or for the victims of accidents in public streets or roads.

We had to cultivate the feeling that such enterprises were something necessary and desirable, especially since the use of anesthetics and the great improvement in surgical antisepsis have tended to make the hospital the regular place for surgical treatment of the rich as well as of the poor.

We had also to show the wisdom of isolation by the removal, even from the houses of the rich, of the patient afflicted with a contagious disease, in order to save the rest of the family as well as to offer a greater chance of recovery to the patient.

CHAPTER XXVIII

By resignation of the resident physician, Dr. Zakrzewska is obliged to resume entire charge of Hospital and Dispensary and she again shows symptoms of over-fatigue and strain while awaiting Dr. Sewall's return from Europe to fill the vacant position—Illustrations of the application of Dr. Zakrzewska's humanitarian instincts and intellectual convictions to the treatment of her patients, in addition to technical medical care— "A Lesson"—"Another True Story." (1863.)

As Dr. Sewall accepted the offer of the position of resident physician at the Hospital, to take effect on her return from Europe in September, Dr. Zakrzewska continued to fill the duties of this position both at the Hospital and on the two added days in the Dispensary.

The most robust health and endurance have their limits, and she has already been noted as giving many symptoms which showed that she had been presuming on hers ever since the over-strenuous days of establishing the New York Infirmary. Repeated notes of overfatigue and strain creep into these letters to Dr. Sewall.

Specializing largely, as she did, in that branch of medicine (obstetrics) which is most regardless of convenience and most inconsiderate as to sleeping hours, she worked literally day and night. And feeling the whole burden of responding to the demand for the trained woman physician which she

314

had so largely helped in awakening, she refused no patients.

Her humanitarian instincts and her admirable ability to enter into the feelings of her patients, and to recognize their limitations and their struggles, prompted her to send no bills until they were asked for. She writes:

If you could see my office day after day full of school-teachers, dressmakers, mill operatives and domestics, all too proud to go to the dispensary and yet not rich enough to pay a large fee, you would agree with me that the prescription for good meat, wine or beer would be a farce if I took the money with which they ought to buy these instead of taking the small fee which allows them to keep their self-respect.

Not content with reducing her fees to a minimum or to zero, she always added the constructive work which from her point of view belonged within the province of her profession. This was not done by giving charity regarding which she had definite and very modern views. She writes:

It is not *Charity* which we must cultivate and practice: it is *Justice* to one another. Charity is what an opiate is to a patient: it soothes for the time but the same bad consequences result as follow the drug. We must teach ourselves that the Golden Rule must be actually practiced in order to reach and raise those who need to be helped.

And again she emphasizes:

The Golden Rule must be practiced every day and not merely formulated as a pious recital on Sunday.

Investigating the routine of the patient's life, she would help her to reorganize it along the lines of hygiene, of economics, and of a balanced perspective; and then would follow a reëducation not only of the patient but of the patient's family and even friends. In this way, her influence extended to the men of the family and of the community. And these vied with the women in acknowledging their indebtedness to what they called her "common sense." She depicts this aspect of her work so clearly in a couple of sketches written in later years that they are inserted here to add to the definiteness of the outlines of this phase of her history. The first of these (*Souvenir of the New England Hospital Fair,* 1896) is:

A LESSON

I will a round unvarnish'd tale deliver.
—SHAKESPEARE.

Mary was the third child of five in a family in humble circumstances. The father, an industrious journeyman carpenter, aided by the thrifty mother, managed to keep all the children in attendance at the free public schools of Boston until they graduated at the age of about fifteen years. Soon after leaving school, Mary obtained a situation as child's nurse in the house of a rich family, with whom she remained nine years in the varying capacity of nursemaid, chambermaid and seamstress. She then married a journeyman plumber twenty-six years of age, he being thus two years her senior. He had laid by from his earnings a sum of money about equal to what Mary had saved from her nine years' wages, and these combined were amply sufficient to set them up in respectable housekeeping in a neatly furnished tenement having a kitchen, dining-room, living room and chamber, also a storeroom and bathroom.

In due time, the baby made its appearance and found awaiting it a handsome cradle, and a ward-robe not only comfortable but pretty and plentiful. The young father with no small pride carried his son and heir, arrayed in a white cashmere cloak and suitable belongings, while by his side walked his prettily dressed wife, when on Sunday afternoons they went to visit friends and relatives. Thus far, all was well.

After the lapse of five years and a half, four little ones formed the pride and the care of these young folks; and it was just seven years from the time of their marriage that I first entered their home as visiting doctor from the dispensary, the indigent being attended at their homes when illness pre-vented their coming to the free dispensary at the clinic hours.

I found the family of six living in two rooms heated by the kitchen stove. The children were ill with scarlatina. All around was the evidence of poverty, although not destitution nor degrading squalor. By observation and subsequent inquiry, I soon learned the cause of this changed condition. It was simply this—Mary, who had gradually adapted herself with grace and intelligence to the comforts of the rich house in which she had lived from her fifteenth to her twenty-fourth year, could not now conform herself to the smaller means and ways of living of a wife and mother in moderate circumstances.

She had learned to cook delicate, expensive viands, had a sure belief that tenderloin is the only steak fit for eating, and had great skill in the pretty and dainty ornamentation of the babies. These tastes which she acquired in the rich merchant's family could not be gratified with the workman's means; she had unlearned the thrifty habits among which she had lived as a schoolgirl in her parents' home and she became confused in her methods of work, while the steady increase in her family reduced her in strength and added to her cares and labors, a condition not inclined to promote the good temper of the naturally amiable woman.

Ofter now, the husband, returning home from his work, found no table laid for dinner, and still oftener must he start out early in the morning to find a breakfast in a neighboring eating house, which is always the first step towards finding rest and companionship in the saloon.

This was the condition as it unfolded itself to me during my brief attendance. The children recovered, and with the aid of cod-liver oil and tonics provided by the charity of the dispensary, soon regained full health.

A little more than a year passed when one day in October, 1876, Mary presented herself in my private consulting room. She looked haggard and pale, was poorly clad and in a desperate frame of mind. Her husband had gone from bad to worse. He paid the rent for two shabby small rooms in an old house and provided weekly the coal for the kitchen stove. All the rest of his earnings he spent for his own meals. Often, if he came home at all at night, it was in a state of partial intoxication. Naturally, no firm dared give him regular employment and he supported himself by odd jobs.

The poor woman had resorted to needlework for support, this being the only means for her to earn money and look after her children, whom she could not send to school for lack of shoes and decent clothing.

It was Friday afternoon. She had just carried her work to her employer and received her pay of one dollar and sixty cents. She laid it on the table before me and said, "This is all I with my four children shall have to buy food with until next Friday—it is not enough to buy even bread and tea and that is all we have lived upon for the last three weeks." She looked wan and hungry and cried bitterly. I sent for a little luncheon, and while she ate it, I devised the following plan:

"Mrs. S——," said I, "take this money and spend it as follows:

Buy 7	lbs.	corned beef	$0.35
21	"	potatoes	.25
14	"	cabbage	.28
7	"	Indian meal	.21
1 qt.		molasses	.15
7		loaves bread	.35
Salt		....	.01
			$1.60

"Boil the meat in twelve quarts of water until very tender. Divide the meat and broth in seven parts, also the potatoes and cabbage. Cook one portion of cabbage and potatoes each day in the portion of broth. Divide this stew into five equal parts for you and your four children. Do the same with the

Indian meal, cooking one part every morning. Salt it well, and pour on it one-seventh part of the molasses—that is for your breakfasts. Use one loaf of bread each day for supper. Come again next Friday and let me know the result.''

She promised to follow this written prescription, and did so. The ensuing Friday she again presented herself before me, looking less distressed having earned $1.70. She said she ''was glad to have done so, as the children could eat more than the seventh part of the purchase, and it was hard for her to eat it herself and deny the children.'' However, she had obeyed and was able to do more work having earned ten cents more that week, although she and the children ''felt sorely the lack of tea.'' I advised her to make a change in her purchases, spending the same amount of money for a fresh shin of beef and turnips or a salted shoulder of pork, and to use the ten cents for extra molasses.

After two weeks, she came again to report to me. The change in her appearance was remarkable, and her account of her children's condition was good. Also, she had been able to earn two dollars per week, which, however, was the utmost she could do in the time she could spare from the family work. At the end of another two weeks she came to me and asked permission to give to her husband a share of the dinner on the coming Sunday. He had smelled the stew when occasionally coming home and desired to partake of it. It was therefore agreed that he should add fifteen cents as his share for the cost of the dinner, which he did, and when Christmas came, she told me had done so regularly every day for the previous three weeks.

I made them a Christmas present of a piece of roasting beef, fifty pounds weight of apples, and the same amount of potatoes, while former friends to whom I had spoken of their destitution, sent tea, sugar and milk, also shoes and stockings for the children.

After this sumptuous holiday feast, severely cold weather followed. Careless housekeepers in all ranks of life allowed their water pipes to burst, and great was the demand for plumbers' work, especially in the suburbs of Boston. Mary's former friends were willing to employ her husband again, under his promise of strict sobriety, as they would not risk the danger of house-burning by the carelessness of a tipsy plumber. Mary cooked him substantial dinners of the description given above, and he felt like a man again in his home.

Being skillful as a workman and very obliging in disposition, he gained friends while jobbing in the different houses. Those who had known him before encouraged him to persevere and finally persuaded him to remove to one of those suburban towns where his business would be in good demand and where he would escape from the temptation of eating house and drinking saloon. Meantime, Mary had learned good lessons during these sixteen weeks. She now knew how to provide and cook good, cheap and wholesome meals, and soon adapted herself entirely to such ways and means as his earnings would provide.

It is now 1896, and the twenty years are completed since the beginning of that time of misery in that family, who now own three houses, in one of which Mary's husband carries on a fine, thriving business, over the entrance door of which may be read the sign "John Smith & Son." Another house is occupied by them as a dwelling, and the third, an investment of their earnings, is rented to their daughter's husband who is foreman in their business.

Their life is simple and plain but comfortable, and when I met Mary recently, she told me that she had taught all the children, two boys and two girls, how to cook and how to mend clothes, and with great pride she assured me that corned beef and cabbage is their favorite dish, "although the children will often make ice cream for Sunday dessert."

The second sketch alluded to (*The Woman's Journal,* May 13, 1893) is:

ANOTHER TRUE STORY

Some years ago, the wife of a farmer living not many miles from Boston came to my office to consult me, because she feared she was suffering from a disease such as can only befall a woman and which she fully believed was "killing her by inches." With sunken cheeks, dull eyes, sallow complexion, pale lips and no more flesh on her limbs than was necessary to make locomotion possible, the woman sat there and told of her ailments—sleeplessness, utter lack of appetite, backache, depression of spirits, etc.

After listening and taking notes of her story of misery, I made a careful examination and then told her that she was entirely free from all disease, but that she was simply worn out and needed six months of rest and good living.

She sighed deeply and said it was impossible to follow such a prescription as their pecuniary means would not permit it. She said further that their two children had outgrown the district school of the town, and she had, with true Yankee ambition, persuaded her husband to send them to a relative in the city that they might have the advantage of came, she told me he had done so regularly every extra dollar of their earnings, although from motives of economy, the children spent Saturday and Sunday at home.

She said she felt sure a tonic would restore her appetite, and that the relief to her mind in knowing that she was free from disease would aid in curing her. So, carrying in her hand the valuable recipe for a tonic which might or might not be of use, she left me, promising to report herself in ten days.

At the end of that time she appeared, looking more dejected and forlorn than at her first visit, so much so that I was startled, and thought that I had made a mistake in my diagnosis as well as in my prognosis. With sobs, she informed me that a great misfortune had befallen them. This statement at once explained to me her appearance.

It was at the time when the first Jersey cows were imported into this country from England, and they were held at a great price. She told me that her husband, about six months before, had invested all the money they had in the savings bank in the purchase of one of those valuable creatures. On the day following the woman's visit to me, this precious cow had begun to be ailing. The trouble increasing, a veterinary surgeon had been consulted, and he told them if they would save the health and life of the cow, they must procure a faithful, intelligent man to take charge of her from morning to night. This sad event made it necessary for them to take for attendance on the cow the services of their best hired man, while the hiring of another man in his place would prevent their expending money for the charwoman who gave the good farmer's wife an occasional lift with the housework. She sobbingly ended her story by saying, "I must work even harder than a week ago—you must give me a stronger tonic."

The case looked so sad and hopeless that I sat silently thinking for a moment, when suddenly a bright thought sprang into my mind, and I said, "Why don't *you* nurse that cow and let the char-woman do your work in house, kitchen and dairy?"

As when a sunbeam bursts through heavy black clouds, so did a light flash over her face and into her eyes as I said these words; but in a moment it darkened down again as she began to think of all the objections to such a plan. But the idea was born; it grew; and with my vivid power of imagination, I overthrew all her objections one after another, until her conversation became really animated, and the plan appeared so plausible to both of us that the good woman went out of the office with no stronger tonic than hope and courage can bestow.

The whole affair was forgotten by me in the pressure of business and in listening to more stories of moral and physical misery. The summer with all its joy and beauty slipped away, and brilliant October brought a new flood of professional business and cares.

On one of these autumn days, a plump, sunburnt, cheerful-faced woman entered my sanctum, holding in one hand a huge bouquet of gorgeous dahlias, in the other a little jar of cream, and on her arm hung a small basket with a dozen fresh eggs.

"Don't you remember me?" she said. Of course I did not, although the voice was familiar.

"Well, I am Mrs. F——, whom you advised to nurse her cow."

I could hardly believe my eyes, even after her

repeated assurances of her identity with that miserable wreck of the May before. She gave me an animated description of what followed her leaving my office; of all her doubts and misgivings during her journey home as to what her husband would say to such a proposition for both a sick wife and a sick cow; and of how she had timidly introduced the subject to him by telling him that I was a queer doctor who did not believe much in medicine.

All this prepared him for the account of my plan to which contrary to his usual habit when women proposed anything, he listened gravely, and then said thoughtfully, "Well, my dear, we might try it." She at once called in the charwoman who had supplied her place that day and made arrangements with her to come daily.

The next morning she went to the field, with her rubber waterproof, her husband and the cow. The latter was tied to a stake, and my patient seated herself near on the waterproof (as I had suggested to her) while she watched the cow and petted and talked to her. The two took kindly to each other. One day's experiment proved that she could keep the cow in such subjection and quietness as the surgeon had ordered, plucking the fresh grass for her and feeding her as needed. All went well. Let me give a part of her story in her own words:

"My husband was satisfied with the first day's result, and made the few arrangements necessary. And you, Doctor, ought to have seen me as at sunrise, day after day, rain or shine, I walked to the pasture, with a big basket on my right arm full of my mending work; in my right hand a large white umbrella which my husband had bought for me; and in my left hand the rope to which my bossy was tied, and which, by the way, I did not need after a fortnight, she following me at my call and lying close beside me when not walking a few steps for a bite of the rich grass.

"My charwoman brought me all my meals and a pail of water for bossy. I soon had a keen appetite, almost impossible to satisfy; even the abundant provisions brought me and eagerly eaten with such good relish still seemed to leave a hollow unfilled; and after my walk home at sundown, I slept sweetly as I had not done for months.

"The cow got well; she is now followed by a strong, beautiful heifer six weeks old for which my husband has already had an offer of just half the money that he paid for the cow. And I—I feel strong, well and happy, can do all my work, and have taken none of the tonic. Besides all this, both my children are equally well, because when they came home for their weekly sojourn, they felt that they must spend Saturday and Sunday out in the field with poor mother who had no other diversion than the company of a cow. I really believe that their being with me out of doors has done them more good than they would have got from the change we had planned for vacation, a visit to relatives up in the mountains.

"So I thought I had better come and tell you of all the good you have done to our whole family by your excellent advice, although it seemed so queer to us all and, you may well believe, to our neighbors too."

"How many months did you do this?" I asked. "Was it not tedious to be all day in such dull company?"

"I did this same thing," she replied, "every day, from the time that I left you until the calf was three days old. And as for tediousness or loneliness, I

never felt it, for I have done a heap of sewing, old
and new, which had been accumulating during the
past year when I could not sew because I was so
miserable. Besides, I always took some reading
matter with me, especially on rainly days when I
could not use my needle. And as my bossy liked to
have me talk to her, I read aloud the Boston *Journal*
and our town paper. These she seemed to enjoy
as much as my chatting with her, even when it
came to the obituaries, death notices and quack
medicine advertisements.''

She assured me that she had not had a single
cold, although she had several times been drenched
by thunder showers that had overtaken her when
she was unprotected. She said also that she had
learned the great lesson of the folly of carrying self-
neglect and self-sacrifice to such an extent as to
bring trouble not only on one's self but also on all
the family.

If this little tale should be read by the family
described, I wish one of them would send name and
address (which I have no right to betray) to the
Woman's Journal.

CHAPTER XXIX

Question of escort in night practice—Expansion of Hospital by purchase of four houses on Warren (Warrenton) and Pleasant streets—Professional recognition slowly growing—She buys a horse and buggy—For first time in America the name of a woman is listed officially as specializing in surgery, Dr. Anita E. Tyng being appointed assistant surgeon—Resignation of the consulting surgeon (Dr. Samuel Cabot) and the attending surgeon (Dr. Horatio R. Storer), the latter the only man ever appointed on the attending staff—Dr. Cabot continues to act unofficially. (1863-1866.)

Boston had already extended itself in all directions into suburbs which still kept their dependence upon the center, but the means of communication remained primitive, as already described in the outpatient work which Dr. Zakrzewska established at the New England Female Medical College. And the isolation was most complete at night, the hour when the cry of suffering humanity rings most insistent.

So the Doctor was obliged to walk long distances to answer the calls of those patients who could not afford to send a carriage for her. Her familiar itinerary was from Roxbury to South Boston, to Dorchester, to West Roxbury, to Brookline, to Cambridge, and so around the circle. Temperatures of all degrees from below zero to up in the nineties were never allowed to discourage her.

As in New York, she was unmolested in her

travels. But she never took unnecessary risks. She always went with the messenger who called her, and who was generally a man. She writes:

If he could not accompany me on my return home in the night, and no accommodation for me was possible in the little apartment, I walked with the policeman, and waited at the end of the different beats for the next one to take me to his limits. I was well known among them, and was not at all surprised when a Franklin Park policeman recently accosted me as a friend well remembered in the night walks of former years.

The second year (1863-1864) of the existence of the New England Hospital, and of this phase of Dr. Zakrzewska's life, was marked by such increased growth of the institution that it was decided to purchase the former residence of Rev. Charles F. Barnard, No. 14 Warren Street (later Warrenton Street), to add to it three small dwelling houses in its rear (Nos. 13, 15, 17 Pleasant Street), and to connect them by a covered passage. The large house was described as "well built and convenient, airy and sunny, with a pleasant outlook on the Chapel yard and greenhouse" (p. 331). It seemed prudent to continue to lease two of the Pleasant Street houses to tenants but even so the increase in accommodations was marked.

The result of this expansion [says Dr. Zakrzewska] was enabling us not only to enlarge our work, but also to divide it into three distinct departments —Hospital for medical and surgical cases; Lying-in Department and Dispensary.

Had our work not been wanted [she continues], had our help not been needed, here and throughout the country, we should not have found so many patients asking for help and advice; nor have had so long a list of names of students waiting for a vacancy; nor have met with that response from the community which provided the means for carrying on our institution and enabling us to enlarge it.

Professional recognition was slowly growing, but even slight advances helped to lighten the almost overpowering mental strain of isolation. In such conditions, every slight word or act of indorsement, even though with reservations, was like a ray of hope that at last the dawn was breaking.

Referring to this period of professional loneliness, Dr. Zakrzewska writes in a letter to the editor in 1900:

In looking over these reports, there come back to me the many hours of fear and anxiety when I really was the only person who stood before the world responsible for our work in the Hospital.

The few brave men who supported my efforts were advanced in years and had a large practice; they were often not available for consultation when requested to come, or they came too late, when the danger was over or had ended in death.

My co-workers were young and inexperienced, looking up to me for wisdom and instruction, while the public in general watched with scrupulous zeal in order to stand ready for condemnation; this zeal being stimulated by the profession at large who wanted to find fault but did not dare to do so openly so long as the two or three professional men stood as a moral force behind me.

I remember how twice—once in New York and once in Boston—a man colleague told me I was foolish to take to heart the death of a patient which I saw coming as a natural event. Such consolations helped to uphold me.

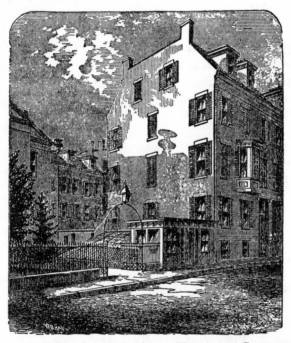

THE NEW ENGLAND HOSPITAL FOR WOMEN AND CHILDREN

This hospital was first housed in a dwelling house on Pleasant Street further along than the rear houses here seen (1862-1864). This was soon outgrown in favor of the one front and three rear houses here shown or indicated (1864-1872).

This professional loneliness must have been peculiarly poignant to her, since it contrasted so painfully with her recollections of the cordial fellowship which she had enjoyed with Dr. Schmidt and other leading medical men in Berlin.

An appeal issued by the directors in June, 1864, asking for funds for the purchase of the new buildings, contains a letter by Dr. Horatio R. Storer giving cogent reasons for the desirability of a special hospital for women and noting the particular conditions which made the New England Hospital peculiarly suitable for such purpose. This appeal was signed also by Drs. Walter Channing, C. G. Putnam, Henry I. Bowditch, and S. Cabot.

And about this time, Dr. Walter Channing writes to Dr. Zakrzewska:

I regret I had not made my visit later as I was too early to have the pleasure of seeing you. I was desirous to do so to express to you my entire satisfaction in regard to the operation you performed the evening before. It was a very difficult operation and was done under circumstances most unpromising of success. I do not think it could have been done better.

I write also to say that if at any time I can do anything to aid you in the performance of your important duties, I shall be always ready and happy to do so.

Very respectfully & truly yrs.,
WALTER CHANNING.

Boston, 39 Mt. Vernon Street,
June 2, 1864.

Remembering the financial difficulties of both Dr. Zakrzewska herself and this young, struggling enterprise of hers, one may well wonder at the second annual report (1863-1864) stating:

Half of our beds are always filled by patients who pay nothing, and the resident physician has the right to receive at half price those whose circumstances require this indulgence.

And realizing how the prices of the necessities of life must have advanced with the continuance of the Civil War, one is not surprised to read elsewhere:

We have been reluctantly forced to double our price of board, placing it at eight dollars per week.

The third year (1864-1865) of Dr. Zakrzewska's new life of freedom, of the longed-for opportunity for expressing her ideals, and of the attaining of sympathy and support for the forms of such expression, found the Hospital continuing its growth, like a manifestation incarnate of her soaring spirit.

This growth compelled the addition, with alterations, of the remaining two houses on Pleasant Street; and the housewarming which dedicated this further enlargement of its opportunities netted a precious six hundred dollars.

The Legislature of Massachusetts now voted the Hospital five thousand dollars for the purchase of the new site, on condition that a similar amount should be raised by subscription. And the Boston Lying-in Hospital Corporation increased its donation to one thousand dollars.

For the first time Dr. Zakrzewska, as attending

physician, presented to the board of directors a formal report which she thus introduces:

Before this year I had never considered that a lengthy report given by me was a necessity. Hitherto our Hospital had been so small and so simple in its management that it was easily understood by the directors and friends.

This is now changed: for after four years of exertion the Hospital has assumed from a simple ward the form of a complicated institution, with its resident and assistant physicians, its consulting, attending and assistant surgeons, and its attending and consulting physicians. Such an institution must necessarily attract the attention of the community; therefore inquiries are constantly being made as to how this institution is carried on. Nothing can answer all these different inquiries better than a minute report.

The most striking feature in its character is that it is designed to give to educated medical women an equal chance with their professional brethren to prove their capacity as hospital physicians, and to admit only female students to its wards—all other hospitals closing their doors to women as physicians and students.

The increase in the number of patients seeking daily advice soon gave a reputation to the institution, and the liberally inclined part of the community as well as of the profession began to look upon it as a test of female capability in professional life.

In this report Dr. Zakrzewska notes that the increase in the number of patients had become so great that Dr. Storer offered to share the dispensary work

with her and Dr. Sewall, taking two mornings a week
and making an even division of the time.

Referring to the raising of the question as to
whether it is not an inconsistency to have a gentleman in attendance, as it has always been stated that
the advantage of our Dispensary is that women can
be attended by physicians of their own sex, she
continues:

In reply to this, I can only say that there is a distinct notice given on the Dispensary cards as well
as in the waiting room, when Dr. Sewall or I, or when
Dr. Storer is in attendance, so that patients can have
their choice.

Interesting features of the annual meeting of the
Hospital for this year and of a levee which followed
it, were an address by Dr. Elizabeth Blackwell on
"The Culture Necessary for a Physician," and a
reading of some charming poems by Mrs. Julia
Ward Howe.

Hand in hand with the growth of Dr. Zakrzewska's
Hospital work progressed the growth of her private
practice. And the year 1865 was notable in that for
the first time she felt able to set up a carriage in
proper medical style. She thus describes this felici-
tous occurrence:

In 1865, I bought a second-hand buggy and a horse
for two reasons: one was that I could not accomplish
and do justice to my professional work by using public conveyances; the other, that it became a matter of
necessity to uphold the professional etiquette and
dignity of a woman physician on equality with men.
The effect was marvelous. Even the newspapers
took notice of the change.

At the Hospital further advance was made by the creation of the staff position of assistant surgeon, Dr. Anita E. Tyng[11] receiving the appointment. Thus for the first time in America the name of a woman is listed officially as specializing in surgery. This year was also notable for the addition of a second consulting physician, Dr. Henry I. Bowditch accepting election.

Dr. Henry I. Bowditch was always an earnest supporter of the education of women as physicians. He befriended Dr. Harriot K. Hunt and Dr. Nancy Clark, and then Dr. Zakrzewska herself when the latter came to Boston in 1856 soliciting money for opening the New York Infirmary. He remained the steadfast champion of medical women and continued as consulting physician to the New England Hospital until his death in 1892.

Dr. Zakrzewska realized the necessity of having on the consulting staff of the Hospital men physicians of the highest standing in the profession, such men serving as vouchers to the community for the medical women and their hospital.

But aside from this vital consideration she also believed that the best results follow when men and women work together. In this conviction she was ably supported by Dr. Henry I. Bowditch, who wrote to her at one time:

In regard to having a full corps of well-known experts, male and female, connected with the hospital, I still have no doubt. As I think there should be women physicians and surgeons in the other hospitals, so I think it important for the fullest success to have a joint corps at the women's hospital. Also,

I cannot but think it would be beneficial pecuniarily to all the hospitals if such arrangements were made.

Indeed, Dr. Bowditch was prepared to go even further, for in another letter he expresses the opinion that all three hospitals—the New England, the Massachusetts General and the City, should throw open their clinical instruction to both men and women. Though he was still conservative enough to advise that the clinics should be held at different hours for the two sexes.

In spite of the increasing support given the Hospital, its financial situation continued to cause anxiety. This was due to the need for paying for the four buildings purchased, to the increased expenses of the expanded institution, and to the disproportionately large amount of service given free or at only nominal rates.

The acuteness of the problem continued to increase and in the following year (1865-1866), although the mortgages had been paid off and the general debt reduced, the institution was unable to pay its current expenses.

To meet this situation a more conservative course was felt to be imperative, and it was decided, except in Maternity cases, temporarily to discontinue receiving any patients at a reduced rate except in the free beds, those which were endowed or definitely subscribed for.

Dr. Tyng continued as assistant surgeon, and her progress was so satisfactory that Dr. Storer writes:

During July and August, I shall be able to visit the Hospital only on Saturdays. During my absence, I wish Dr. Tyng, in accordance with her duties as assistant surgeon, to take my place as concerns both the Dispensary and the Surgical Wards. Of course, operations of any magnitude will be reserved until the days of my attendance.

In the midst of this peaceful development and orderly progress, clouds suddenly gathered and a tempest broke forth, with much lightning though with little thunder. This was followed by the clearing of the air characteristic of the passing of tempests in this latitude but, as sometimes happens, a marked change in the local landscape was the result.

The storm center seems to have been Dr. Storer. It is often difficult to explain misunderstandings and disagreements. Frequently, no one person seems to be definitely responsible. Electric conditions develop from many causes; minor frictions occur; an accident produces a spark; and an explosion follows.

Dr. Storer was connected with the Boston Lying-in Hospital before that institution suspended operation. He later became connected with the New England Hospital as already related, beginning then to specialize in the diseases of women. He worked assiduously in his department, and he accepted the letter of his obligations to the Hospital.

Subsequent history shows that this acceptance did not include the convictions of the spirit. Perhaps a psychoanalyst of to-day would trace the ultimate explosion to the "complex" resulting from conflict between this letter and spirit.

Or, perhaps (as suggested by the primary resignation of Dr. Cabot) it was a technical disagreement as to the limits of the respective domains of attending and consulting staffs—always a subject filled with delicate potentialities.

Or, perhaps, as claimed by Dr. Mary Putnam-Jacobi (*Woman's Work in America*, published in 1891), a most careful and conscientious observer with the true scientific spirit, it was because the successful outcome of Dr. Storer's operations fell too often below the boldness of his conceptions of them. (Dr. Sewall in this year says in her report as resident physician, "Only three deaths have occurred among our patients, and all these took place in the surgical wards after hazardous operations.")

Be the explanations—one or all—as they may, the first outward manifestation of the storm was the receipt by the board of directors of the following letter from Dr. Samuel Cabot, the early and long-tried friend of the Hospital who had from the beginning served as consulting surgeon:

Boston, June 2, 1866.
To the Board of Directors of the New England Hospital for Women and Children.

LADIES AND GENTLEMEN:

Feeling as I do the very warmest interest in the cause of female education and advancement, and believing as I do that the path of medicine and surgery, as well as every other path to honor and profit, should be open to women as well as to men—still, I feel constrained to send you my resignation of the office of Consulting Surgeon to the New England Hospital for Women and Children with which you have honored me, and to request you at your earliest convenience to accept it and to appoint my successor.

I cannot enter into any explanation of my reasons for this step, and can only ask you to believe that it is from no loss of interest in the cause you represent nor from any dissatisfaction with the ladies connected with the Hospital.

Very respectfully
Your obedient servant,
S. CABOT.

This resignation was accepted with great regret when after consultation it was found to be irrevocable.

This letter having brought the subject of consulting physicians to the attention of the directors, after much thought and inquiry the following preamble and resolutions were unanimously passed at their regular meeting on August 13:

WHEREAS, the confidence of the public in the management of the Hospital rests not only on the character of the medical attendants having its immediate charge but also on the high reputation of its Consulting Physicians and Surgeons, and

WHEREAS, we cannot allow them to be responsible for cases over which they have no control, therefore,

Resolved, that in all unusual or difficult cases in medicine, or where a capital operation in surgery is proposed, the Attending and Resident Physicians and Surgeons shall hold mutual consultation, and if any one of them shall have doubt as to the propriety of the proposed treatment or operation, one or more of the Consulting Physicians or Surgeons shall be invited to examine and decide upon the case.

Voted, that a copy of this resolve be sent to all medical officers connected with this Hospital

On September 10, the board of directors received from Dr. Storer a letter containing his resignation as attending surgeon, and on this letter the report comments, ''Its tenor left the Board no alternative but its acceptance, which was unanimously voted.''
The report then continues,

The Directors would, however, take this first public occasion to express their sense of the value of Dr. Storer's professional services and of the aid which he has rendered to the Treasury of the Hospital. Cheerfully bearing witness to his talent and active zeal in his profession, they offer him their best wishes for his future success.

Dr. Storer's letter containing his resignation was remarkable for its expressions of misunderstanding of the resolutions quoted above and for its misrepresentation of the general charitable policy of the Hospital. But it was chiefly remarkable for the needlessly offensive manner in which the writer revealed his personal disapproval of the study of medicine by women. Yet he condescended on second thought to qualify the latter statement, by adding:

For certain of the professional ladies whom I have met, I have personally the highest respect and esteem. Miss Zakrzewska, the beauty and purity of whose life as already published to the world I have long seen verified, may well challenge comparison in

practice with a certain percentage of my own sex.
Miss Tyng, now for two years my assistant in private practice, has such natural tastes and inclinations as fit her, more than I should have supposed
any woman could have become fitted, for the anxieties, the nervous strain and the shocks of the practice of surgery. And there are others not now
officially connected with the Hospital whose names
I would mention in terms of similar commendation.

Such are, however, at the best, but very exceptional cases, and I am driven back to my old belief,
the same that is entertained by the mass of mankind, that in claiming this especial work of medicine
women have mistaken their calling.

An interesting by-action of the writer was his con-
current sending of this extraordinary letter of resignation to the *Boston Medical and Surgical Journal*
for publication. This journal has already been
quoted as being opposed to the entrance of women
into the medical profession, and at this time and for
many subsequent years, it still continued its attitude
of opposition.

It is of a certain interest to note here that Dr.
Storer once more emerged in public to express his
sex-peculiar views regarding women physicians.
This was in San Francisco in 1871, when, at the annual meeting of the American Medical Association,
the question of women as delegates and members
was brought into the debate upon a related subject.
In the discussion, Dr. Storer spoke in opposition,
saying:

. . . We will grant that some exceptional women
are as interested in our science as ourselves; that

some of them have those peculiar qualities, that
especial temperament, that gives them not merely
a taste for anatomy and surgery but courage to
face the greatest dangers and anxiety in surgery;
and that there are some women who are able to go
out in inclement weather and brave the storm. We
may grant that women, some of them, may have had
peculiar means or favorable opportunities which
allow them to get this same education that men have.
We may grant, and grant it freely, that in some matters, women intellectually, are as completely mis-
tresses of their subject as we are masters of ours.

But, beyond this there is a point that is fundamental to the whole matter. . . and that is, this inherent quality in their sex, that uncertain equilib-
rium, that varying from month to month according
to the time of the month in each woman that unfits
her for taking these responsibilities of judgment
which are to control the question often of life and
death . . . women from month to month and week
to week vary up and down; they are not the same
one time that they are another.

To this, Dr. Gibbons of San Francisco replied:

If we are to judge of this proposition by the arguments of my friend from Boston, I think it would
prove conclusively the weakness of his side of the
question. . . . Is it not a fact that a large majority
of male practitioners fluctuate in their judgment, not
once a month with the moon, but every day with the
movement of the sun. . . .

Thus are some of the humorous pages of history
made.

However, this seems to have been the last time
that the subject of women as members was discussed

in that Association. In 1876, the first woman delegate (Dr. Sarah Hackett Stevenson, from the Illinois State Medical Society) was seated amid cheers. And in 1877, Dr. Henry I. Bowditch of Boston, in his presidential address, congratulated the Association that women physicians had been invited to assist in the deliberations.

CHAPTER XXX

*New England Hospital students granted the privilege of
visiting Massachusetts General Hospital—Letter from
University of Zurich stating women are admitted on
equal terms with men—Extracts from letter by Dr.
Zakrzewska to Dr. Sewall on vacation in Europe—
Sophia Jex-Blake collects endowment for four free
beds—Dr. Samuel Cabot resumes his position of consulting surgeon—Dr. Zakrzewska resigns from service at the Dispensary, being succeeded by Dr. Helen
Morton—Dr. Zakrzewska shares her service at the Hospital with Dr. Sewall who is appointed second attending physician—Land bought in Roxbury for new
Hospital buildings. (1866-1871.)*

RETURNING to our chronicle of 1866, the immediate
consequence of the foregoing tempest was that the
Hospital remained for the rest of the year without
either attending or consulting surgeon, the surgical
cases being treated by the assistant surgeon, with
the aid of Dr. Samuel Cabot (acting unofficially),
and by the attending and resident physicians—Dr.
Zakrzewska and Dr. Sewall.

The annual report of this year notes the receipt
of the first annual report of the Chicago Hospital
for Women and Children, founded by Dr. Mary Har-
ris Thompson.[12] This institution may be called the
oldest hospital daughter of Dr. Zakrzewska, a previous attempt by Dr. C. Annette Buckel[13] to open a
woman's hospital being obliged to yield in its infancy to the greater interests excited by the out-

break of the Civil War, Dr. Buckel giving her services to the Sanitary Commission.

An important event of the year 1866-1867 was the granting to the New England Hospital students of the privilege of visiting the Massachusetts General Hospital under certain restrictions.

The house at 14 Warren Street (changed to Warrenton Street the following year) was now used for the medical and surgical wards and for the offices of the assistant physician and the matron. Of the Pleasant Street houses, No. 13 was the house of the resident physician, No. 15 contained the Lying-in Wards, and No. 17 was given over to the Dispensary.

Once more the course of the Hospital becomes the uneventful one of quiet, continuous growth, and Dr. Zakrzewska as attending physician concludes her report for 1867-1868, as follows:

The Hospital and Dispensary are established; many physicians who a few years ago were opposed to female practitioners have not only become convinced of their professional capability, but several have been willing to give instruction and aid in any way possible.

The Massachusetts General Hospital has been admitting the few students whom we consider under our guidance and instruction. We have good reason to hope that this friendly relation will continue. Harvard College is still closed against us for theoretical instruction, but I do not think that free, liberal America will remain long behind another republic across the ocean—I mean Switzerland.

One of our students who made application to the University of Zurich, received the following reply:

Zurich, May 6, 1868.

DEAR MADAM:

I reply to your letter of March 17 which has just come to hand. I have the honor to inform you that there exists in this University no lawful impediment to the matriculation of female students, and that female students enjoy equal advantages with male students.

There is here full liberty, and every one may attend the lectures as long as he may desire. The majority of the students need from five to five and a half years' course before taking their degree.

In answer to other questions of yours, I send you some printed regulations of the University.

I am, with great esteem,

Yours,

BIERMER,

Professor and Dean of Medical Faculty.

The University of Zurich is known as one where only men of the highest standing in the profession are employed to instruct the students. Such names as Moleschott, Griesinger, Breslau, von Graefe, Horner, Mayer, and Billroth are familiar as authorities in the medical world, and these men have been, and still are, the most influential teachers there.

In Paris, also, women can have the same advantages as men. And in America the time is rapidly approaching when through the deeds and words of women the profession at large will be convinced of the wisdom of following the same course.

A breath of encouragement was at this time wafted from New York in a speech by Dr. Willard Parker, this noted physician saying at the opening of the Woman's College of the New York Infirmary, which took place on November 2, 1868:

Woman has always been a helpmeet to man and to a great extent is a co-worker with him, and as such in medicine, I bid her Godspeed. If it is charged that women who study medicine are sometimes unfit for practice, I would answer—so are many men. A doctor is born, not made, and is, naturally, found in both sexes.

In the summer of 1868, Dr. Lucy E. Sewall, who was continuing as resident physician, took a vacation of three months in England and France for recreation and study. In a letter to her, dated July 16, Dr. Zakrzewska writing from her new address, No. 1041 Washington Street, says:

I have hardly anything to report except that we have had intensely hot weather since you left, such as I have not experienced since the first year of my arrival in America. The thermometer stood at ninety-six degrees in our parlor in Roxbury, and we felt that we were cooling ourselves when we entered there. Yesterday, it was one hundred and three in the shade out of doors. . . . I envied you very much when I read how cool you were in Halifax and thereabouts. I am sure I would have been very glad to play the lady with you. You will now understand how pleasant it is to be away from business for a while.

Dr. Buckel will write you all about the Hospital. You need not worry in the least as all is going on well. At our last Hospital meeting Mrs. Cheney reported, ''I feared very much for the Hospital when

I saw how heartbroken the patients were after Dr. Sewall's departure. But a day after they sang the praises of Dr. Buckel as loudly as if they had never known Dr. Sewall."

To this report I added, "It is the old story although a very unsatisfactory one. Our places are filled just as soon as we leave them. And we all have to learn that lesson and feel comforted by it because it is thus that the world does not get off its hinges."

The day before yesterday, we had our house-warming—I missed you very much. . . . The heat has prevented me from going to Melrose [Dr. Sewall's home] so far; all we can do is to live and to fan. . . .

Within the two years just closing, the financial pressure began to be relieved and four free beds were established in the medical wards. About the same time, it was decided to charge at the Dispensary a fee of twenty-five cents to such of the patients as were able to pay this amount. The results exceeded all expectations. The patients acknowledged the fairness of the rule and yet the really poor were not shut out.

Nevertheless, it was at the close of this year, as already noted, that the Hospital was obliged to borrow money to meet its outstanding debts.

This was truly the darkest hour and it was followed by the dawn of which the proverb speaks. As the sunshine of help from the community grew stronger, it was possible steadily to extend the ministrations of the Hospital to the more dependent, so the report of 1898-1899 was able to state:

Nearly (if not quite) two thirds of all our work is given in charity . . . though we are slow to give charity indiscriminately but would have each one make some return, however small, for benefits received, thereby aiding her to keep her self-respect.

The treasurer's report for the year of 1868 notes the receipt of one thousand dollars which was collected by Miss Sophia Jex-Blake for supporting four free beds. Sophia Jex-Blake came to this country as a student of Dr. Sewall and was a resident student at the Hospital. She went later to the newly opened Woman's Medical College of the New York Infirmary, and still later she returned to Great Britain and became the leader in the struggle which attended the attempt to open to women the medical course at the University of Edinburgh—reference to which has been made by Dr. Zakrzewska in a previous chapter. The attempt failed and she went to Switzerland where the men students at the University of Berne seemed to find no difficulty in permitting women to study medicine with them.[14]

The year of 1869 was especially noteworthy for the burden which was lifted from Dr. Zakrzewska's mind by the official return of Dr. Samuel Cabot to the consulting staff of the Hospital, though ever since his formal resignation in June, 1866, he had continued to advise the women who, against almost insurmountable obstacles, were struggling to give the surgical help called for by the increasing numbers of their patients.

If one requires expert teaching and constant practice to learn to diagnosticate and prescribe for medical ailments, it is much more difficult for one to learn to diagnosticate and prescribe for surgical ailments, since a surgical prescription demands trained skill of the hands as well as of the brain. And opportunities for acquiring this trained skill of the hands are at the best very limited in number and very expensive in detail, while they also require a very exacting environment and an entourage trained to the highest degree. And they are, further, beset on all sides by dangers which are momentous and immediate as well as more remote.

It is a fine index of the essential quality of these earlier women that they were not daunted by the difficulties of the situation, and that the conservative spirit of the sex was not too much affrighted by the dangers which on every hand confronted them and their patients.

Under the necessities of the situation, a friendly surgeon of the eminence of Dr. Samuel Cabot was a veritable tower of strength. Well might Dr. Zakrzewska, with gratitude that failed of words to express itself, say year after year in her annual report as attending physician, "To Dr. Samuel Cabot, we are again indebted for advice and instruction in all the important surgical cases which have occurred during the year."

Dr. Anita E. Tyng who had spent her apprenticeship as assistant surgeon to the Hospital, had been obliged to resign her position there, but Dr. Zakrzewska and Dr. Sewall were ably assisted in this branch of practice by Dr. C. Annette Buckel who had been assistant physician for the past three years and who, having particular ability for surgery, de-

sired to specialize in that direction. They were now
aided also by Dr. Helen Morton [15] who had returned
from Paris and had become connected with the
Dispensary.

With the arrival of such capable assistants among
the younger women who had all been her students,
Dr. Zakrzewska felt justified in relinquishing some
of her arduous duties. And now her leading assistant, Dr. Lucy E. Sewall, resigned as resident physician (a position which she had held since 1863) and
was appointed second attending physician. She
thus divided the Hospital service with Dr. Zakrzewska, each being on duty every alternate three
months.

Dr. Zakrzewska continued to serve on the board
of directors as she had done since the beginning of
the Hospital, but the added freedom gained by being
released from work at the Dispensary and in being
able to share her Hospital duties, gave her greater
opportunity to elaborate and press forward her
plans for building a hospital which should be more
suitable for its purposes than any altered dwelling
houses could possibly be Writing of the successes
achieved by the Hospital and of the satisfactions
derived from its possession of the four houses in
Warrenton and Pleasant streets, she continues:

But after a few years, we found that even these
accommodations were becoming too small. Also, the
character of the neighborhood was changing from
private residences to retail trading stores, and it
was easy to foresee that the time was coming when
this location would be entirely unsuitable for the
sick.

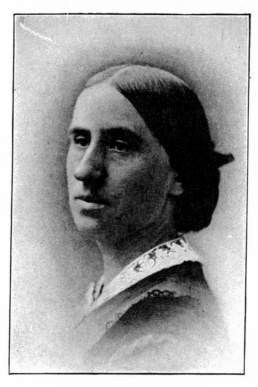

MARIE E. ZAKRZEWSKA, M.D.
(About 1870)

As it was neither my intention nor that of the Directors to carry on simply a charity, but rather to make this charity at the same time a school for educating women physicians on the European plan before mentioned and for the training of nurses for the benefit of the community, we felt that confidence in the value and need of our work had now been sufficiently established to warrant our erecting a building which would serve all these purposes and which in its arrangement might become a model hospital among the charitable institutions of the country.

About this time an especially interesting bequest of two thousand dollars was received by the Hospital from the estate of Mrs. Robert G. Shaw, the language of the bequest stating that the money was "to be used by Dr. Zakrzewska in aid of any Hospital or Infirmary for the poor and sick which may be under her superintendence in the City of Boston at the time of my decease."

The accumulating demand for a children's ward in the Hospital was so strongly felt this year that one of the physicians took into her own household for care and treatment a child patient whose case was particularly urgent.

This pressure for a children's ward was an additional factor in making Dr. Zakrzewska and her associates begin a still more definite campaign for the erection of new hospital buildings which should be especially suitable for the varied demands made upon them. Alterations in the streets and increase of business in that part of the city had enhanced the pecuniary value of land in that vicinity, so it was hoped that the sale of the present property would supply the money needed for building the new structure. It was planned to hold a Fair in December in order to raise the money needed for the purchase of the new land.

And one may judge of the courage required to attempt to carry such ambitions into execution when it is noted that the institution had just held its own financially, the year closing with the same amount of debt as that with which it began.

The Fair in December, 1870, justified the ardent hopes which breathed through every detail of its preparation and completion, and over twelve thousand dollars was realized.

A committee was immediately appointed to select a site, and after much investigation this committee recommended the purchase of an estate in Boston Highlands (now Roxbury), on Codman Avenue (now Dimock Street), between Shawmut Avenue (now Washington Street) and Amory Street (now Columbus Avenue).

With the formation of a building committee (which included all the medical officers) the new venture was definitely launched. The skies were lifting, favoring breezes prevailed, and the year closed with all running expenses met, all debts paid, and only the new building expenses to confront the treasurer—but it must be admitted that these were formidable enough, since they were on such an expanded scale.

The report of the resident physician, Dr. Buckel, for the year of 1870-1871 reflects so clearly her association with Dr. Zakrzewska and contains such interesting pictures of some phases of the social life of the period that a few paragraphs may be quoted, especially as some of them bear upon variations of a question which to-day is still perplexing our community, and which has at last reached legislators all over the United States in a concrete and radical form.[16]

CHAPTER XXXI

New Hospital buildings completed—Description of build-
ings and interior arrangements—Children's Depart-
ment established—First general Training School for
Nurses in America definitely organized under the
direction of Dr. Susan Dimock; one of the graduates
of its first class (Miss Linda A. Richards) later help-
ing to organize the training schools of the Bellevue
Hospital of New York, the Massachusetts General
Hospital and the Boston City Hospital—New England
Hospital medical women invited to attend some of
the Clinics at the Massachusetts Eye and Ear Infir-
mary—Though delayed by the epizoötic epidemic and
the great Boston Fire, the new Hospital buildings are
finally formally dedicated—First Hospital Social
Service in America organized in connection with the
Maternity. (1871-1872.)

ARCHITECTS, contractors, builders and workmen,
all took a personal interest in the plans of the new
Hospital buildings, and all made larger or smaller
contributions to the enterprise. With such a spirit
the structure grew apace, and even early in the
spring of 1872 a few patients were moved in—some
who especially needed the advantages of the good
air, sunlight and almost country quiet. But all the
patients were transferred before the end of September.

Dr. Zakrzewska writes:

At last we were able definitely to inaugurate the

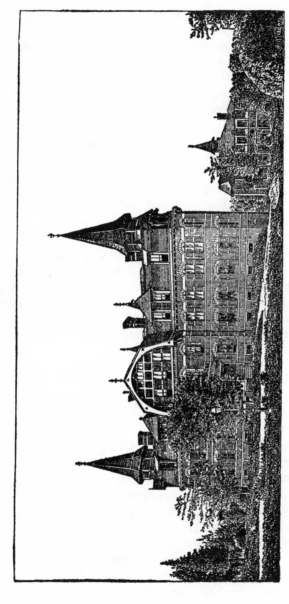

FIRST BUILDINGS OF THE NEW ENGLAND HOSPITAL FOR WOMEN AND CHILDREN, ERECTED 1872.

The main building was later named in honor of Dr. Marie E. Zakrzewska.

work for which we had been preparing during the previous ten years, namely, to dedicate our own building to our threefold object—a clinical school for women physicians and students; a training school for nurses; and a charity, especially for lying-in patients.

For this latter purpose a cottage, the "Maternity," was expressly built, while the medical and surgical patients occupied the main building. Some rooms were reserved for private patients, who paid fully for all they received. This latter department is very desirable in all hospitals, not only for the accommodation of travelers who may be taken ill while sojourning in a strange city, but also for those who when boarding cannot have the comforts of a home; while it likewise gives to our nurses a fair chance to be trained in attendance upon the sick of all classes and conditions of life.

Thus we had arrived nearly at the point at which we aimed, only that the means needed to carry on the work were not yet secured. We had no endowed wards and we had only a few endowed beds in the Maternity; therefore, we had no *Funds* but must depend upon the daily interest of the public to sustain the institution.

We now offered to the public not only the idea of reform, as we comprehended it, but also the visible embodiment of it in brick and mortar. Our vision had become materialized, and the work done within its walls spread the tidings of its success among the suffering and the needy.

The Drs. Blackwell, Ann Preston and myself stood no longer alone as the bearers of an idea—hundreds of young women had joined us. The path had been broken, and the profession had been obliged to yield, and to acknowledge the capacity of women as physicians. The argument that we few were exceptions to our sex has ceased; medical societies in different parts of the country admit women as members; hospitals begin to open their doors to women; men physicians endeavor to be polite towards their women colleagues; and their women colleagues certainly stand on a level with the men as regards good education.

And last but not least, society admits that it is highly respectable for a woman to become legally a physician, and offices and houses are now rented to medical women without fear of injury to the reputation of the neighborhood.

Thus, the world does move! But I am sorry to be forced to say that it is not the Republic of America which has given the proof that "science has no sex," only in so far as that it has furnished the largest number of women students. But it is the Republic of Switzerland which has verified this maxim. Our best women physicians have been educated there as well as in Germany and in France—for even these two latter countries have received women into their schools more on an equality with men than has America. And not less than six of our pupils from Boston are at present receiving the benefits which the opportunities for medical study and research offer in Vienna.

The United States still hesitate to allow to their women that education which they offer to their men. The result will be that talented women will go abroad and seek for the better medical education which Europe offers them and, returning with a higher standard of scientific learning, the men here will not only be obliged to acknowledge such women as their equals but they will be compelled to raise their own professional standards.

So far as my knowledge extends, this will be the first instance in history where through injustice to women, men themselves will be benefited.

The plan was to have one large brick building which should contain all the administrative offices of the Hospital as well as a small number of medical and surgical wards, the intention being to add later a wing entirely devoted to wards. But the Lying-in Department was to be housed in an entirely separate structure.[17]

Quite as essential and desired a policy of expansion, but one which had waited on the new building, was that of the training of nurses.

We have seen the importance which Dr. Zakrzewska attached to this question ever since her first hospital control, back in the days when she organized the practical details of the New York Infirmary. And we have noticed the recurring references to the difficulties which delayed the full development of her plans. But she continued to exercise her choice of individuals as best she might, and she endeavored to give the most thorough training for as long periods as she could make practicable.

Thus, writing of the opening of the New York Infirmary on May 1, 1857, she says:

We kept true to our promise to begin at once a system for training nurses although the time specified for that purpose was only six months.

She began with two nurses, one of whom remained for several years, becoming invaluable as head nurse. But she was evidently not satisfied with the success of this first system for, eight months later, she says:

We now began to make more positive plans for the education and training of nurses. The first two who presented herself and who after four months' superior women, one a German, the other an American, but neither was willing to give a longer time than four months. During this time they received no compensation except their keeping and one weekly lesson from me on the different branches of nursing.

After these left, it was again a German woman who presented herself and who after four months' training remained for several years. The second pupil nurse was sometimes of American, sometimes of Irish, descent and nothing remarkable.

When she removed to Boston and opened the hospital (Clinical Department) in connection with the New England Female Medical College, she there also attempted to carry into execution her conviction of the necessity for training nurses. But in Boston as in New York, women who wished to be nurses were unwilling to give time for training, and applications were few. Nevertheless, she succeeded in training six nurses.

When she founded the New England Hospital, the act of incorporation expressly stated that the training of nurses was one of the fundamental purposes of the new institution. And the first annual report says:

We offer peculiar advantages for training nurses for their important duties, under the superintendence of a physician.

In 1865, the term of six months is again emphasized. In 1868, it is stated that the Hospital offers to candidates board, washing and low wages after the first month of probation but it insists on an attendance of six months. And it adds that few women are willing to give the requisite time.

But now, at last, she found the desired opportunities opening before her. Aside from the influence of European experience, and especially that of Florence Nightingale and of the subsequent writings and utterances of the latter, undoubtedly the agitation which demonstrated the necessity for practical hospital training for the medical profession, had its effect in preparing the minds of both men and women for the realization of the fact that the same necessity existed for the training of members of the sister profession of nursing.

And the lectures to the New England Hospital nurses (which, under certain conditions, were open to women from outside) were steadily attracting women who were better and better prepared to study a profession rather than merely to practice an art.

But Dr. Zakrzewska had still found herself hampered by the narrow quarters which restricted her plans for nurses as well as for doctors, students and patients. She had been still further limited by the human impossibility of even her vigorous strength and endurance being equal to the superhuman demands developed by the successful materialization of her vision. And the training of assistants and colleagues required primarily a sacrifice of the time and energy already imperatively mortgaged.

Now, not only was the material building ready for

the Hospital, but also there was there incarnated the spirit of a common purpose, a spirit into the creation of which she had so literally incorporated her own self.

Hence, as the executive Head, she now had at her command not only a commodious structure but also director associates; a corps of younger physicians, trained theoretically and practically in both medicine and surgery; a supply of patients, always beyond the possibilities of accommodation; and a promising reservoir of aspiring women accepting and demanding training in nursing.

Immediately then, upon the opening of the new building, steps were taken for the expansion of the New England Hospital Training School for Nurses, and for its establishment as the "first general training school for nurses in America," organized and equipped to give general training along the then most modern practical lines, with a full corps of instructors in all branches, and with a hospital service that included medicine, surgery and obstetrics. This change was described in the annual reports of the year of 1871-1872, by Dr. Sewall in the medical report and by Mrs. Ednah D. Cheney as secretary of the corporation.

In addition to performing her duties at the Hospital and attending to her continually expanding private practice, Dr. Zakrzewska served on both the building committee and the furnishing committee for the new hospital. But while, among the staff of medical instructors, she delivered the greatest number of lectures, the details of organizing the new Training School for Nurses were delegated to Dr.

Susan Dimock,[18] who became resident physician in August when Dr. Buckel received leave of absence to go to Europe for rest and study.

During the first year of the new Training School for Nurses ten applicants were accepted after probation, two of these completing the year and being graduated. One of these first graduates was Miss Linda A. Richards who later helped to organize the Bellevue Hospital (New York) Training School, and still later that of the Massachusetts General Hospital and that of the Boston City Hospital.

During this eventful year, two important financial losses shadowed the high light thrown upon the foregoing successful working out of the far-reaching plans which Dr. Zakrzewska had for so long labored to develop. These were the loss of the annual donations of one thousand dollars each from the Legislature of Massachusetts and from the Boston Lying-in Hospital Corporation—the former having voted against any appropriation to private charities, and the latter having decided to reopen a hospital under its own control, in the overcrowded part of the city. Hence, it was again considered expedient to plan for a December Fair. But many days of doubt and hesitancy were to precede the opening of this Fair.

It had been planned to have the formal dedication of the new building take place at the time of the annual meeting of the board of directors. As this day approached it was found that it would be impossible for the friends of the enterprise to reach the new location of the Hospital. The great epizootic epidemic was prevailing; horses were everywhere succumbing to its virulence, and all the activities of the city which depended upon these necessary animals were almost paralyzed.

A fortnight later traffic was more controllable, but in the meantime every one had passed through the calamity of the great "Boston Fire," and Mrs. Cheney spoke the language of restraint when she said, "It was not easy to go to men whose warehouses and offices were in ashes, or to women who had lost their investments in insurance, and ask them to give us the money that we needed to complete our building and to carry on our work."

Under such circumstances it redounded to the credit of both the hospital workers and the community of Boston that the formal opening of the Hospital was not longer delayed, that the Fair was held in December as planned, and that it resulted in a sum exceeding five thousand dollars.

It is important to note that it was also during this year that the first Hospital Social Service work in America was begun. This was organized in connection with the Maternity—Dr. Dimock, Miss Lilian Freeman Clarke, Miss Elizabeth Greene and Miss Mary Parkman coöperating.

And this year was further marked by the opening to the New England Hospital medical women of some of the clinics of the Massachusetts Eye and Ear Infirmary.

CHAPTER XXXII

Dr. Zakrzewska goes to Europe for her first vacation in fifteen years—Letter to Dr. Sewall from Switzerland —Dr. Helen Morton is appointed third attending physician to the Hospital (in charge of the Maternity) —Tragic death of Dr. Dimock—For the first time the Hospital has a woman on the staff as attending surgeon, Dr. C. Annette Buckel being thus appointed— The Hospital is represented by exhibits at the Centennial International Exhibition, the plans and elevations of the new buildings receiving an award— Mrs. Cheney writes from Europe of the interest taken over there in the Hospital, and the looking toward it from England, Scotland and Germany for encouragement and help. (1872-1877.)

THE addition of a third attending physician at the Hospital (Dr. Helen Morton who took charge of the Maternity) and the continued increase in the number of younger doctors still further relieved Dr. Zakrzewska and enabled her in the summer of 1874 to go to Europe for a long-deferred but much-needed vacation. The constantly growing demands in both Hospital and private practice upon her professional skill, and in the community at large upon the many gifts of her broad personality, became at last a breaking strain upon the vitality so grievously depleted by the pioneer work of these first fifteen years in Boston.

Midway in this resting time (August 19, 1874) she writes to Dr. Sewall:

My vacation is half over, and just now I am enjoying a short stay in the queerest little old town and ditto hotel between the Bernese and Wallis Alps. Such a rest from work and care I have never had in all my life! My head is getting steady once more and, although I am not yet as quiet in my upper regions as I ought to be if I want again to work hard, I am certainly very, very much better than I was at the time I started from Boston. I have had only slight headaches, never sufficient to lie down, and I am much less confused, in spite of the three languages around me.

We travel in a very leisurely way, different from tourists, for we stop and sojourn wherever the fancy happens to take us. In this way, we have seen a great deal of Switzerland, and have enjoyed the usual places of interest as well as the out-of-the-way places such as where we are now.

I have so often thought of you and of what you are doing and have followed you in your summer's work. I suppose just now you are away on your vacation. What I am most curious about is whether you succeeded in selling your present house, and whether you bought that nice one on Boylston Street. It would be such a beautiful situation that I wish I could find you settled there on my return

. . . However beautiful all around me is here, I long for home and my friends. My home in Roxbury is, after all, the most desirable spot for me, and the few but true and kind friends I have made in America are far dearer to me than all I could possibly find here in Europe.

After this journey, I shall be more positive in my love for my American home than I ever was before. The very freedom one breathes in the air there is refreshing and stimulating compared with the air of servility, destitution and depravity which an observing person sees everywhere here. How Americans can prefer to live over here is to me incomprehensible.

. . . Miss Sprague has hardly yet got over the effects of her seasickness, and in four and a half weeks we shall undertake the journey again. We hope to be in Boston by the 2d of October ready for work. Please tell Dr. Dimock of the very pleasant call I had from Professor Meyer and that he gave me his picture to bring home to her. I hope she is doing well and can wait for my help till October.

I have little time for letter writing, as I am too tired to write at night and, besides, my eyes have given out. For the past few weeks, I can neither read nor thread a needle by candlelight, and often even by daylight everything is in a blur.

But tell Dr. Dimock I am thinking a good deal about her and hope she will not work too hard, so that she can bear the winter's responsibility and have her turn here in Europe next summer.

In the spring of 1875 as planned in this letter, Dr. Dimock who was acting as attending surgeon, in addition to her duties as resident and attending physician, obtained leave of absence and sailed for Europe to undertake additional surgical study, but she had the misfortune to be a passenger on the steamer *Schiller* which was wrecked on the Scilly rocks early in May. Her loss was felt keenly, not only because of the charm of her personality but also because she had been a representative of the hopes of the Hospital for a woman who would be broadly fitted and trained to serve as attending surgeon. The name of Codman Avenue, a street which ran through the

hospital grounds, was later in her memory changed
to Dimock Street.

Later in the year, Dr. C. Annette Buckel, newly
returned from two years of study of surgery in
Vienna and Paris, was regularly appointed as attending surgeon. This was an important event for
both Dr. Zakrzewska and the New England Hospital
because now for the first time since 1866 an attending surgeon reappears in the annual report as a
member of the staff. And this event was especially
noteworthy because for the first time the name of
such staff member was that of a woman.

Although Dr. Buckel did not retain her position
beyond that first year (removing to California on
account of ill health), yet her appointment seemed
to end the surgical vicissitudes of the Hospital.
Never since then has there been a time when the
position of attending surgeon has been omitted from
the annual report. And never has there been lacking a qualified woman to carry on this work. Indeed, it soon became necessary to appoint a second
attending surgeon, then a third, and then a fourth.
And to these have been added from time to time
one or more assistant surgeons. And with this con-
quest of the surgical field was surmounted the last
difficulty in filling staff positions with qualified
women.

Dr. Zakrzewska's vacation in Europe had lasted
only a few months, though it should have been a
year or even more. Recuperation from brain and
nerve fatigue is much slower than from muscle fatigue, a lesson we all learn only by bitter experience.
Her wonderful physique once more drew upon its

vital reserves and responded to the spur of her call to duty, and she returned to work with apparently renewed vigor.

Fortunate it was that she was able to resume the helm at the Hospital in this eventful year of 1875, following Dr. Dimock's untimely loss and the necessity which had arisen for Dr. Sewall's taking a long vacation.

For eight months it must have seemed to her almost like a reversion to earlier days. But there was the incomparable difference that Dr. Helen Morton now took entire charge of the Maternity, having developed at the Paris Maternité, according to Dr. Zakrzewska, "unusual skill and special fitness for difficult and surgical obstetric cases." And later Dr. Elizabeth C. Keller [19] came from Philadelphia to serve as resident physician, she succeeding Dr. Buckel the following year as attending surgeon and occupying this latter position for many years.

Writing of this time to Dr. Sewall in Europe, Dr. Zakrzewska says:

I think we shall all like Dr. Keller. And it is a very good thing to have a fresh and new element come into Boston, as we tend to renew ourselves too much from and through ourselves.

In the autumn the return of Dr. Sewall and the arrival of Dr. Keller once more released Dr. Zakrzewska and permitted her to resume the wide relations which she held outside the Hospital. She was constantly called upon to express her views on the questions regarding women, questions which were more and more appealing to the increasing number of medical women as well as to the community at large. She responded to these calls both in speech and in writing.

Realizing how much the interior arrangements of the new buildings were due to the advice and planning of the medical women, it was a great satisfaction to her that in the following year (1876) at the Centennial International Exhibition held in Philadelphia, the plans and elevations of the new buildings of the Hospital, together with photographic interior views of the wards, etc., were exhibited in the names of the architects, Messrs. Cummings and Sears, and received an award for "well-studied design securing economy of service, good distribution of various parts for ventilation and cheerful accommodation."

Also that at the Centennial, a history and description of the Hospital was displayed in the Massachusetts Exhibit in the Department of Education and Science, and in the Woman's Department.

In 1877 Mrs. Cheney writes to her from Europe:

All that I have seen and heard of the work of medical education for women in Europe has deepened my sense of the importance of our Hospital work. It is known in every circle that I have entered where there is any interest in woman's progress, and in England and Scotland and Germany they look to us for encouragement and help.

There was a great improvement in the financial condition of the Hospital during this year (1877); and among other items in the treasurer's report occurs the following which speaks for itself as an in-

teresting commentary on the policy developed by
Dr. Zakrzewska in the Hospital, as we have already
seen it developed in her private practice:

The executors of the late Mr. Augustus Hemenway
devoted to us the liberal sum of fifteen thousand
dollars from the sum left by his will to charities
not promoting pauperism.

CHAPTER XXXIII

Dr. Zakrzewska and the other pioneer medical women find a new foe in an increasing number of medical women who are poorly educated and otherwise unfitted—She addresses the New England Women's Club on the "Medical Education of Women"—Unsuccessful attempt to persuade the New York medical colleges for men to accept scholarships for properly prepared women—Opening of the Woman's Medical College of the New York Infirmary—Further movement to open for women one of the great medical colleges for men —Dr. Zakrzewska's comment on this proposition, with special reference to Harvard—The New England Hospital Medical Society—Action taken by Harvard University in 1879 on the question of admitting women students of medicine. (1865-1880.)

THE pioneer medical women (Drs. Elizabeth Blackwell, Marie E. Zakrzewska, Emily Blackwell, and Ann Preston) to whose successful struggles are due, for the first time in the history of the world, the real opening of the profession of medicine to women equally with men, had no sooner begun to take breath after their first stupendous battle, than they found themselves confronted with a new foe.

This foe was within the ranks of their own sex, and its development threatened an undermining campaign which seemed almost more disheartening than the militant one from which they had just emerged. This new foe was the increasing number

of women doctors, poorly educated and otherwise unfitted, who began to appear all over the country.

Because the evil was so insidious and was cloaked
by the necessity and the desire for competent medical women which had been demonstrated and
aroused throughout the country, it was most difficult
to meet.

The Philadelphia women met it by striving even
harder to bring up the standard of the Woman's
Medical College and to expand the field of the
Woman's Hospital.

The more eastern women, meaning those of New
York and Boston at the New York Infirmary and the
New England Hospital, met it by trying to establish a standard and by trying to educate both the
profession and the laity to accept nothing lower
than such a standard.

To these women, the simplest as well as the wisest
procedure seemed to be an attempt to persuade some
of the best of the already existing medical colleges
to accept a number of properly prepared women
students.

To this end, it was proposed to inform the community at large of the situation (the subject being
really as vital to the laity as to the profession, since
doctors can practice only through patients), and to
collect a large sum of money which might serve to
endow a number of scholarships for women in some
of the leading medical colleges of the country.

As early as 1865, a fund of fifty thousand dollars
had been collected for this purpose, but all the colleges refused to accept women as students, even under such auspices. As the situation was particularly

pressing in New York, the Drs. Blackwell were then so urged to take the next best step (the best having proved to be beyond their power) that they consented to add a college to their Hospital. And thus, in 1868, was opened the Woman's Medical College of the New York Infirmary.

This college set a standard which was never surpassed by any of the colleges for men. But one small college insisting on a high standard could not compete numerically with rivals offering apparently equally desirable advantages and with standards easier of attainment. So the campaign continued!

In 1877, Dr. Zakrzewska being invited to address a body of leading nonmedical women (the *New England Women's Club*), brought this problem to them for conference. She said in part:

At first the study of medicine appealed only to earnest women who felt a decided calling in that direction and who really thought to benefit their sex by acquiring information which would serve others through their advice. Very few, if any, of these first women combined with this idea that of vindicating their rights as Women.

It was no easy matter at that time to become a doctor of medicine. The great obstacle, want of schools, sifted out the weaker elements; and those who succeeded in obtaining teachers and in being admitted into the colleges then open to women were, as you will conceive, possessed of unusual perseverance and firmness of purpose.

But soon there appeared among the candidates for medical honors another purpose, the desire to gain these honors through simple study during a prescribed course without any laborious work.

The first suggestion of this came through some men physicians who, becoming alarmed at the movement and perhaps conscious of their own mediocrity, felt instinctively that there was danger of their being overshadowed by women, who are by nature sympathetic and more caretaking in sickness.

These raised the cry of "competition." Many women believed the cry was caused by alarm at a real danger, that of the women making money of which the men desired to retain a monopoly, and they imagined that a new field especially adapted to their sex was opened—one in which, with a short course of technical study, they could more easily and rapidly than in other vocations open to them acquire a name and abundant means of support, if not a fortune.

The laity then awoke to this movement, and that portion of them whose head and heart were interested in the "rights" of women began to establish schools and colleges for the purpose of educating women physicians. And in a short time such institutions sprang up in several cities.

After years of struggle and gradual improvement, the Philadelphia medical school for women (Woman's Medical College of Pennsylvania) has acquired deserved value when judged by the standard of men's schools.

And the Drs. Blackwell were later compelled to open a medical school in connection with the Infirmary (Woman's Medical College of the New York Infirmary), in order to stem the flood of inferior physicians which was pouring forth, especially in New York, from schools which were far below mediocrity.

Thus to-day, of all the institutions open to women for medical study, only these two and the University of Michigan even try to reach the standard of medical education necessary to compare favorably with that of the men.

I say, *try* to reach that standard. By this, I do not wish to imply that the teachers and professors in these schools are always less capable than those in the male schools. No, the fault is in the students themselves, and so it will be for some time to come. Here, allow me to state why this is so and has been so for many years.

As I have said before, in the beginning of this movement women who persisted in the study needed uncommon perseverance and firmness of purpose. For the acquisition of these qualities, a certain amount of educational training and concentration of thought and will were requisite.

At present, such uncommon perseverance and determination are not so indispensable. It is now very easy to become a physician. If the higher and better medical schools will not admit women, the lower and the less strict are willing to do so. Socially, the woman doctor is respected and in some circles even lionized and ranked far above the teacher; therefore, two great obstacles are removed.

All that a young woman needs is the permission of her parents and the means of support while studying. Both of these are now more easily attained, since her social position is likely to improve rather than to decline as it formerly did.

Also, the number of schools and colleges has increased and they require a certain number of students in order to exist. Hence arises a rivalry among these institutions, and instead of elevating their standard to make good women physicians some lower it in order to fill their classes.

The effect of this sort of education is that the

country is rapidly being swarmed with women physicians of very doubtful ability as regards either preparatory or medical education.

At the same time, the need for well-educated women physicians becomes the more pressing, as is manifested by the ready employment they all find, though there is no chance for discrimination between the real and the sham article denoted by the sign "Doctor."

Hence, in many places the movement is beginning to be again viewed with distrust by communities which have again and again been disappointed when hoping to find scientific education and practical talent among the women practitioners who were offering their services to the public.

In a word, the so hopefully sown good seeds are in danger of being suffocated by the still more thickly sown weeds.

It is against this danger that I feel I must warn you. And I wish to call upon every educated woman within my reach to aid in destroying this evil.

Every individual can assist in this great reform; first, by trying to get clear ideas on the subject in order to discriminate and to judge; and then, to assist in every possible way those who are striving to elevate the educational and moral standards in medicine.

Some highly educated physicians have said to me, "We see no reason why a woman should not study medicine. If she can become wiser and her practice better, then we *must* have her, for our aim is the *better;* if she cannot do this or cannot even do as well as men, she will work her own destruction in her endeavors."

Women should be willing to accept this or any

other just test, but in order that the experiment shall be a fair one, they must have preparation and education and subsequent opportunity, equal to those given to the men.

The continued refusal of the larger medical colleges to admit women, under endowed scholarships or in any other way, led to the development of a more ambitious plan, this being. the idea of purchasing direct partnership rights for women in one of these colleges.

But this required the raising of a much larger amount of money. In this direction there was made in 1880, a tentative proposition which involved the formation of a central organization with State branches, for the purpose of collecting such large fund and then arranging for its wise use.

The statement was made:

All sectional jealousy must be laid aside. Neither Boston, nor New York, nor Philadelphia must insist upon being the seat of the medical school. If Harvard would accept our conditions, it might possibly present certain guaranties which would give it a first claim in spite of the greater clinical advantages of the larger cities. But the College of Physicians and Surgeons in New York, and the University of Pennsylvania and the Jefferson Medical College in Philadelphia, must also be considered.

In making the large united effort which seems desirable in order to take an advance step in the education of American medical women, we must secure that great impersonal enthusiasm for a cause which shall be far above purely sectional pride.

When this proposition was submitted to Dr. Zakrzewska for consideration, she replied as follows:

In order to answer your letter of July 27 carefully, I must dictate it because an affliction of my eyes prevents me from writing myself. My health is pretty good, and the very best of oculists declare my eyes to be good, still the least use of them for reading or writing gives me so much pain that it prevents sleep and unfits me for thinking business.

The proposed crusade against the mediocre medical colleges has been recognized as necessary, not only by myself but by all the physicians connected with the New England Hospital. Perhaps the fact that we are working independently of all colleges has given us a more impartial opinion in regard to these schools. We have, I think, the best chance to judge of the results which these schools produce because we receive the young graduates for the practical training.

Perhaps you will remember that I wrote you four or five years ago how discouraged I felt about the manner in which the different female medical colleges educated and inspired their students and how derogatory the result was to the whole movement.

. . . The proposition to raise one hundred thousand dollars for the purpose of securing admission into a male college could be carried out quite easily, comparatively speaking. In Massachusetts alone, it could be done if Harvard would consent to add a small class of women to its medical department. The fact is that when a few years ago the New England Female Medical College here in Boston was broken up, there came unofficially from some one in authority in Harvard the proposition to take it, provided the public would endow it with one hundred thousand dollars.

In such case, the female students would be educated in their own building which was two miles from the building for men. However, the examinations of the women students for entrance into the college were to be the same as those for the men, and the instruction was to be given by the same professors—in fact, Harvard Medical College repeated for the benefit of women alone.

I did not favor such an arrangement but actually discouraged it, because it seemed to me disastrous to the whole spirit of woman's work in the profession.

I feared that after trial professors of acknowledged rank might declare that teaching six or twelve women was not satisfactory, although it might recompense them financially, and that therefore they would either give it up entirely or leave the instruction to the younger teachers.

I could not advocate a school exposed to such a risk because if the instructors of Harvard Medical College should become more prominent in the woman's branch while the professors took the lead in the men's branch, it would give both the students and the public the impression that the women were of secondary importance.

Another attempt to open Harvard to women has been made within a year or two by a lady who proposed to give ten thousand dollars towards a fund which would pay for a class of women in the medical department.

Many discussions concerning this proposition came up in the different meetings which were held in consequence of this offer. The result was always the same, namely, divided opinions—entirely against the admission of women at all; against their admission with men; and against the formation of a small class of women alone.

The only encouraging part of the discussion was that those who were entirely opposed to women's studying were a very small minority, while those against coeducation were less firm in their opposition. Besides, I am perfectly sure that if the younger men who now hold positions as instructors at the College could cast their votes and could influence the Directors' decisions, there would be more chance for the admission of women.

The New England Female Medical College was absorbed into the Boston University Medical Department, an inferior school and a homeopathic one, which has no other merit than that it admits men and women on equal terms to all its advantages; therefore, it does not injure the movement for women any more than it does the profession at large.

Our Hospital does as good a work as any hospital carried on by medical men. We have now two good women surgeons, and all kinds of operations are performed as a matter of course, without being considered extraordinary occurrences, as was formerly the case.

I can safely say that the Hospital work, which we enlarge as fast as our means will permit, has become a power throughout the country, and the Hospital in all its appointments is more or less acknowledged as the most complete of any under the control of women physicians.

This is as good a picture of the situation here in Boston as I am able to give you. If we had gained admission into the Massachusetts Medical Society, we would stand on equal footing with the best part of the profession.

In some of the smaller towns of Massachusetts, young women physicians have been admitted into the county societies, and these being a part of the Massachusetts Medical Society have thus opened a discussion which will eventually lead to the admission of women into the parent society, which is another step towards getting admission into Harvard Medical Department.

On October 1, Dr. Smith who was graduated in Zurich will take the position of resident physician with us, and we shall try to persuade other educated women to study in Zurich so that we can fill this post with such graduates and thus overcome little by little the opposition to coeducation.

Can you not see from these statements that the raising of money alone will not suffice to bring about the equally good education of women and men? To be sure, if I had a sum large enough to endow a medical college, I could bring about coeducation and thorough scientific study by getting men of the best talent from both Europe and America, but one hundred thousand dollars would be only a drop in the bucket towards such an enterprise.

Meanwhile, we have another bright prospect in the admission of women to the University of Michigan, at Ann Arbor. Although the medical students are not in the same classrooms, yet the lectures and the opportunities for women are precisely the same as those for men.

The lectures are given in separate lecture rooms, except in chemistry. The students of both sexes work together in the laboratory and are present at most of the clinics. The work in the dissecting-rooms is quite separate, and occasionally the women are not present at some special operations.

The movement for educating women as physicians

has become so widespread that I think it impossible to work for the elevation of the standard of their medical education in any other way than by having the leading women of each state keep in view as their final aim the opening on the basis of coeducation of the best medical colleges.

The number of persons now interested in the whole movement is so great and the labor to raise money to maintain the institutions, even such as they are, has required so much nerve and strength that even to hint at their abolition or their absorption in male colleges might have a detrimental effect in dispiriting the public who, taken as a whole, are not yet settled on the question of coeducation.

The American people, both men and women, have to work out the different problems of advancing their interests without having them favored or opposed by a fixed social class whose prerogative it is to exercise a controlling influence on any standard set up.

The medical education of women must now take its chance for growth like all the other questions of woman's rights, yes, even of men's rights, politically speaking. We are, with all the rest, passing through the phase of crystallization, and only the merit or the capacity of the individual can act to bring about a good and lasting effect.

We must grow at present by every one of us doing her utmost best from day to day; and if the principle is a correct one that it is within women to exercise their faculties according to their inclinations the same as men do, it cannot be overthrown. I do not want to give you the impression that I wish to be pessimistically indolent; on the contrary, I want you to understand that I include in that "utmost best" criticism as well as denunciation of the imperfect or mediocre and readiness for any crusade for the better, for the higher, and for the perfect ideal.

The physicians connected with our Hospital have formed a Society,[20] and have framed a constitution which admits to membership both men and women. So far we have only women members, and there are only a very few in the society who are not connected with the Hospital, because we mean to be as careful and as stringent as possible.

I wish I could visit you this winter and talk all these matters over, as I really need a rest of a year, not because I am sick but because I feel that I may be, as the strain upon my nerve power has been so intense for thirty years that relaxation is needed if I want to end my life in usefulness.

For the present, I cannot do anything more than to plan for such a recreation, but when the moment comes to carry out this plan, I shall write to you in order to make arrangements for us to meet in a way which will give us time and comfort.

The ten thousand dollars referred to in the above letter was offered in 1878 by Miss Marian Hovey toward the new building which Harvard was about to erect, she making the condition that women should be admitted as students.

According to Dr. Chadwick, the Corporation referred the communication to the Board of Overseers who in turn referred it to a committee consisting of President Eliot, Alexander Agassiz, Dr. Morrill Wyman, J. Elliot Cabot and Dr. LeBaron Russell. In 1879, majority and minority reports were presented, the latter by Dr. Russell alone.

The majority report recommended acceptance of the trust offered by Miss Hovey, and presented an outline of conditions which were thought to be desirable to govern the admission of women students.

It further stated that of twenty-one members of the Medical Faculty who expressed their views in writing, six were in favor, with restrictions; three were in favor of making the experiment but had strong doubts of its expediency or success; five were opposed, but were willing to try the experiment under certain conditions; seven were strongly opposed. Thus, fourteen were at least willing to try the experiment conditionally, while seven were unconditionally opposed.

The minority report opposed acceptance of the trust and advised that the medical women should establish their own school, modeling it upon the Harvard school.

A vote of the Board of Overseers was immediately taken upon the adoption of the majority report, the vote standing seven to nine. It was then voted to reconsider the motion two weeks later.

Meantime, a meeting of the Medical Faculty was held and the admission of women was negatived in *two* resolutions, one by a vote of thirteen to five and one of fourteen to four.

Following this action of the Medical Faculty, the Board of Overseers at their next meeting voted (17 to 7):

That the Board of Overseers find themselves unable to advise the President and Fellows to accept the generous proposal of Miss Hovey.

It then voted (16 to 10) for the following motion which was proposed by the President:

That in the opinion of the Board of Overseers it is expedient that, under suitable restrictions, women be instructed by Harvard University in its Medical School.

CHAPTER XXXIV

Opening of the Massachusetts Medical Society to women—Letter on the subject to Dr. Zakrzewska from Dr. Henry I. Bowditch—She declines to present herself for examination for admission, having already twice prepared herself and been refused examination because she was a woman—Dr. Zakrzewska's reply to the question "whether to enforce obedience medicines should be administered to refractory prisoners in reformatories and prisons." (1879-1884.)

It was in this same year of 1879, however, that the cause was heartened by the beginning of the tardy capitulation of the Massachusetts Medical Society, the council of which following in the wake of ten or a dozen of the other State medical societies, finally voted to admit women to membership on equal terms with men.

This society differs from most of the other State medical societies in that its membership does not consist, as does theirs, of delegates from the constituent county societies. Members join the Massachusetts Medical Society as individuals, and it aims to include all reputable members of the profession.

It had previously refused to recognize homeopathic and eclectic physicians, holding these latter as "irregular" practitioners of medicine, even though their diplomas were legalized by the same authority as that which had legalized those of its own members.

Its refusal to admit women to membership showed its intention to classify women also as "irregulars," even women who had received their diplomas as regular classmates of men who were acceptable.

The *Boston Medical and Surgical Journal*, of October 9, 1879, expressed itself characteristically in an editorial:

We regret to be obliged to announce that at a meeting of the councilors, held on October 1, it was voted to admit women to the Massachusetts Medical Society. . . . Enshrouded in her mantle of science, woman is supposed to be endowed with power to descend from that high pedestal upon which we men have always placed her, and to mingle with us unscathed in scenes from which her own modesty and the esteem of the other sex has hitherto protected her.

The editor seems to have forgotten that women had long mingled in those "scenes" as patients and as nurses; it was only as physicians that they were being "protected" from them.

However, the "protectors" were loath to discontinue their gallant services and, following the protest of the Suffolk District branch of the State Society, the Council rescinded its vote, thus relegating the medical women to their pedestals.

But the Society continued in a state of unrest, friends of the admission of women gaining in strength and their opponents losing proportionately, though by-issues were also injected. Eventually, the inevitable was foreseen; the question remained only as to the form which it would take.

The handwriting on the wall was visible when in
1883 the Pennsylvania State Medical Society (!)
sent a woman (Dr. Alice Bennett) as delegate to the
annual meeting of the Massachusetts Medical Society. She was accepted officially, and she sat
through the proceedings, and nothing happened.

At the annual meeting of the following year, 1884,
the By-Laws were amended so as to permit of the
admission of women on an equality with men; and
then that storm center cleared.

An editorial in the *Boston Medical and Surgical
Journal*, June 19, 1884, loyally accepts the action
of the Society but it cannot forbear a little over-
flow of emotion in the following words:

. . . We believe that women in this particular
community are already aided and abetted in too
many foolish fads and fancies. There is too much
bad piano playing and too little good cooking and
sewing taught them. . . .

[Many years later, the editor of this book met
the editor of the *Boston Medical and Surgical Journal*, and in discussing the subject of medical women,
she is glad to say he admitted that he had "read-
justed" his "point of view."]

Dr. Henry I. Bowditch viewed the action of the
Society in a different light, as is shown in a letter
written to Dr. Zakrzewska after the details of this
advanced step had been arranged and the women
were preparing to take the Society examinations:

Boston, June 15, 1884.

MY DEAR DOCTOR:

I thank you for the letter received yesterday. The result was entirely unexpected, and I can only thank God and take courage for the future days and for opportunities to fight for simple right and justice.

For I assure you that all through these years since I have advocated the examination of women by the Massachusetts Medical Society, I have myself stood upon the eternal foundations of justice to every human being. My old anti-slavery warfare and its principles, with the experience gained in that fight against prejudice, have been of immense support to me.

. . . I have always consulted with honorable, educated women, in spite of all By-Laws. At first I believe some of the bigots thought I ought to be punished. But I cared not a farthing for the dark hints of discipline impending, feeling sure as I did that light would appear the next day and that with the element of Time and simple justice on my side, Right would certainly prevail.

But as I now look back upon this final victory, and mark the various tyrannical rulings of our presidents and the stupid arguments urged by the opponents and their victories up to the present hour, with their final and, if not graceful, certainly good-natured and boorish submission to the fact of being in a hopeless minority themselves—I marvel, and, as I said above, take courage for any future fight for the True and Right.

Some of the arguments by our opponents in the council were so weak that I think they injured their own cause.

For example, Dr. —— says: "Our fathers never meant that women should be members, and how

absurd it would be for us to admit them! They
are different from men and cannot properly become
our associates in medicine, etc.''

Dr. ——, with becoming pompousness of manner
after duly twirling his gray mustaches, said: ''I
am not in favor of women being admitted because
they have never done anything original.''

Dr. Wyman suggested that the names of Mrs.
Somerville, Mesdames Boivin and Lachapelle in
France and Jacobi in America certainly proved
that women were capable of high intellectual work.

''*I* do not admit that they are exceptions,'' replied
Dr. ——.

I was fool enough to forget to ask what original
work had ever been done by members of the Massachusetts Medical Society, and especially by the
speaker himself. That would have floored our an-
tagonist very effectually.

But let us not think of the past, but prepare ourselves for the future that is opening so brightly
before us.

I am glad that the young students are preparing
for the race. As for yourself, I do not wonder at
your decision. You do as I think I should do.

Your ''pioneer'' race and energy will always command the respect of the community and of the professional men who know you and who are not bigots
to a ''Code.''

I remain
Very truly yours,
HENRY I. BOWDITCH.

The reference at the end of Dr. Bowditch's letter
is to the course upon which Dr. Zakrzewska had decided, after mature consideration of the question of
taking the examination for admission to the Massa-

chusetts Medical Society. She expresses this decision and the reasons for reaching it, as follows:

The Massachusetts Medical Society has within the last three months decided to admit women. The perseverance of women in the practice of medicine and surgery, their professional competency, the increase in their numbers, and the impossibility of ignoring them any longer, have led to the result that physicians of this Society acknowledge women in daily practice and have thus broken the rule which binds them to friendliness and coöperation with members only. Necessity, not acknowledgment of the principle of the right of woman to practice, has finally conquered, and the Massachusetts Medical Society is willing to allow women to present themselves for examination with the view of admission.

On the other hand, the regular women practitioners have found it necessary to protect themselves against being confounded with charlatans of every description, and have formed themselves into a society which adopts the name of the Hospital in which their practice started and now centers.

Besides the physicians living in Boston, a few scattered over the New England States are members of this society. Thus a union of reliable women practitioners is begun and promises to be of interest and usefulness. If a union with the Massachusetts Medical Society can be effected by them, it would be beneficial to both and, no doubt, to the profession at large.

The obstacles to such a union consist chiefly in the fact that any one wishing to become a member of the Massachusetts Medical Society has to present himself or herself for examination before a number of censors chosen by the Society, and at

present in the Suffolk District Medical Society consisting of five of its youngest members, who have
to examine the candidate in Obstetrics, Histology,
Anatomy, Physiology, Pathology, Materia Medica,
and Chemistry, that is to say, precisely in those
branches for proficiency in which the candidate has
received a diploma years ago.

It is well known that wisdom and experience acquired in practice push into the background text-
book knowledge, and that most physicians after
ten years of practicing life have gained a great deal
of knowledge which is not in the textbooks and
have forgotten a great deal which is.

It is therefore a question whether the amount of
benefit gained by admission into the Massachusetts
Medical Society is worth the waste of time necessary for reading and studying books which we have
long laid aside and simply use occasionally for reference.

To young beginners, I would advise the seeking of
this privilege but as for myself, I feel constrained to
make the following statement:

When I came to Boston in 1859, eight years after
my graduation in Berlin as *accoucheuse* and three
years after graduation as physician from the Western Reserve Medical College of Cleveland, Ohio,
and having been regularly employed in teaching
classes and private pupils in medicine, consequently,
in the full life of a student—I made application for
examination to be admitted into this society and
was refused.

Again, five years later, that is, in 1864, I made
the same application, and was not so decidedly refused. Thinking there was a possibility of my
being admitted, I set myself to work reviewing some
of my studies in order to prepare myself to meet

the high dignitaries in the shape of the young men members and censors of that venerable society; but after several months of discussion, I again received a refusal.

This last refusal I met with the declaration that "when the time comes for women to be received into this Society—and I know it will come before I have passed out of this existence—this venerable Society cannot have me as a candidate for examination but must give me an honorary membership if it wants me at all."

To-day, its condescending proposal for my examination for admission has been made, and I am only a little more than fifty years old. But after twenty-six and one-half years of practice (that is, nearly at the end of my career), my only personal interest in this affair is that I am happy that the younger women can have the benefit of an association which is very desirable for all beginners, and most desirable in assisting women to gain the position for which they strive.

I have done my part, and I feel satisfied with the results achieved. I have aided the women of this country by word and deed, by example and sacrifice, and I am willing to retire, leaving them the field in which to sow and to reap where I have helped to plow, associated as I have been with the pioneer women of the medical profession.

It was about this time that, at one of the meetings of the New England Hospital Society, that body was asked to give an opinion upon a question which had arisen in reformatories and prisons, that is, "whether medicines which cause anesthesia, emesis or prostration should ever be administered to refractory prisoners to enforce obedience through their action.''

A unanimous ''No'' expressed the instinctive feeling among all members present of the absolute wrong in the use of such remedies to compel obedience. The discussion of this subject was continued to a subsequent meeting, and Dr. Zakrzewska was requested to prepare a written statement of her views upon this point. She writes:

I. From the medical standpoint, the administering of a pharmaceutical preparation for any other purpose than to aid in the restoration of health is malpractice. An emetic or an opiate might be easily given to a culprit who is in perfect health but who refuses obedience to the prison regulations; this could be done by deceiving the offender. But the administration of ether or chloroform would meet with opposition for the overcoming of which an application of force would be needed, which would be as much in the nature of corporal punishment as would the use of the rod.

No physician could sanction the use of remedies for any other than their legitimate purpose and must refuse such demand from the prison superintendent or warden.

II. From the legal standpoint, no prison official has a right to order for the purpose of enforcing obedience the administration of powerful medicines to a healthy individual, thus rendering her ill for hours or days, shocking a system otherwise in harmonious action, and thereby also possibly producing bodily injuries, internally or externally, which may after the release of the prisoner easily lead to a complaint in a court of law, a complaint which could well be sustained.

III. From the moral standpoint, the deception which is necessary either by disguising the medicine in some usual beverage or by false statement, pretending a necessity for some medical remedy, such as hypodermic injection of morphine, would at once awaken distrust of the whole official management and would thereby destroy the very principle upon which all prisons should be conducted, that is, the reformation of those intrusted to their care.

If we once admit that medical remedies can be used by the physician under the orders of the superintendent in order to enforce obedience or as punishment, where shall we stop? The physician and the superintendent can become in time accomplices in such practices as may lead to even fatal results, for such officials have almost absolute power in these institutions which are subjected to only occasional examinations by State committees.

CHAPTER XXXV

Association for the Advancement of the Medical Education of Women—Coeducation or segregation—Dr. Zakrzewska leads another attempt to persuade Harvard to admit women to its Medical School (1881-1882)—Failure takes from Harvard final opportunity to be first great medical school to admit women on equal terms with men, this honor passing to the Johns Hopkins in 1890—Massachusetts Legislature directs that a woman physician be appointed in each State Hospital for insane patients—Dr. Zakrzewska takes a vacation in Europe—Letter to Mrs. Cheney and others—The New England Hospital requires all resident students to possess the degree of M.D., and changes their status to that of internes—The Hospital establishes District Nursing in its out-practice—Letter from Dr. Zakrzewska to Dr. Sewall who is on vacation in Europe—Dr. Zakrzewska compares earlier and later women medical students. (1879-1886.)

As a further move in the campaign for opening the larger colleges to women, there was formed the Association for the Advancement of the Medical Education of Women. This association had a membership of medical and lay men and women from different parts of the country, and Dr. Mary Putnam-Jacobi was its president for many years.

Mary Putnam, one of the earlier students of the New England Hospital, and a graduate of the Woman's Medical College of Pennsylvania, was the first woman to be admitted to the *École de Médicine* of the University of Paris, from which she was graduated in 1871. Later, she married the noted Dr. Abraham Jacobi of New York, becoming herself one of the most brilliant members of the profession in America. It will be remembered that in 1876 she was awarded the Boylston Prize of Harvard University, the identity, and consequently the sex, of the competitors for this honor remaining unknown to the judges until after the verdict was rendered.

The above association not only carried on an educational campaign, but for several years it assisted the Woman's Medical College of the New York Infirmary by paying part of the faculty's salaries and by helping to enlarge the College and the Hospital.

Although continuing the support of such separate women's colleges as maintained their high standards, the leading medical women and the well-informed men and women of the laity still realized that these were (and in the nature of things, must be) only the lamps which are kept trimmed and burning as additional guaranties that the sacred fire shall never be extinguished.

The main temples and the central fires are found in the large medical schools which were then monopolized by men, and the struggle must continue till these temples and fires are acknowledged to be human possessions, and hence open to women equally with men. Only then will it be possible to maintain the high standards to which both men and women physicians should be held, and which are required for the safety of the communities in which they practice.

Hence the persistence in seeking entrance to the

men's colleges. Not because they are colleges of men, no, but because this is still so largely a man's world, with men so often holding possession of the Best.

And it is the Best in their chosen profession that medical women have always been seeking—the best teaching; the best laboratories; the best libraries; the best facilities for training all their faculties; the best clinical opportunities; the best hospital advantages.

Aside from valid reasons for not segregating women students and physicians as a separate group, all the conditions enumerated above have an economic basis. They require money as well as scholarship—and scholarship itself requires money or it will starve—and no community can afford to duplicate the expensive plants required for proper medical education, so as to have twin institutions in which medical men and medical women shall be separated.

The answer and the advice always given by the men who happen to be in possession of these legacies of the ages and of the race—for the great medical schools owe their continued existence to the money and the help of the women as well as of the men who have gone before—has always been, "No, we cannot let you enter our colleges. Build your own colleges!"

It is as though the great universities of the country should decline to admit any but their local students, telling all others to build their own universities. Do Harvard and Yale Universities refuse students outside of Cambridge and New Haven, or even outside of Massachusetts and Connecticut, saying, "No, you cannot enter here. Build Harvards and Yales for yourselves!"

Illogical as has been this advice, women have been driven by desperation to attempt to follow it for both academic and professional studies. A certain measure of success has been attained in the academic institutions, owing to the large number of women desiring education of the kind there given. In the field of medicine, as well as in that of the other technical professions, the situation is far different. The number of women desiring such education is small when compared with the number of those desiring academic education and, as has been well-established, the expense for properly equipping professional schools is much greater proportionately as the number of students is smaller.

So, in 1881, another attempt was made toward persuading Harvard to admit women to its medical department. The New England Hospital Medical Society, through a committee of which Dr. Emma L. Call was chairman, had asked the assistance of the leading medical colleges for women toward making a combined appeal for the opening to women of the medical school of Harvard University. And in September, the following communication was formally presented:

To the President and Overseers of Harvard University:

GENTLEMEN:

Would you accept the sum of fifty thousand dollars for the purpose of providing such medical education for women as will entitle them to the degree of Doctor of Medicine from your University?

This sum to be held by you in trust, and the interest of the same to be added to the principal, until the income of the fund can be used for such medical education of women.

If such an arrangement cannot be made within ten years, the fund to be returned to the donors.

This letter was signed by Drs. Zakrzewska, Emily Blackwell, Lucy E. Sewall, Helen Morton, Mary Putnam-Jacobi, Elizabeth M. Cushier, Alice Bennett, and Eliza M. Mosher—the Woman's Medical College of Pennsylvania feeling unable to join, but writing:

. . . While we are in hearty sympathy with the object of your efforts, it seems impracticable at present to offer any active coöperation.

After a delay of several months, the following reply was received from Harvard University:

Treasurer's Office, Harvard College,
No. 70 Water Street, Boston, May 2, 1882.

DEAR MADAM:
I have the honor to enclose a copy of a vote recently passed by the President and Fellows of Harvard College, in relation to the Medical Education of Women in Harvard University.

Yours very respectfully,
E. W. HOOPER, Secy.

Marie E. Zakrzewska, M.D.

(COPY)

At a meeting of the President and Fellows of Harvard College in Boston, April 24, 1882.

Upon the question of accepting the proposal contained in the communication received by this Board on September 26, 1881, from Marie E. Zakrzewska, M.D., and others, in relation to the medical education of women in Harvard University.

Voted, that while the President and Fellows of Harvard College recognize the importance of thorough medical education for women they do not find themselves able to accept the proposal contained in the communication above referred to.

A true copy of Record
Attest: E. W. Hooper, Secy.

To Marie E. Zakrzewska, M.D.,
for herself and others.

Thus did Harvard lose its last opportunity to become the leader in the opening to women of the great medical schools of America, its misfortune in this respect being due to what appears to have been a certain indecisiveness.

It showed the perception and the conviction of the justice of the women's claim as early as 1850, or even 1847 (away back when Oliver Wendell Holmes was dean of the medical school), and it seems to have had, then and afterwards (1879), the desire for performance but it appears to have failed in resolution, and so it was at the mercy of minor cross-purposes.

At any rate, the result of its vacillation was that eight years later the honor was taken by the Johns Hopkins University of Baltimore.

Meantime, Dr. Zakrzewska had in 1881 spent another vacation in Europe, and this time she particularly inquired into the progress of medical women in England. On May 28, she writes:

DEAR FRIENDS:

I shall mail this letter eventually to Mrs. Cheney, but I intend it to be of the same interest to Miss Lucy Goddard and Miss Peabody.

After a very rough passage, we arrived in London on the 17th of May at 4 A. M. My companions desired to begin sight-seeing at once and so, as is customary, we proceeded to Westminster Abbey. You all know how little appreciation I have for Fame; but whenever I go to places like this Abbey, Fame presents to me another aspect. It is entirely impersonal—names are of no consequence, but the reasons why these landmarks of civilization are placed there for the beholder are of intense interest.

You all know that every shade of greatness is here represented in the monuments to men. There are some to women also, but only because these women happened to be queens or wives of royalty, though a few have been erected to high-stationed philanthropists. In no other capacity could I discover the name of a woman.

Query: Before long, will there be erected a monument to a woman physician? We find the names of men physicians here, for no other reason than that they were eminent in their profession. Will there ever be a monument to the first woman physician because she was the leader of the movement; because she had the energy, will and talent, as well as the education, which would make her worthy of imitation; and because she is a landmark of the era marked by women's freeing themselves from the bondage of prejudice and from the belief that they are the lower being when compared with men?

These are the speculations which follow me wherever I go and wherever I find the monumental display to and for talent. I did not find Mrs. Somerville's name on even a tablet in the Abbey. Why is it that women do not start a movement for placing one there and in other significant places?

We need such landmarks of civilization not because those who died have lived for fame, no, but because the now-living, as well as those who will live long afterward, need encouragement for utilizing their capabilities, and monuments of this sort suggest to them the possibility of their so doing. The person who is covered by a monument is of no consequence, but the fact that a "woman" can work and make an impression upon civilization needs to be made known and to be remembered.

Apropos, the word "woman" reminds me of the custom of speaking here in London. I have not heard a single time the word "lady" used as we use it in America. The Queen is spoken of as "a good woman," the Princess Louise as "a sickly woman," Mrs. Somerville as "an eminent woman," the Duchess of Blank as "a fashionable woman." Nowhere do we hear a dressed-up cook or chambermaid mentioned in the streets as "that lady there," but as "the woman in the velvet gown," etc. I wish some of our prominent women in America would make a crusade against the habit of applying the word "lady" to every woman under every condition.

But now I must speak to you of what interests us most of all, namely, the work of the medical women in London. There is no doubt but that the position here of the woman physician is, professionally and legally, a far better one than with us in the United States. By the indomitable will and energy of Dr. Sophia Jex-Blake, the women who study medicine have been placed fundamentally on the same level with men. The method of study, theoretical and practical, is precisely that of the men.

And although the Royal Free Hospital has only one hundred and fifty beds for the medical school of women, while the medical school for men of St. Bartholomew's Hospital has six hundred and that of St. Thomas' Hospital has one thousand, five hundred, that makes no difference in the mode of study nor in the amount of knowledge which the woman student can acquire. One reason is that the number of women is only about forty while at either of the other hospitals, the number of men runs as high as seven hundred. Besides, I am told that women are more ready to gain knowledge through dispensary practice, which is entirely outside of the hospitals.

There is, however, one branch which is very much neglected, both theoretically and in clinical instruction, Dr. Charles Drysdale being my authority for the statement that this neglect is just as great in the men's course, namely, the instruction in higher midwifery and obstetrics as taught in France and Germany. He assures me that if there are English men of eminence in this branch, they have laid the foundation by going to Germany to study. Alas, these opportunities are not open as freely to English medical women.

Dr. Drysdale, as well as some of the most prominent women practitioners here, expressed the wish that Boston or some other large city in the United States which has a hospital for women would so develop this particular branch as to induce the educated medical women of England to go thither in order to perfect themselves therein. The opinion of those who express such a wish is that money would gladly be paid to its full value for such opportunity for study.

Such an opening for the English student would react very beneficially upon our American medical student, for there is no doubt but that the English medical women and students have in every respect a higher average education than we have. And the standards of education and civilization can best be raised through international intercourse.

We now have in Boston decidedly good women surgeons and the beginning of a good department in surgery. This is of momentous importance for the reason that surgical work tells best both in the profession and among the laity. We also have in Boston excellent women obstetricians who do a great deal of obstetric surgery, but who give instruction to only the few privileged students of our Hospital.

This branch could easily be enlarged and developed by our Hospital Staff if through larger means, greater opportunity for practice could be afforded them, and thus make it worth her while for the attending physician to give more thorough instruction both to our own students and to students from abroad. By saying making it worth her while, I mean allowing her compensation for time and labor.

On the whole, we must begin to think of compensating our staff of women physicians. Now that the woman physician is an accepted fact in America, it becomes our duty to compensate those who have spent time and money in study (and especially those who have gone to the continent of Europe) for the labor which they expend upon the students not able to follow such a course.

After introducing the woman into society as a physician, we must now take the next step, namely, see that those who follow are well-educated; and, therefore, we must utilize the knowledge of the former by giving her the chance to spread it among the new disciples. In other words, every physician with a good education who comes to us must be well paid, so that her time and strength will belong to our patients and to the students of the Hospital. And if other students who are not inmates of the Hospital wish to avail themselves of our instruction, they must be made to pay for it, whether this instruction be given by the resident physician or by one of the attending physicians.

This has been my view for some years, and I am now very much confirmed in it through talk with the friends of medical education here, where I see most clearly that work without money value set upon it is not expected nor is it considered to be of the first class.

The students here pay £80 for the theoretical instruction and £40 for the hospital instruction, besides paying for their board outside of school and hospital, for they do not reside in either. Our institutions in the United States would not permit such a rate, nor do I wish to suggest it, but I wish that the friends of the movement for the medical education of women would come forward, as have those here in England, and provide us with means so that we can afford to pay an ample salary to our physicians, or at least to our resident physician, and thus secure her services for some years to come for the benefit of all concerned.

The English generosity in this respect seems marvelous to me. For instance, the Royal Free Hospital would not connect the medical school for women with its work, saying that it had not room for them. The governors of the hospital were asked how much money was needed, and the enormous sum of £5,000 was set for a limited number of years, namely, five. At the expiration of this time, a similar sum, or even more, or perhaps nothing at all, might be needed. In a very short time the sum was raised, the money being used to build another wing to give room to the women for study.

Out of the funds of the school, towards which the student contributes £40 for three years' study, a large sum is paid to the physician who gives the instruction in this hospital. The funds of the school are raised by private subscription, and the fees charged to the students, although high, do not suffice to pay for the instruction given. In so far as the fees do not suffice, the situation is similar to that in our American colleges and schools; it differs in that the instructors are fully paid for the time and knowledge given to the students. The result is a higher education in medicine and a higher grade of individual physician than in the United States.

In the two branches, surgery and the medical treatment of general diseases, the woman student has now in London ample opportunity. Plenty of material is provided, not only by the Royal Free Hospital but also by the New Hospital for Women, as well as by the dispensary attached to the latter. The latter hospital is carried on precisely as is our New England Hospital for Women and Children except that it has no maternity department. It admits patients for as little as four shillings a week but only a few are entirely free.

The attending physicians are all married women of high social position, mothers and housekeepers and quite rich. It is thought by the English women that these prominent women should work in order to live down the prejudice, which seems to be very strong, that if women study or do anything they will

cease to be willing to become mothers and housekeepers. This explained why in the medical school
the "Mrs." was always introduced to me before the
"Miss" was spoken of.

I think this is all I have to communicate to you
about the work which lies so near to our hearts, and
as my London visit closes to-morrow I think I shall
have nothing more to add, but shall see what the
women in Germany are doing.

But I may tell you that I attended a small, public,
woman suffrage meeting held to consider Mr. Hugh
Mason's proposition in the House of Commons to
give the franchise to women. The meeting was
a rather select one. The audience was admitted only
by cards, which, to be sure, any one could procure
beforehand, but which forms more or less of a hindrance to attendance.

The speakers were all women and in favor of the
measure. They were seven in number and each
spoke for about ten minutes. They were fluent, elo-
quent, concise and modest. Their dignity was su-
perb. There was a great deal of applause, and happiness over what had been gained was expressed in
many a face. But the whole affair lacked vitality,
enthusiasm, and breadth of feeling and fellowship.
And, compared with even our smallest meetings, no
matter whether held by women alone or by both men
and women, it made me homesick for Boston—for
America!

Should you see any of our Doctors (for instance,
Dr. Morton), ask them whether they care to read
this epistle. Perhaps Dr. Smith will decipher it and
read it at one of their meetings. But let Miss G.
have it first, and tell me in a few words what you
think of it, and how you are doing and whether
your health and that of our friends is good and

strong and ready to carry our work a little farther on.

I am getting rested, and while my two companions are going sightseeing I am writing this. If you want to recommend our lodgings here, do so. They are in every respect desirable and recommendable. Be sure to give my love to all inquiring friends—Miss Farnham, Miss Cary, Mrs. Boardman, and a number of others whom I have no more paper to mention.

Faithfully yours,

M. E. Zakrzewska.

In 1880-1881, the New England Hospital took the important step of requiring all resident students to be the possessors of the degree of M.D., and of changing their status to that of *internes*.

In 1881, plans were made for having a nurse always on duty at the Dispensary to respond to calls in the out-practice, but these plans did not materialize until 1883, the New England Hospital thereby becoming the leader in establishing the service of District Nursing. This form of service has since additionally expanded, under other auspices, into an organization which on a large scale renders valuable assistance to patients at their homes.

The year 1884 was marked by the setting up of another milestone along the upward path of the medical woman, this being that the Massachusetts Legislature not only permitted but directed the appointment of medical women in the State Hospitals for insane patients.

In February, 1886, Dr. Zakrzewska writes to Dr. Sewall, who was then in Europe:

. . . In ten weeks from to-day, I shall start on my Western tour, and I suppose you will start by that time for the United States.

My health is very good. I am better than I have been for thirty years and a great deal better than when I went to Europe five years ago. Nevertheless, I look forward to a five months' vacation with a great deal of pleasure and feel sure that it will add years of health to my life.

The Hospital work goes on well. I suppose Dr. Call informs you of the different legacies we have received. Even if they are not yet handed over to the treasurer, we can now be sure of the solidity of the institution as far as money is concerned.

Now comes the professional standard and the question as to whether in the course of time women as physicians will prove themselves to be organizers and creators or simply handmaids. So far we cannot boast of much originality among our corps of women. However, we can feel sure that all the women physicians of the Hospital are above the average of the men physicians. Genius, after all, is rare.

Apropos of sister Rosalie. It occurred to me that you with your usual generosity might think of her and bring with you some present for her. Now I honestly beg of you not to do any such thing, because the poor thing is sick and tired of all the bric-a-brac and vases which she has received, in spite of our not sending out invitations.

Last Sunday morning when I called, she showed me a whole closet full of stuff which she had packed away in the attic because it is beyond human thought and possibility to place these things and take care of them in her little house. When I told her in consolation that she might use these things as presents

again in the course of time, she replied in her usual
way, "No, I shall never inflict them on people. If
I make presents, I shall give flatirons."

My nephew Herman is engaged to be married to a
young German-American lady who visited me for
a week. She is handsome, an accomplished singer
and pianist, a good housekeeper, and a sensible
woman. We are very happy about his choice and
feel grateful to her that she selected him.

On the 22d at twelve o'clock, I shall give a great
lunch party to the students and doctors. About fifty
people will come, I hope. The snowdrops in Washington Street are in bloom since the 9th.

In line with her questioning in this letter of the
achievements of medical women of the then present
date, is her estimate of the quality of the women
students of the later times as compared with those
of the earlier days. She writes:

I am frequently asked whether the quality of medical students among women is not much better now
than formerly. This question is a very subtle one
to reply to justly. There is no doubt but that the
educational standard among all youths, female and
male, has been greatly raised; that accomplishments
are not so universally considered all the education
that girls need; that the increase of colleges for
women alone, as well as the coeducational institutions, has promoted a thoroughness of training
which was unknown fifty years ago in the schooling
of young girls; and that all these advantages have
promoted thought and earnestness of purpose in deciding upon a profession.

But that the student of either sex is in consequence
of this education of a better quality and promising

more marked ability, especially in the medical profession, by no means follows.

In the early decade of this movement, the woman who entered upon professional study had to possess qualities which no school, college or university can bestow. Originality, perseverance, persistency, self-abnegation, industry in study, and a certain amount of practical knowledge, as well as perception of human nature and social conditions, were absolutely necessary for each and every woman student in order to succeed even in going through the medical colleges then at their disposal, to say nothing of later attempts to enter into general practice.

The help then offered by professional men was not based at all upon the principle of right nor on the suitability of the woman to become a physician. No, it was offered only by such men as stood head and shoulders above their colleagues in the professions. They were men who could afford to make enemies in and out of professional circles and who could afford to be pleased with a talented "exceptional woman"; intellectually to pet her, as it were; to teach her; to indulge her; yes, to speak in high terms of her and compare her with historic women of the past, feeling even proud that they had discovered such an exception to womankind.

They seemed entirely unaware that the woman student perceived their delusions but nurtured in the depth of her heart the conviction, "What I am able to do now, hundreds, yes, thousands, will be able to accomplish after me." Meanwhile, the women were grateful for all favors, advantages and teachings, utilizing them but industriously aiming higher and higher so as to gain all that could be gained through the qualities enumerated above.

Such a schooling trained the women far better

than all the colleges do now, in spite of their excellence; on the other hand, the complaints of the women students of to-day as to the disadvantages yet to be overcome are greater than they were then. Yet at this present time, almost every chance exists for women if it is in them, to become original investigators, workers and practitioners.

CHAPTER XXXVI

*Twenty-fifth anniversary of the New England Hospital—
Drs. Zakrzewska, Sewall and Morton resign as attend-
ing physicians and are appointed advisory physicians
—Presentation to the Hospital of portrait of Dr.
Zakrzewska painted by Miss Ellen E. Hale—Address
by Dr. Zakrzewska before the Moral Education Asso-
ciation—Her reply to the question "Should Women
Study Medicine?"—Her opinion on "What's in a
Name?" (1887-1890.)*

In 1887, the Hospital celebrated its twenty-fifth anniversary, a pleasant feature of the event being the
presentation to the Hospital by the graduates and internes of the portrait of Dr. Zakrzewska. This was
painted by Miss Ellen E. Hale and was placed in the
directors' parlor. The occasion was also marked
by the resignation of all three of the attending physicians, Drs. Zakrzewska, Sewall, and Morton. So
many qualified women were becoming available for
hospital service and were asking for opportunities,
that these three women who had borne the burden
and heat of the earlier years felt they could now
stand aside and make room for their younger sisters.

Their resignations were accepted and they were
immediately appointed advisory physicians, thus remaining in a position where their knowledge and
skill continued to be available to the Hospital and
to their successors, those immediately following

them being Dr. Emma L. Call [21] and the Drs. Augusta and Emily Pope.[22]

The additional time thus available to Dr. Zakrzewska gave her greater opportunity to respond to the many demands upon her for public speaking and writing.

An address delivered before the "Moral Education Association of Massachusetts" about this date is so timely, and so pertinent to the problems which still beset us to-day, that it is here inserted:

The question is often asked me by persons not attending these meetings, What is this Moral Education Association? and What does it intend to accomplish?

When I reply, I always construct my explanation as I myself comprehend the motives of this Association and the purposes toward which we intend to work.

I am naturally an optimist. I fully believe that the world—by which I mean the human beings on this mighty planet—is constantly improving; that we, as a people of to-day, are progressing; and that we have reached a condition of physical, mental and moral improvement such as has never before been attained by the inhabitants of this globe. Yet I feel that we are far from being what we might become if each one of us would carry out fully, all the time, daily and hourly, the precepts of the Golden Rule.

In order to attain such a state of perfection, workers are constantly needed who, with deeper insight or stronger convictions or warmer hearts, shall lift the banner high over all our heads, and thus summon followers from all directions.

Now I call this Moral Education Association such a banner.

During the thirteenth century, after the knights of Middle and Western Europe returned from their crusading expeditions in the Holy Land and settled again in their homes, they formed an association, the chief object of which was to raise the "standard of honor." A spoken word was an inviolable contract; an ignoble deed, however slight, was considered so dishonorable as to relegate the perpetrator from the order of knighthood.

To many, it may seem to have been an unmeaning pastime, this cultivation by these men of an ideal honor in themselves and in others. Yet this movement ushered in a grand era of poetry, both lyric and dramatic, of chivalry, and of learning. It formed the nucleus of right in many directions and created a new code of morals.

In this same sense, and applying it to the elevation of the honor of woman, I joined this Association because I know that it is a good field in which women can work by helping to create a code of morals befitting our enlightened age, a code which shall govern our relations to all mankind, to our children, to each other as women, and to the State.

The increase of wealth and the increase of an intelligent population producing more and more wealth—this is the bright side of our progressive age. But there is also the dark side of the picture—the increase of luxury and its twin brother, sensuality.

In nature, as a rule, it is the female who nurses the young into maturity; in this case, it is the female who must stifle these twin brothers while they are yet in their infancy, so that they may never reach their dangerous maturity.

Luxury carried beyond a reasonable degree of comfort vitiates human strength and thus enervates both body and mind; then temporary stimulation and relief are sought in the excitements of sensuality. By sensuality, I understand all indulgences which carry to excess the natural physical appetites. Man, with his greater physical force, is the aggressive element in this strife for gratification, and woman with her slighter physique, the passive.

If we first make these points clear to ourselves, it will be easy to make them clear to others and to show to every woman the necessity of being on the defensive against these twin brothers, Luxury and Sensuality. All history teaches us that they have been the destroyers of nations in ancient times. Let us not deem that we are proof against their omnipotence. The defensive weapon can be none other than a code of morals as high and as idealistic as our present state of education and development will produce.

Further, this code ought to be in accordance with the political form of life in our country. We cannot afford to imitate any other people, any other nation. The women of this continent, and especially of the United States, enjoy a place in social life such as no women of any nation ever held before, or hold now. They can have all the power they want if they will simply take it, and if they will make themselves equal to all the responsibilities such a power involves.

Especially do I wish to speak of a danger to be avoided. We need to create and to foster among women a realizing sense that we *are all alike* and that the *worst* women belong to *us* as much as do the best. We cannot feel proud of the virtues and talents of one woman without feeling an equal degree of shame at the vices and the degradation of another.

There is no *third sex;* and we must see to it that this feeling—I cannot call it an opinion—that there exists a class of *animal women,* shall never take root in this country. In order to effect this, we must create a code of morals in accordance with our free institutions. Never should we look across the ocean for a guiding rod. Nowhere has woman been so poetized and so idealized, nowhere have music and the plastic arts so celebrated her as on the continent of Europe—yet everywhere there woman can be bought! She is legalized merchandise, and is inspected as such for the purpose of purchase, *which is prostitution.*

Among the nobility and the aristocracy the men hold it below their dignity and honor to be traders or even merchants because they consider that all commercial enterprise tends to make men mercenary, so lowering their character. Yet these same men do not hesitate to purchase women; while the aristocratic and noble lady thinks it right and just that there should be a special class of women for this purpose.

This is no exaggerated statement; it is a fact that women of education and of high standing speak of a certain class of women as if there were a third sex—a creature resembling woman in all outward appearance but sterile in propagation, sterile in morals, and sterile in intellectual capacity, a slave to men, and a creature of contempt in the eyes of women.

The word by which these women are designated when spoken of is "creature." In Europe, in common conversation and in everyday literature, this word "creature" has become a legitimatized desig-

nation for prostitutes. It is therefore deplorable
to hear women in their superior position as employers speak thoughtlessly of honest, virtuous women—
their nurses, seamstresses, servants and the like—
as "these creatures."

I say, therefore, that one of the laws of our moral
code should be, "Respect the *woman* in every
woman."

This respect for all womankind leads us to consider next the moral relations to children. The
highest ideal code cannot be too high here, and example should take precedence of teaching.

I would advise a whole code, explanatory of modesty, purity, chastity, truthfulness, obedience, self-
denial, and self-control, clearly to be comprehended
and strictly to be practiced by every woman—married and unmarried, mothers and grandmothers—so
that example shall teach the virtues to the boy as
well as to the girl.

Moral precepts and admonitions, repeated daily
in words are listened to with indifference; but from
a living example are drawn good draughts of healthful moral strength. For instance, speak before a
boy, no matter how small (in fact, the smaller the
more dangerous), with contempt of a woman, and
you may be sure the seed of contempt toward all
womanhood is sown and will grow and mature and
bear fruit for another generation. The same is
true if, in the hearing of girls, contempt for men
is expressed; yet here the effect is less bad for, as
I said before, the girl is the passive, not the aggressive, element in nature.

Next, we need a moral code in relation to men.
Here, the first principle should be, what is wrong
in woman is wrong in man. There is no special right
for the man. Although we cannot demonstrate an

absolute Right, yet the Golden Rule will always serve as a test where there is doubt. Men are born as pure and innocent and good as women. *We develop* qualities in them from a false conception of the aggressive impulses inherent in the masculine constitution. This is the point which we must bear in mind—man is not willfully nor intentionally vicious; but we allow him to practice a pernicious code of morals from early childhood, when we begin to say, "Oh, a boy will be a boy."

Of course, we want a man to be a man, but we also want a woman to be a woman. And we cannot make any advance toward the standard of a true man and a true woman if we give one set of morals to the man and another to the woman. Our constitution should be alike for both sexes, although from natural causes some of the by-laws must differ. This is the only way by which we can establish such relations of men to women and of women to men as shall be honorable to both and elevating to mankind in general.

Let us now consider the last but not the least point in our code of morals, that which concerns our relation to the State. This is, of course, the broadest and the most comprehensive theme with which moral education has to deal. Here again we shall see that we have our own code to make. For by "State" we mean in this country a different thing from that which Europe so designates. We do not mean a government given to a people by an aristocracy established centuries ago. We must learn to understand that when we speak of "the State," we mean the voluntary association of a free people which governs itself through and by the individual exercise of both intellectual and physical powers. Hence, there arises at once the need of a full com, prehension of our duties as members of such a State.

These duties are of two kinds—the duty of the normally endowed members (those having moderate or superior physical and mental qualities) toward each other; and, secondly, the duty of this fortunate class toward the less favored—the weak, the feeble in mind or in body and the crippled—those born or later afflicted with less capacity to take up the struggle for existence. We have all seen how the man born rich may become poor; and on the other hand, how the child born a pauper may yet lift himself to the position of the millionaire or to the highest office.

Here, then, lies our duty. Especially must we women educate ourselves and the young in regard to our relations to all humanity—particularly to the suffering, to the frail, and to the poor near our own doors. We have to create a code of morals strong enough to be just toward all the unfortunate—men, women and children; yet it must be free from that sentimentalism which cannot discriminate between an honest poor person and a criminal. On this point, endless illustrations could be given to show our lack of moral education. How difficult it is to preserve the righteous balance without being harsh to the criminal, the drunkard and the female vagrant! We have this great lesson to learn—that the poorest, the lowest, even the most degraded, when honestly striving to keep out of the almshouse or the prison, stands far higher in the scale of humanity than the reformed or the reforming prisoner; and that justice ought first to be done toward these poor degraded ones before sentimental charity is bestowed upon the criminal.

For here comes another part of this code as regards the State. What is charity? What is benevolence? What is the best way for their application? What is justice?

I would advise that all the members of this Moral Education Association, and nonmembers too, form classes where these subjects may be discussed, not simply where morality is preached to the moral, but where we enlighten ourselves by an interchange of opinion and by faithful investigation of moral questions. We need to know what is the real moral requirement in our peculiar state of American society. We are a State which has not been produced by propagation of one and the same race, so we have thus formed a nation with its own peculiar characteristics. We are an aggregate in a free country of many races and of many nations, a country where it is possible for the slave to step at once into self-sovereignty, or for the pauper from any foreign race to rise in a few years to the position of a well-to-do trader or merchant or artist, according to the intellectual capacity which he possesses. On the other hand, even with us these people may go down and form the center of a proletarianism unless they are prevented by education both of the intellect and of the morals.

A similar opportuneness characterizes her answer to the question which continues to be asked to-day as it has been asked down the ages:

SHOULD WOMEN STUDY MEDICINE?

So many women, both young and of mature age, appeal to me for information concerning the profession of medicine that I have thought it desirable to express my opinion thus publicly. The principal points inquired about are How to study medicine? and What are the prospects in practice?

There are so many medical schools now open to women, both in the East and in the West, that the selection of one for the purpose of study need depend only upon individual convenience and the pecuniary resources of the student. A student needs to have means for her support during three full years of college life and, if possible, for an additional year's residence in some hospital before entering upon practice.

Next comes the question, What can she expect in practice? Many young women enter the profession because it seems to them a lucrative business. Yet for a young person to choose this path in life because she thinks it leads invariably to success— by which she means a plentiful purse—is a mistake.

Success in the practice of medicine may coexist with small pecuniary gains; the money gain should be incidental, not primary, in the thought of the physician. A well-educated physician, who has passed through the regular course of study and who conscientiously works within the legitimate sphere of her knowledge, must allow about ten years of indefatigable labor before her practice brings a competency worthy the name of independence, by which I mean a comfortable living free from the anxieties of petty economies and allowing occasional relaxations from duty. Many a young woman has gone out of my office excited and indignant because I have expressed doubt that the medical profession would be the best career for her to choose, and her final exclamation as she left me is very significant, "You have been successful; why should not I be so?"

This "why not" is just the hard point to explain. On April 5, 1888, it was just thirty-six years since

I began to seek practice. Young (twenty-two and one-half years old), full of enthusiasm and self-reliance, willing to work, ready for self-abnegation in every direction, I felt sure that I should succeed in life, but this success never presented itself before my mind in the shape of a plentiful purse.

Besides the moral qualities I have mentioned, I started with another great advantage, namely, a good physical constitution. In no profession is sound steady health so requisite as in the medical, for the practitioner must be ready night and day, and at the beck and call of patients—whether paying or charity. Thus this profession demands a body free from annoyances of all kinds and a clear, sound head, to enable one to be decisive in judgment, firm in advice, and kind in sympathy.

Another step in the ladder of success is a good business training from early youth. By this I mean correctness in listening to every word spoken, accuracy of observation, and logical deduction. Every faculty must be, as it were, on the alert and yet kept under the control of judgment.

Yet there may be sound health, good education, and carefully trained faculties, and still a something lacking for success in life as physician. I call it a power of adaptation to the various temperaments and conditions of humanity; a moral courage; an ability to step forward and seek opportunities for practice; a kind of self-confidence and fearlessness in entering every class of life.

Thus equipped, and backed by friends or pecuniary means to sustain the respectability of the beginner during the first few years of her attempts to seek practice, a young woman has still to overcome prejudices and obstacles which are not easily described, for they are of an intangible nature, relating sometimes to personal appearance and oftener to that indefinable quality—tact.

Yet notwithstanding all these difficulties, it is far easier to-day for a woman to establish herself as physician than it was thirty years ago. The annoyance and tribulations which we pioneers had to endure were far greater than the natural ones which have always to be overcome. For women physicians were then looked upon not only as intruders upon the field hitherto occupied by men alone, but also as disreputable persons and they were constantly confounded with the women who, prefixing "Dr." to their names, carried on a foul and illegal practice.

So great was the prejudice against the first women physicians that friends and acquaintances hesitated to invite them into their social circles. Yet in spite of this hostility, I was inclined to encourage other women to study medicine; for, inexperienced like all young people and more enthusiastic than most, I imagined that every one who expressed a desire for some active work was as willing and as well prepared to undergo hardships and privations as I myself was. Years have made me wiser and, consequently, more cautious in advising these young seekers.

Every physician, man or woman, who has acquired prominence through ability, finds himself or herself placed in the position of adviser to youth. No one claims infallibility in judgment; great talent is not always recognizable to the wisest counselor; but the duty is the same for all—a conscientious statement of what the medical profession demands. Its difficulties and the various obstacles should be stated clearly to the young man or woman who is so often dazzled by the brilliant success of the few, forgetting the many who are plodding along in economical, modest paths or have retired entirely, and who are therefore unknown.

Yet while I have thus shown the darker side, I can see that the study of medicine is full of opportunities for women, and that there are so many ways of becoming useful, if not as practitioners then as teachers and resident physicians in female schools and colleges, that no truly talented woman need fear want of success in some branch of the profession.— *The Woman's Journal, June 23, 1888.*

Less weighty but not less serious, and again as though a response to another question which is agitating us to-day, is the following article reprinted from *The Woman's Journal* of April 5, 1890:

WHAT'S IN A NAME?

It may be true that "a rose by any other name would smell as sweet." But even Shakespeare does not convince us that a Montague would not still be a Montague though called by another name. No, the name becomes a part of the individuality. A name has two distinct qualities—the lighter, social and emotional; and the graver, legal and representative. Pet names denote affection and are usually applied to infants as expressive of their helplessness or diminutiveness in contrast to our superiority to their small persons. The continued use of these pet names when their bearers fill active and responsible positions in life, indicates thoughtlessness if not real inferiority of intellect.

To explain my meaning fully, I will illustrate from my own experience both conditions—the social and the legal value of names. Quite recently I was asked whether I knew a Dr. Carrie S——, of ——town, whom the inquirer wished to consult on arriving there. Instinctively I replied that I should not care to know a "Dr. Carrie" or "Hattie" or "Maggie," etc., and I certainly would not ask the advice of any physician who had not more sense than to advertise herself by sign or word as a diminutive person. How can a woman think deeply on any subject who has not brains enough to object to such pet names?

A short time ago, a friend who was visiting me handed me two letters to be posted. One was addressed "Mr. C. Albert ——" and the other, "Miss Nellie ——." Glancing at the addresses, I remarked, "I thought your son's name was Bert as I have always heard him called so, and why has your sister changed her name from Ellen?" This sister was then forty years old and had been teacher to her sister's sons who lived in the country where there was a lack of schools suitable to prepare lads for the Latin school. Yet my friend said in reply to my remark, "No, my son's name is Albert and we called him Bert or Bertie, but since he entered Harvard College, he has forbidden our using those names, because," she added, "boys, you know, have more pride than girls. My sister likes to be addressed as Nellie." Thus the teacher, twenty-two years older than her nephew, was denoted by spoken and written word "a girl" without "pride." I wish all girls and women would comprehend this fact— that as long as they are pleased with a diminutive name, so long will they be classed in the category of diminutive human beings.

Again, consider the ludicrous side. Here enters a woman twenty years old, six feet tall, addressed as Maggie. Now, must such a woman reach a height of eighteen feet before she attains the dignity of

"Margaret"—that is, the name of a full-grown woman?

I once had under my medical care a girl whose face was greatly disfigured by an eruption. She had a dark complexion and dark hair, yet her name was Lily. When a little more than fourteen years old, she came to me, her eyes sparkling with delight. "Oh," she said, "I have found out that my real name is Lucy; I was called so for an aunt who died last week and who left me one thousand dollars in her will because I am her namesake. I cried for joy, not about the money, but because I have got rid of that horrid name of Lily." Seeing my astonishment at her excitement, she added, "You do not know how I have suffered from my schoolmates; they nicknamed me Tiger Lily on account of my face, and now, see, Lily was only a pet name; it is not my real name!" Her mind was relieved, she was at ease and happy to assert her dignity by an appropriate name. She soon recovered from the torment of the eruption, and I have no doubt that the mental relief of having a sensible name aided in her recovery. Again, how would a woman with the dignified name of Margaret feel if she read in the newspaper the notice of her marriage with "Tommy" Smith? A certain amount of etiquette is essential in life—it gives weight and dignity to everyday occurrences, and is, as it were, an expression of a sense of social responsibilities.

The second question is the legal and representative quality. To understand the full importance of this, let us recall the fact that throughout the whole civilized globe, it is customary to give to the child the father's name. It is not necessary to discuss here whether it would be better to change this custom and give to the child the name of both father and mother. The fact is established that the child receives a personal name prefixed to that of the family of which it is the offspring. By this latter name it becomes known, and in the course of years this name becomes a part of the individual, belongs to the character itself, and can no more be got rid of than the blood which flows in the veins and had its origin in the parents. It is a rare thing for a man to admit even the thought of changing his name; if it were Smith, he is and remains Smith, simply denoting his individuality by the prefix *A*, *B*, *C*, or whatever the initial may be. He cannot be addressed by any other name, and he can receipt bills and sign legal papers by no other name without being considered guilty of misrepresentation.

The importance of this individuality of name is nowhere better recognized than in Germany. A girl named at birth Anna Eleanora Miller is and remains Anna Eleanora Miller all her lifetime, no matter whether she marries once or six times in the course of her career. By no other name can she sign a deed or contract; thus only can she bear witness; and she is not summoned by the courts as witness under any other name than that of Anna Eleanora Miller.

If she has a husband, she is addressed in law by her name, Anna Eleanora (or, if she has ten given names, then by all of them) Miller, wife of Brown, or wife of Baron Ketzow, or von Alden. If she becomes a widow and marries again, she is addressed in law (of course not in social intercourse) as Anna Eleanora Miller, widow of Brown, wife of Baron von Ketzow.

To make this clearer, let me illustrate still further by giving the name of a well-known lady who, after she became a widow, studied medicine and now practices dentistry in Berlin, having been dentist to all the children of the Empress Friedrich. Her diploma would be utterly valueless had it been given to her with the name of her first husband; only by her maiden name could she be authorized as a practitioner. Her sign at the door reads, "Dr. Henriette Pagelson, widow of Hirschfeld, wife of Tiburtius," she having, after a few years of practice, contracted a marriage with Dr. Tiburtius. Thus she is, and remains, Henriette Pagelson, and by this name only is she professionally and legally responsible; this stamps her individuality, and the other names of Mrs. Hirschfeld and Mrs. Tiburtius become merely social and conventional designations.

The question of changing names will and ought to become of grave importance before the law in this country. As we now have women lawyers, it should be their special charge to bring up at once this neglected matter—the question of the legality of diplomas as regards the names thereon—before the legislatures in their respective states.

Let me suppose a case in order to show the gravity of this subject. A young woman who has studied medicine receives a diploma under the name of Anna Elizabeth Brown. In a few years she marries, removes the sign from her door and puts up a new one reading "Dr. A. E. Stone." Soon after this she has to sign a death certificate, which she does by writing "Anna Elizabeth Stone, M.D." Such a document has no legal truth in it. Again, suppose the relatives of a patient sue this doctor for malpractice, cannot the lawyer make a good case from the fact that her diploma certifies to the ability of "Anna E. Brown," and that a "Dr. Stone" does not exist? Does not this create a flaw or an irregularity in the indictment executed by the com-

plainants? Still further, the husband "Stone"
dies, and in a year the widow marries McIntosh and
again changes sign and signature to "Dr. A. E.
McIntosh," while no diploma, and therefore no such
doctor of that name exists, but only the original
"Anna Elizabeth Brown, M.D."

What is thus true in the medical profession is
true in commercial pursuits and in all professions.
Annoyances also arise in social relations. A short
time ago, I was asked if I knew a Dr. Alice Smith
of a certain city, she having referred to me for
professional recommendation. I at once declared
the woman to be a fraud. A few months later, Dr.
Alice Smith, having been informed of my not very
complimentary appellation, sent me a letter expressive of much injured feeling. In this letter, she
gave her maiden name under which she had served
as interne in our New England Hospital where we
had valued her as one of our best assistants.

Now, if men cannot see the importance of this
demand for a settlement of the question of women's
names, I wish that our women lawyers would bring
the subject before the legislatures, requesting some
decision on the legal qualifications as to names for
any professional or business relation of women,
whether they are single, married or widowed. If
the woman cannot call her name her own and will
not drop the diminutive pet name, she does not deserve to be considered a full human being.

Let me be understood—I do not mean to say that
in social life a woman should not accept the name of
her husband. I do not desire to overturn existing
customs, and I think it is far more sensible to be
"Mrs. Smith" in common social life than to be "Dr.
Brown," which may be the title on the diploma, but
all this could easily be left to personal decision.

Princess Louise of England will not be called Marchioness of Lorne. Baroness von Essmarsch prefers to be called Frau Doctor (having married Dr. von Essmarsch), and objects to the title of Princess Mecklenberg to which she is entitled, and by which she is addressed, as aunt of the present Empress of Germany. Here love casts aside all titles; nevertheless, it is only as Princess Mecklenberg that she can legally be addressed, or legally be empowered to sell or to give away even a few feet of land. The only signature valid in law is "Princess Mecklenberg, wife of Dr. von Essmarsch."

Throughout Europe, the women in all classes cling more closely to their family names than we do. On visiting cards, one commonly sees "Mrs. Brown, née Miller." If one wishes to be specially respectful, one addresses in the same way, mentioning both names, the envelope which incloses even a friendly letter to a married woman. And, finally, on the gravestone placed above a deceased married woman, the maiden name is always conspicuously inscribed before the married name.

CHAPTER XXXVII

Opening of the Medical School of the Johns Hopkins University to women on equal terms with men—Consultations with Dr. Zakrzewska by women interested in the event—Her report of the attitude of the community towards women surgeons—New building for the Maternity Department of the Hospital (the Sewall Maternity and, later, the Helen Morton Wing)—Opening of the Goddard Home for Nurses—Because of misbehavior of men students, Columbia University of Georgetown closes its doors to women—Dr. Zakrzewska writes on "the Emancipation of Woman: Will it be a Success?" (1888-1894.)

THESE were eventful days (1888-1890) for all friends of the advancement of the medical education of women, leading up as they did to the opening to women of the medical school of the Johns Hopkins University in 1890.

The same fear of beguilement and subsequent disillusionment which Dr. Zakrzewska had felt regarding the proposed opening to women of the Medical School of Harvard University, away back at the time when the future of the New England Female Medical College hung in the balance, haunted the minds of all workers for the cause of medical women.

So many colleges had been opened to women and had then been closed to them, in response to the storm raised by one or another protesting group, that experience had made women feel they must always be on their guard.

One of the prominent women of Worcester wrote to Dr. Zakrzewska in 1890:

Our Women's Club has been urged to contribute to assist the Medical School of the Johns Hopkins University, with the idea that women shall have there all the advantages which men have, and as I have seen your name with other well-known names, I desire to ask if you really think that they will act in good faith if the $100,000 should be given them.

We are told by parties in Baltimore who ought to know that the whole policy of Johns Hopkins is conservative in spite of its high rank, and that women would never be admitted on the same terms as men.

As one of an investigating committee, I am to report on October 22d. Will you be so kind as to tell me what you think of the scheme? If the money is raised and offered on condition that women shall be so received, we are told that it will be refused. In that case, it would not seem worth while to give anything towards it.

This must be a matter which would greatly interest you, and I venture to hope that you will find a moment to reply.

In the course of her correspondence with Dr. Zakrzewska, a leading woman of Baltimore who was one of those foremost in the present movement, writes:

I will bear your cautions in mind and watch very carefully. I myself have not much confidence in the willingness of many men to give women a fair chance, but since out of the four women who began this movement, three of them have fathers on the

two boards who are deeply convinced of the righteousness of the cause, I cannot help feeling hopeful.
Moreover, the physicians at the Hospital have been
most cordial and helpful to every well-qualified
woman who has sought its advantages.

I inclose a copy of the trustees' resolutions. I do
not see how, although they reserve the right of making "such rules and regulations as they may deem
necessary for the government of its School of Medicine," they can possibly ignore the paragraph that
"in making such rules and regulations, the terms of
this minute shall always be respected and observed"
—and these terms we insisted should be *the same,*
not equal.

However, I agree with you that we must watch
carefully, and if there should ever be a sign of trying to evade it you may depend on us to fight it out.

It is interesting to note that half of the $100,000
was given by one woman, Miss Mary Garrett,
daughter of one of the original trustees of the Johns
Hopkins University. Also, that the $10,000 previ-
ously offered by Miss Hovey to Harvard, on condition of its admitting women and which was declined
by its medical faculty, was transferred to the Johns
Hopkins.

When, in 1888, Dr. Zakrzewska and her two earliest
co-workers on the Hospital staff, Drs. Sewall and
Morton, resigned as attending physicians and became advisory physicians, Dr. Sewall had in the
state of her health an additional reason for relinquishing her arduous duties. And Dr. Zakrzewska
suffered keenly during the next few years in realizing the approaching loss of this particularly dear

colleague, who had always been to her as her own
child though her junior by only a few years. Dr.
Sewall died in February, 1890.

At the annual meeting at the close of the Hospital
year, 1890, Dr. Zakrzewska again was called upon
to present the report from the resident physician—
this position being temporarily vacant.

Referring especially to the increasing work of
the Hospital under women surgeons, she says:

The results thus far are so satisfactory that no
other hospital can show a greater percentage of
recoveries. Our reputation for successful operations increases; and the request is often made by
patients that no men shall be present.

An old lady of seventy-nine years, the prolonga-
tion of whose life depended upon the immediate removal of a large ovarian tumor—an accidental fall
having caused inflammation—insisted upon having
even no consultation with men, nor any men present
at the operation, saying, "I am old enough anyway
to die, only I don't want to suffer as I do now; and
if the women can save my life for a while longer,
I shall be grateful." She was saved, and went
home well in just four weeks from the day of
operation.

Another change has come with this advance in
the medical women's world. Women now express
the strongest confidence in women's skill, entirely
refuting the fears and opinions of former years
that "women would never have confidence in their
own sex." The opposite condition has now become
so manifest that when in a first consultation a patient decides at once and unreservedly to employ
a woman surgeon, we are frequently obliged to re-

mind her that her friends or her family may prefer to have a man perform the operation.

A patient was brought into my office from the carriage before the door. She seemed so weak and exhausted that I did not venture to speak frankly to her but called the friends into an outer room and informed them of the need of the removal of a large abdominal tumor without delay. After a short deliberation, they considered it best for me to inform the patient. I did so. A few moments of silence ensued, and then came the response, "Where can it be done? Will you do it?" Answering the latter question in the negative and the former by proposing our Hospital, she replied, "Well, take me there and I will have it done to-morrow."

We did take her there, but the case was too grave for an operation on the morrow as important preparations were necessary. But in a few months the patient left the Hospital well, and when a half year later she came into my office, I did not recognize the changed woman.

Such cases are not infrequent now, and the gratitude of many a mother, wife, and daughter spreads throughout our land the fame of our Hospital, the skill of our surgeons, and the kindness of our nurses. The number of women surgeons is but few as yet, but I do not care to compete numerically with men. I simply repeat the claim which I made thirty-five years ago when pleading the cause of women physicians, namely, give to women whose qualifications and tastes lead them to study the healing art, the opportunity to develop such talents to the utmost on an equality with men.

It is due to the perseverance of woman's nature and to the freedom of this country that such comparatively great results have been achieved in so few years. I, who saw at most a possibility in the dim future, am permitted to behold an idea realized —an idea for the materialization of which I expected simply to plow the ground before I passed away from this life, leaving it for others to cultivate. But see! Already, under the sunshine of free institutions and the favoring breezes of universal progress, we reap the fruits of our labor.

In June, 1892, a new Maternity Building was completed and dedicated. It was named the Sewall Maternity, in memory of that early and devoted friend of Dr. Zakrzewska and the Hospital, Hon. Samuel E. Sewall, and of his daughter, Dr. Lucy E. Sewall, who was, successively, Dr. Zakrzewska's first student, assistant, and staff colleague.

The old Maternity was renovated and transformed into a home for the nurses, and it served this purpose until replaced by a new building in 1909. It was named the Goddard Home for Nurses in honor of the Goddard family—Miss Lucy Goddard, one of the incorporators of the Hospital and first president of the board of directors; George A. Goddard, for many years the devoted treasurer of the Hospital; and his mother, Mrs. M. Le B. Goddard, one of the earlier directors.

Some years later (1906), a wing was added to the Sewall Maternity, the Helen Morton Wing. This was named in honor of Dr. Helen Morton, classmate of Dr. Sewall and Dr. Zakrzewska's second student, assistant, and staff colleague.

In the midst of the congratulations and rejoicings which followed the opening to women of the Johns Hopkins Medical School, the distrust which Dr.

Zakrzewska had already voiced was, in 1893, given another justification by the action of the Columbian University of Georgetown, D. C. (now the George Washington University Medical School), which decided to close the doors that it had opened to women.

For at least ten years the medical department had been graduating women on equal terms with men. But there had always been three members of the faculty who were bitterly opposed to allowing women to study medicine on any terms. These three professors made the path of the women students as rough and stony as possible; and the male students, taking the cue from these professors, added discourtesies and affronts to hostility.

Finally, in the dissecting room, some of these students so debased themselves by offering insult, not only to the women medical students but also to the helpless bodies of their fellow beings who had been given to them for scientific study, that the faculty and trustees were obliged to take official notice of the occurrence.

Now, mark the administration of justice. The male students committed the offense which no one attempted to condone. Were the offenders punished? No. Neither were the innocent victims of the offense, the women medical students. But the whole sex of the innocent victims was selected to make vicarious atonement. The verdict was that the women then in the Medical School should be permitted to complete their course, but after that no more women should be admitted to the school.

After this demonstration can any one doubt that the story of Adam and Eve and the Garden of Eden has biologic foundation and, as the good old books say, "is in the nature of man." But we can rejoice that this is a nature which man is steadily moving upward to modify and correct, hence the increasing number of men who are willing to do justice to women.

It remains to add that the trustees were said to have been almost unanimous in their opposition to the exclusion of women but to have been overborne by the financial control exerted by the three professors mentioned.

The indignation of a large portion of the lay community was aroused by the injustice thus done to women, and an appeal for advice was made to Dr. Zakrzewska, whose views on such a situation have already been stated. Fortunately, the Johns Hopkins Medical School is not far removed from Washington.

The era of the "emancipation" of woman as an all-inclusive phrase had not yet passed, though it was approaching its eclipse by more specific terms. Using it as an antithesis of "oppression," Dr. Zakrzewska writes in *The Open Court,* June 21, 1894, on "The Emancipation of Woman: Will it be a Success?"

This article was in reply to one on "The Oppression of Woman," evidently written by a man who voiced his protest against the subjection from which women have suffered for so many centuries, and who claimed for women freedom to develop along their own lines. His plea was apparently similar to Tennyson's when the latter sings:

. . . "Leave her space to burgeon out of all
Within her—let her make herself her own
To give or keep, to live and learn and be
All that not harms distinctive womanhood.
For woman is not undevelopt man,
But diverse."

Perhaps, as is so often the case, an undercurrent
of masculine patronage had crept into the plea of
the advocate. Or perhaps Dr. Zakrzewska merely
felt the weariness that comes to all normal grown-up
women when their normality and growth are com-
mented upon as phenomena, instead of being accepted as the thing to be expected. On a very hot
day, the chirr of even a friendly katydid may seem
too obvious, repeating (what should be) "an undis-
puted thing in such a solemn way." At any rate,
she responds:

I admit that the writer of this article is right,
positively right, logically right, sentimentally right,
to the end of these reasonings which are lucid and
clearly stated.

Then I ask, What is the value of this new point,
this proving that the evolution of woman's activity
cannot be otherwise than feminine? If twice two
make four, no exertion of either man or woman can
make it five. Let us leave it as a positive fact, and
not worry when we see any individual trying to
prove that twice two make five.

Why are all these mental somersaults and capri-
oles in men's writings needed? Will their attempts
at prophesying or illustrating the future effects aris-
ing from the activity of a yet unknown quantity
alter or check the present phenomenal awakening
of woman's ambition?

Allow me to elucidate my meaning by a true story of what happened in my native city, Berlin, about fifty years ago.

In a courtyard lived a poor family. The father was a locksmith by trade. His eldest son, a boy of twelve, bright, industrious and smart, spent all his time either in the schoolroom or in his father's shop. Not even on Sundays could this poor family enjoy rest but worked in the dreary shop. The boy was very fond of eating string beans which the mother could seldom afford to buy.

He therefore decided to raise them in a box before his window. He used some old pieces of boards for the construction of his window-garden, and all the inmates of the front as well as of the rear houses became interested in his experiment, everybody feeling it to be his or her duty to express opinions on the subject.

Thus it came to pass that the boy was told that the beans planted would rot because the boards were not porous enough to allow air to pass; that the soil in the box could not be regulated as regarded the daily moisture needed; that the rain could not be discharged after flooding the window garden; that the heat of the sun reflected from the window glass would burn the tender growths; that not more than two stalks of beans could be raised if the seed turned out to be dwarf beans, and if pole beans, he could not fasten them high enough; that no good growth could be expected if there were not a flow of air all around to favor the plant; that the already dark room (this being the only window) would be darkened too much by the growing plants and thus the three children who slept in it would not awaken in time for school, which commenced at seven o'clock; that the health of the children would be in-

jured by the exhalation of the plants and the moisture of the earth in the box; that his mother should
be warned not to allow such an experiment as it
would be a moral injury to the boy when he found
himself disappointed in the success of his plan, as
the most valuable of emotions—hope—would thus
be destroyed; that the father ought to realize that
he would lose at least half an hour daily of the boy's
help in the shop; in fact, all the arguments and all
the prophesying were that a complete failure would
be the result and that the boy would be crushed under
the weight of it.

However, the boy prepared his box, took note of
the many suggestions and obviated some of them,
as by perforating his box with small holes, by opening the windows when the sun shone from ten in the
morning to three in the afternoon, etc.

The twelve beans which he had planted grew and
proved to be pole beans, so he tied strings for them
to climb up on as high as the tenant above his room
allowed him to do. He watered and nursed his
plantation with care and love, and lo and behold,
the beans flourished and blossomed and bore fruit
relatively plentifully.

During this time of growth, an old and wise
tenant of the front house, also a professor, joined
the group who for eight weeks had watched and
discussed in the yard this willful boy's experiment.
This critic remarked that he observed a new phase
of which nobody had thus far taken notice and which
might have both good and bad effects, namely, that
a hailstorm might yet come and destroy this garden, although there might also be a good result as
the plants would protect the window panes if the
storm should occur when the windows were closed.

All admitted that this was true, and all admired

the wisdom of the Herr Professor, and went to their respective abodes a little mortified that they had not thought before of this neglected point of the subject.

The boy had the satisfaction of gathering a mess of well-grown beans, sufficient for a hearty meal for the whole family. But while eating his favorite dish, he said, "Well, mother, I did succeed; but to tell the truth, the beans don't taste so good as those which grow in the fields. So next year, I will not try again but I shall sow nasturtium seeds for you to enjoy."

He did so, and his window was a perfect delight and source of cheer to him, to his mother, and to the tenants of the little court. He continued to do this until he had to enter the army, at eighteen years of age. His younger brothers (he had no sisters) followed in his footsteps, and when I left Berlin my last look was at the nasturtium window.

Let me ask, did it matter much which the boy raised, beans or nasturtiums? What use was it to him, or to his family, or to the tenants when the latter all joined in the chorus, "I thought so" or "I told him he could not raise beans"? Let each one try nature's forces and take his chance! And twice two will always remain four.

CHAPTER XXXVIII

*Dr. Zakrzewska's own description of her attitude as a
critic—Her judgments on various details of Hospital
policy: Against the admission to the Hospital of
women students of the Boston University Medical
School (that being then a school of homeopathy); On
the reciprocal relation of the medical staff and the
board of directors of the Hospital; On a question of
Hospital discipline; Letter to an ambitious colleague
whose feelings have been hurt.*

MATTERS of Hospital policy were continually being
referred to her for decision. Before noting details,
it will be illuminating to read what she says as to
her mental attitude when making criticisms:

If I praise, it is hardly ever the person or the relation in which this person stands to me of which I
think—it is simply the praiseworthy thing or deed
which I eulogize.

These very same persons may do or say something
which, according to my comprehension, is not praiseworthy but the contrary, and I criticize and blame
just as strongly as I praised before when many
did not see the praiseworthiness until I drew attention to it.

For the praise, I receive thanks, for human nature
likes far better to hear agreeable things than disagreeable ones.

For the blame, where I pointed out the fault, I
receive double reproach, for human nature likes to

defend, it is vexed because its attention has been drawn to the fact of imperfection and its displeasure tends to fall upon the person who points out this imperfection.

I am fully aware that gratitude and warm friendships are easily gained by speaking well of everything and everybody. Hence it is that secondary, yes, even very mediocre, talents receive a certain amount of fame and appreciation by the multitude.

But to a true nature such kind of appreciation is humbling; and that, too, in just such a degree as to him or her, praise or blame, appreciation or censure, are equally sacred. One who is satisfied with the recognition of the few can calmly wait till the multitude find out for themselves how much of the seed sown among them will grow.

Therefore, when I mention names to you, pray do not believe I speak of them because they are either friends or foes to me, or that I wish either to please or to hurt. Both are far from me—I do not care to please, nor do I want to hurt, anybody.

In answer to a proposal in earlier years to admit to the New England Hospital the women students of the Medical Department of the Boston University (then a school of homeopathy), she decided in the negative. In this connection, she says:

It is my opinion that if we do not intend to lower our aims or to descend from the position which we have taken and which we should uphold, we cannot form any connection, through the admission of its students to our Hospital, with a school which holds itself strictly sectarian and which claims a one-sided knowledge—a faith in medicine which has no warrant, and an advancement in science which neither here in America nor abroad is approved by natural scientists, by chemists, or by microscopists. And which in reality possesses no sound foundation other than that which exists in all new ideas, namely, that of experiment. But this experiment is just as permissible to the regular practitioner who is educated on the broadest terms and who has a perfect right to administer any remedy for the restoration of health.

In stating this opinion, to which I have given thoughtful consideration, I regret personally that I thus exclude women of a school with which I agree as to the great principle of equality in education of the sexes.

At one time, there seemed to be in the minds of some of the later members a question as to the reciprocal relation of the medical staff and the board of directors. On this occasion, she writes:

Our Hospital is utterly different from all hospitals carried on by the City or the State or by private individuals and endowments.

In these latter there exists either a need to provide for the helpless who are dependent on the Commonwealth, or benevolent persons wish to provide a charity and so they establish hospitals. In both conditions, the staff of physicians is employed by those who manage the institutions and, consequently, either money or thanks are due to such physicians as serve.

With us, it is entirely different. None of our original directors wanted a hospital; none of them was inspired by charity or had the means to provide such charity. I, the representative of an idea in its earliest evolution—I sought those Directors that they might serve the purpose of carrying out that idea.

They served then and in the future the women physicians connected with the Hospital. They never dictated as to the number of physicians or internes; they never proposed to enlarge the work; this has always been done by the professional staff. *We* thank *them* for their generous aid, but they cannot thank us for doing much or little.

Of course, the Directors are the corporate body, and they represent us legally before the public; but they carry out our ideas, not we theirs. They simply stand ready to support the principle of giving to women physicians full opportunity to manifest their skill and judgment.

In this connection it is interesting to refer to a letter regarding another matter, which Mrs. Cheney wrote to Dr. Zakrzewska in 1888. Mrs. Cheney says:

I hope you will not think me ungrateful for your inestimable frank criticism, which has been one of the greatest helps in my life even if I cannot adopt all your suggestions, as I must speak my own language—but I am most thankful for the matter you have supplied.

I never know what to say about my relation to the Hospital work. It is not to me what it is to you. . . . I accepted it as blessed work . . . and have thanked you all my life for bringing it to me, but it has never been mine as it is yours.

Other aspects of her mind appear in connection with special experiences, as when she writes to one of the other doctors regarding a question of hospital discipline:

MY DEAR DOCTOR:

I enclose the letter you handed to me and one from Dr. ——. Allow me to tell you how I have managed such letters. I have had precisely three similar experiences. Dr. ——'s patients left in the same way as Mrs. ——, and to this day their relatives are not satisfied that the patients were treated rightly. Still, they are good friends with me in spite of my having acted as I did. This was what I did.

When I received the first letter, I said to myself:

1. There are always two sides to every story.
2. I cannot act at all if I keep this letter secret, as I am requested to do.
3. If there is an accusation, I must have the excuse unless I want to ignore the whole concern and burn the letter.
4. I will not talk, so as not to run the risk of losing my temper.

Therefore, I sat down, wrote a note to the doctor and enclosed the letter of accusation, but requested her not to let either the patient or the student know about it but to tell me what she thought was best to be done.

Now this action seemed right to me, because

1. I investigated the other side.
2. I tried to put things to rights.
3. I gave a chance for explanations.
4. I could not become impatient, because both parties are always more careful when things are put on paper.

After I received the doctor's reply, I took the letters, the patient and the doctor into a private room, and informed them why and how I had acted in the affair. Then I read both letters, and this was followed by an apology on both sides and the matter was ended.

Then, although the patient left the Hospital, she could not say that the doctor was not courteously treated by me. Nor could she say that justice was not done to her.

After this, the doctor and I together had an interview with the student, and we said as little or as much as was necessary to make her more careful, and that was ended.

As it happened, Dr. ——'s patient was one of more education and she saw that she was in the wrong, so she apologized and remained until the doctor discharged her.

I don't think that either you or I are the last authority on such questions. They should be settled with all concerned in harmony and even with polite treatment of the culprit, should there be one.

If you lose your temper with a coworker, it lowers you in the eyes of patients or of others a great deal more than it hurts her. Everybody feels with or for the punished one, and nobody with the one who punishes or condemns.

I find that in going through the wards now, all the patients feel attached to the doctor and are full of her praise, and they hope she will have a good time and come back to her arduous duties with her usual strength, fine spirits and cheerfulness.

As soon as Dr. —— comes home, we shall work out rules for the physicians so that these will be ready for our next meeting. And if they are then properly discussed, I think it might be a good plan to have them printed in our report so that patients may learn their extent and on whom they depend.

Again, one of the doctors was evidently suffering from a wounded *amour propre,* feeling that she had not been treated with sufficient consideration. She had apparently expressed her grievance to Dr. Zakrzewska, and then being dissatisfied with the result of her interview, had tried to express herself more definitely in a letter. Dr. Zakrzewska replies:

My dear Dr. ——:

I will answer the last paragraph of your letter first, because this is the straw which shows how the wind blows, and it also confirms my impression concerning the cause of your manner. I have nothing to forgive in your manner because, personally, you have never offended me. I therefore have nothing to forget either.

But forgetting that we are colleagues and professional women interested in the same work and in the same great cause where harmony is so desirable, you seem to think, or rather you assert, that I should remember your years and your condition of health, which is to account for your speaking without thinking. . . .

Now about your age, I never have thought of you as young even when you were young. At the time we met, I recognized in the instant the genuine talent and fervor of purpose of which you were possessed, and I accepted you not as an inferior but as an equal.

Do you think that I could now make an attempt to throw the mature woman from a past and from a place in my estimation which I let her occupy when she was really a young girl of no experience? Would not this be silly and mean? Do you admit that I am either, or both?

I always saw your weaknesses and faults as clearly as I see them now, and I often spoke plainly of them to you, but I never, never thought of putting you lower on account of them, because weaknesses we all have, and I am glad to bear and forbear with these in people who have something of worth to counterbalance, or else to place these faults entirely in the background.

You say you wish to preserve an opinion of your own on all Hospital matters. Who has ever wished more than I have that you would do this? How often have I said to you when you wished to make changes and have told me that you put these on me and my orders, that my shoulders were broad enough to carry all, but that I thought you should do things on your own authority as this seemed simply right. How often have I referred to you as being a more efficient authority on those points regarding which I thought you were.

And even when you did not agree with my propositions, when did you ever hear that I complained? On the contrary, have I not the more readily yielded and tried to investigate honestly which way would be best? "Do as you please," "suit yourself," "work in your own way"—are not these standing phrases which I have used to every physician?

I am ready to give up the Hospital work at any moment that you all think you can do without me. I have no ambition to *work* in it; I had only the ambition to help women into the position where *they* could work. And this I have accomplished.

In New York I did well, and I am remembered in an honorable and friendly way. And here in Boston I have certainly done my best. And if there are now a hundred women who differ from me and a thousand who know better than I do, I have noth-

ing to say against it. On the contrary, I am glad
and happy about it because this is just the condition which I strove for. My teachings have always
been—you must all do better, far better, than I
have done, because you have far better opportunities than I had. I helped to make those opportunities
and shame upon you if you do not come out better
than your present teacher.

No, no, my dear Doctor, it is not at all anything
of this that is in your manner. In some way you
have got it into your head and heart that you must
play the first fiddle, or still better, be the conductor
and show your importance in every way, small and
big. You want the incense of having everybody
look up to you as the most important person in the
concern; you like to patronize, and so on.

And I, to tell the truth, am very willing that you
should have all this pleasure because I do not care
at all for these things. To me, the answer to one
of the great questions of the time is to assist women
into their right position whether or not they know
me or my name (which, luckily, is so hard that they
won't even take the trouble to learn it).

Now, this will be the last time that I shall write
on this subject. There is no use in trying to make
artificially a harmony which does not any more come
spontaneously. I am very willing, yes, even too
willing, to allow myself to be overruled, because I do
not care at all for the particular minutæ.

You know that I carried on the Hospital quite
differently from Dr. —— or Dr. ——, yes, even from
what you did, but I never tried, nor wanted to try,
to interfere, because it is far better that each individual should do her work in her individual way.
Otherwise, it must fail to be done well. Imitations

are always inferior to the genuine article. But agreeing to a thing is not always liking it.

As for my having wounded your feelings, this is possible—but I daresay it was only in hospital matters when forced out by your hostile manner. I hope I never was rude in my social relations, and if I have been let me assure you that if you will tell me when and where I was so, I will certainly beg your pardon.

CHAPTER XXXIX

Dr. Zakrzewska's private life—Her home—Her friends— Her keeping in touch with the Hospital doctors, students and internes—Her "boys"—Her ethics—Her reading—Men physicians who served as consultants at the New England Hospital.

Concurrently with the public manifestations of Dr. Zakrzewska's life, as recorded in the preceding pages, proceeded her more intimate life of home, family and friends. Allusions to these happy possessions have been made from time to time, but a particular word should be given to one feature which she brought with her from the old world to the new —a feature which enriches life over there, and which would add so much to our American life could we adopt it as generally and as simply.

Reference is here made to the custom of European people of all grades of circumstance in incorporating the outdoors into the daily life of the household, especially for the hour or moment of social relaxation.

Poor indeed the family that has not at least a tiny arbor, or shelter, or shaded spot, where the glass of sirup or other beverage of the country, or the cup of coffee or tea, or the incense of the friendly pipe or the more exclusive cigar, draws the curtain upon the workaday world and releases the spirit for a few moments' dream of content.

457

"Rock Garden" was the name of her most blessed retreat—a large garden with terraces and with the rocks for which Roxbury is famous. There were trees and shrubs, fruits and flowers, tables and seats, and the air was filled with memories of happy hours, hospitable days and friendly meetings. And many groups of Hospital directors, doctors and internes, as well as other friends, gathered there at various times, carefree and festive.

"Rock Garden has always been the Garden of Paradise," comes a voice borne upon the breeze, "but wherever you are or wherever you make your home, that place will soon be ideal to your friends."

Dr. Buckel writes from the gardens of California, her thoughts turned back to Rock Garden:

Oh, what has it not been! You know what it has been to you, but you do not know how dear it is to other hearts. I almost feel as if it ought to be set apart as a place sacred to friendship and to all the sweet memories associated with it.

. . . Christmas at Rock Garden always comes to me as a beautiful memory of generous hearts and joyous greetings. How plainly I can see you holding up the packages and reading off the names in your own inimitable manner, while the big stocking stands yearning to give up its treasures.

And again:

. . . I always think of Rock Garden and the Christmas tree there and how much I enjoyed it, and how dear are the memories. All the Heinzens, Miss Sprague, Dr. Morton, the Prangs, Dr. Berlin, the Drs. Pope, and others, are all fresh in my mind, and I send them kind greetings, with love to Santa and your own dear self.

William Lloyd Garrison at one time described this home which Dr. Zakrzewska had there created for herself and for the friends and patients who were her paying guests. He said:

Dr. Zakrzewska was already settled in her attractive home in Cedar Street, Roxbury, when, in 1864, my father moved to Highland Street near by, and the two families became intimate. Although unmarried, the Doctor rarely failed to have a house full of friends and relatives, making of her home a social center for her German and American acquaintances.

She was a woman of decided opinions and the frankest speech, a circumstance which gave zest and animation to any group in which she mingled. She held firmly to the conviction that personal consciousness ends with death; that so-called spiritual communications are a delusion, that prohibition laws infringe upon individual rights; that homeopathy has no claim to science; and that armed resistance to tyrants is justifiable.

My father held diametrically opposite views, but as both were believers in the utmost freedom of speech, the social clash of arms never engendered a moment's ill feeling. They were closely united upon the questions of anti-slavery and woman's rights, and they were drawn by a common impulse to progressive and philanthropic movements.

Karl Heinzen, who with his wife and son made a part of the Doctor's household, was a striking and remarkable figure. He was a man of massive intellect, possessing a high reputation in Germany as a writer of both prose and verse. His intense love

of liberty and hatred of shams had made him an
exile in America in the tumultuous years preceding
the Civil War. He was of noble stature and frame,
a spacious temple for a great soul, his rugged face
betraying his indomitable and fearless character.
Boston never realized the value or distinction of
this moral hero, for the reason that the English
language was more formidable to him than despots
and monarchies. But in Dr. Zakrzewska he had a
friend who appreciated his noble talents and virtues.

. . . I have dwelt upon this conjunction of the
Doctor with Karl Heinzen because his influence upon
her life was deep and abiding. To see him working
about the ample grounds, trimming the grapevines
and attending to the fruit trees—his recreation and
pleasure—and, when the weather permitted, to
behold the afternoon table-gathering under the leafy
shade at the back of the grounds which rose above
the house, was to receive the impression of a bit of
the Fatherland—a German grafting on a Yankee
hillside. The glimpse was often through or over
the board fence which separated my own house on
the hilltop when, in 1868, I became the Doctor's
closely adjacent neighbor. What animated talk enlivened the coffee, and how many friends enjoyed
first and last the retirement and refreshment!

In the early days, sweet Mrs. Severance and her
interesting family lived also on Cedar Street; the
Prangs were near at hand on Center Street; the
Koehlers and the Elsons were in the vicinity. The
beautiful suburb of Roxbury was then full of natural charm, an object of interest to strangers visiting Boston and at that date untouched and un-
spoiled.

I remember a traveled friend pointing down Cedar Street towards the Doctor's house and asking, "Have you ever been to Versailles?" adding, "The arches of these glorious elms are a reminder of it."

For many years Dr. Zakrzewska had a summer cottage at York Harbor but it is of her busy city homes that her friends wrote most often.

One of the former internes writes to her in later days:

The year spent by me in the Hospital will always be remembered with great pleasure, particularly that part of it when I was quarantined at the Maternity and you used to ask me down to dinner at your house nearly every evening.

She kept in touch with all the doctors and students who had been at any time connected with the Hospital, if writing only at notable times such as the big anniversaries or when some special report or Fair souvenir was published. She always inquired how they were getting on, and whether they received the annual reports of the Hospital which were always sent to their latest address. And so she was kept informed of their changing circumstances, their successes or discouragements, their marriages, their husbands, their children, and their problems of many kinds.

In beginning practice they had the varied fortunes which might be expected from differing individualities, equipment, resources and environment. Some found doors already opened to welcome them;

some had to make places for themselves. One of the latter group writes to her:

I am now doing very satisfactorily but I often think how prophetic you were when you used to warn us, saying, "Five years of waiting and starvation are before every one of you."

Their addresses were scattered all over the world —over the United States from Maine south to Florida and west to California; on the north to Canada; and east and west to England, Scotland, France, Germany, Switzerland, Italy, India,[23] Persia, Japan, China.

In keeping with the breadth of view which characterized her and her director associates, no discrimination has ever been made at the New England Hospital regarding sects, races or nationalities in students, doctors, nurses or patients.

As we have already seen, Dr. Zakrzewska had always a large circle of friends among the famous and high-minded men of her time, and her influence with the men in the families of her patients has also been noted.

It remains to add a word as to the number who were proud to call themselves her "boys." A specimen letter from one of these latter, signed by a name well known in Boston, says:

DEAR DOCTOR:
As no person in the world outside of my own immediate family is dearer to me than yourself, I want you to be one of the first to know of my engagement to —— ——, and I am sure you will approve of my choice.

Trusting that we may meet before long, I am as ever one of your boys.

She had no theologic affiliations. Her clear vision and her keen reasoning powers were unsatisfied with any form of dogma, creed or ritual yet elaborated. And she found these latter unnecessary to the development of a rule of life which reconciled the untrammeled intellect and the highest ethics yet evolved by an upward-struggling humanity.

She was able to organize instinct, training, reason, observation, experience and personal association, and to add to these the communion with the great minds of the race which is to be derived from reading—each continually checking up and correcting all the others. So she developed a mind which she kept in a wholesome state of flux, ready to modify any conclusion as new light rose above the horizon.

She held her course and steered her life as a skilled navigator holds his course, who while he steers by compass and chart yet makes myriad adjustments as required by continually varying conditions of wind and wave and sky.

And pursuers of high ideals in ethics and philosophy were always on her list of friends. This list always included clergymen, and in this connection we may note the observations at a later date of Rev. Charles G. Ames. He says:

Dr. Zakrzewska in speaking of the class of unfortunate women with whom she was often brought in contact in her medical work, once said to me, "I cannot give them money but I always give them my friendship in order to keep them morally alive."

It made me think of Fichte's words, "No honest mind is without communication with God, whether so called or not." After hearing that remark of the Doctor's, I never had any difficulty in giving her my fellowship on the deepest spiritual ground.

Reverend James Freeman Clarke [24] was one of her earliest friends in Boston, their acquaintance beginning back in the days when she came soliciting help for opening the New York Infirmary.

In her address at the opening of the Sewall Maternity new building, in 1892, Dr. Zakrzewska alludes to this episode, saying:

Let me express the gratitude we owe for our existence to a man whose influence secured to us the noble friends who in the spirit of justice to women gave invaluable assistance with their labors and their financial help—I mean, Reverend James Freeman Clarke.

I feel justified in saying that it was among the members of his church that the idea was materialized and that funds for the beginning of the experiment were provided.

We have referred above to Dr. Zakrzewska's wide reading. One of the friends of her Cleveland days, Rev. A. D. Mayo, says:

By an intuitive grasp of what was best for herself in books, she realized the saying of the historian, George Bancroft, "I should as soon think of eating all the apples on the big tree in my garden as to read the whole of any good book. I pluck and eat the best apple and leave the rest." She always knew the best apple on every tree of knowledge, and her mind was stored with the condensed wisdom of many libraries.

And he tells of the renewal in Boston of his friendship with her, some twenty years after its beginning in Cleveland:

Having made Boston my family headquarters, we were brought together in her generously appointed home in Union Park, almost under the eaves of the great church of Dr. Edward Everett Hale. I then verified anew the old truth that a genuine friendship grows even during absence.

Writing at this same date about Dr. Zakrzewska's personality, Dr. Buckel says:

I cannot measure how much I owe to her skillful, energetic, practical instruction as a physician when I was a student in the New York Infirmary; neither can I measure the strength, courage and hope which her bright example has given me throughout my life.

I think, however, that her genuine respect for even the very poorest of the poor immigrants who crowded the most wretched quarters of New York made the deepest and most lasting impression. Others showed sympathy and pity, but she entered into their lives with an appreciation of their difficulties and a coöperation in their honest efforts that stimulated their courage and gave them strength to work on until success finally rewarded them.

She considered the husband, father, son, and brother equally worthy of regard with the women of the family in all her plans for improvement. Although devoted to women's best interests, she never worked for women alone. Her influence over the men in these poor families was most remarkable, considering their supposed opinions as to the proper sphere of woman.

Not a few educated, intelligent men owe their first start in the world to her suggestive counsel. The spirit of comradeship she felt with high-minded, intellectual men greatly strengthened my own convictions as to the true relations of men and women to each other and helped me to enjoy more freely the friendship of men whom I honored and admired.

In her social life, gentlemen were always most cordially welcomed, and they seemed sincerely to appreciate her kindness and highly value her esteem. The picnics and excursions she planned to the suburbs and parks of New York, which were then easily accessible, are among the most delightful memories of my life. Grave professors, exiled philosophers and learned doctors ran with us in our merry games and forgot for the moment all but the gladsome spirit of the play.

During my long association with Dr. Zakrzewska in hospital life, both in Boston and in New York, I do not remember a single misunderstanding. I always had her cordial support in the hospital and a bright, warm welcome in her home. And I knew that any of our students whom I might take to her house would also receive a cordial welcome and realize that she was their friend.

For so many years after its beginning the New England Hospital was so largely regarded as a personal expression of Dr. Zakrzewska, and its place in the estimation of the profession was so largely based upon appreciation of the standards of which she stood as a representative, that the acceptance by a man physician of a position on the consulting staff was really a personal tribute to her.

For this reason it seems desirable to publish here the names of all the men who during her life served the Hospital in a consulting capacity—whether as physician, surgeon or other specialist—the names being placed in chronological order.[25]

CHAPTER XL

In 1896, Dr. Zakrzewska again refers to the confidence of the community in women surgeons, illustrating it by an experience which she relates in her address at the opening of the new Dispensary building (Pope Dispensary—donated by Colonel Albert A. Pope and named for the donor and his twin sisters, Drs. Augusta and Emily Pope) which was located on the site of the old one at No. 29 Fayette Street. She says:

Our Dispensary in especial serves another purpose, namely, to convince rich and poor, educated and uneducated, professionals and nonprofessionals

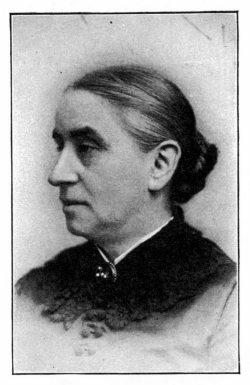

MARIE E. ZAKRZEWSKA, M.D.
(1896)

that women physicians can serve the community at large as well as can men physicians.

Said an Irishman to me a few weeks ago, when I pronounced it necessary for a member of his family to undergo a serious operation and advised further consultation with other physicians, "Can't we have one of the women surgeons from your Hospital?"

Seeing my surprise at this proposition, as the man was by no means an educated person, he said, "Well, Doctor, when I came to this country with my wife, we were very poor and knew nothing. The good women of the Pleasant Street Dispensary attended to us and taught us to take care of ourselves. All our children were born under their care, and they watched that we did right by them, all without any charge. Now that we can afford good pay, I am sure we want the same, for I swear by the women doctors." This speech, delivered in good broad Irish brogue, made me laugh most heartily. I soon had the case in the hands of the proper attendant, and all went well.

So, friends, let us be proud of all we have done, with the promise to do more and better work as science advances.

In June, 1899, on Mrs. Cheney's seventy-fifth birthday, the cornerstone of the new surgical building (the Ednah D. Cheney Surgical Building) was laid. In an address made at that time, Dr. Zakrzewska says:

After fifty years of experimental agitation and practical work, we now are completing the third department of the medical art in laying the cornerstone for this building. The medical pavilion,[26] the maternity, and now the surgical pavilion are the proofs in brick and mortar of woman's independent and faithful performances in the medical profession.[27]

The confidence of the public which generously provided the means for this cause, the confidence of the sick who sought relief at the hands of the women physicians, and the attitude of the profession in general towards the woman practitioner—all these have been acquired through skillful and patient labor.

It would be affectation if we women physicians did not feel proud of the result which we now see materialized, grateful as we are to all those who in earlier years bore with us not only the doubt and opposition but also the ridicule of our attempts. While we remember those who have done their part so valiantly, we do not forget those who have passed away without having had the satisfaction which we now enjoy in the success of our early effort.

On September 6, 1899, she celebrated her seventieth birthday, and on October 24, as stated in the annual report:

The Hospital tried to do honor to the one who, more than all others, deserves to be honored—its senior physician, Dr. Zakrzewska. In her thought, the New England Hospital was born. Because of her zeal and untiring energy and the aid of a few earnest friends, it became a fact. And from that day to the present one, as wise woman, skillful physician, and faithful friend, she has been an inspiration to all.

A reception was tendered her by the Hospital at the home of Mrs. Thomas Mack and there, with Mrs.

Cheney to assist, she greeted her many friends, old and new.

That the Hospital shall always bear an evident sign of its originator, it has been decided to name the main building which was the first one built, "The Zakrzewska Building," and to have it suitably marked by a tablet.

The exhausting excitement of this celebration aggravated the nerve fatigue which had been hanging out warning signals for many years, and to which attention has been called in these pages. At last these admonitions had become peremptory, and at last the high-spirited physician was obliged to confess herself subject to the laws regarding which she had so often cautioned her patients.

A study of her symptoms would in these days lead to a diagnosis of arteriosclerosis, that sad, sure reaction that waits inevitably upon the over-strenuous life, whether this follows the spur of the inward urge or the whip of circumstance. In the earlier days of medical practice, when symptoms of this condition were most in evidence through cerebral manifestations, the diagnosis of an obscure and fatal nervous disease was made, and so it was in this case.

The keen-sighted patient realized that her ailment was progressive, that it might be palliated though not cured, and that the imperative treatment lay in a simplified mode of life with avoidance of care, anxiety and excitement.

So she retired from the last detail of private practice, put her affairs in order, even arranging her funeral service, and then she cheerfully turned her mind to bearing her discomforts philosophically and to making the best of the time which remained.

When the realization of the finality of her situation came to her, she was undoubtedly shaken (when the final summons comes, every normal-minded human being quivers, even if it be only for the moment), but she was not dismayed. Subconsciously her physical condition must have aroused compensatory instincts, as it does with all of us, for at one time she wrote:

Death is to me a good friend. Whenever it comes, it is welcome. So many of my contemporaries have gone and are going into Nirvana, the world becomes young daily and new to me, into which newness I can hardly find myself. So that, when I say, "I have enough," I say the truth.

But additional acceptance of her position was favored by the serenity which comes to a mind which had long recognized the inevitable limitations which time would some time bring, for she writes:

For some years I have been saving money for old age, and in fact, I have done what I have so often encouraged other women to do—become independent of friends and charity. I have arranged to be independent until eighty years—to which age I sincerely hope not to live.

She seldom spoke of herself or of her feelings, but at one time she wrote:

If it were not for my poor head, I would say I was in better health than for years. But, alas! the nervous centers refuse to recuperate and the least excitement renders me sleepless, and a host of regrets, reproaches and condemnations rise up like demons to torment me.

Then, in one of the characteristic remissions of the condition, she writes, with one of her customary glints of humor:

I intend to live another seventy years because life seems so well worth living.

Once she wrote more in detail to Mrs. Cheney, because, as she said:

. . . It seems to me right that my dearest and oldest friend should understand me and not misjudge my actions. . . . Years ago some confusion of mind warned me of trouble to come, and it finally set in in the form of noises in my head. I scolded myself for being so nervous in my behavior while being irritated by these sounds, and I went gladly to California, hoping to get benefit by diversion.

However, the two distinct noises on the top of my head kept increasing so that even the noise of the cars did not drown them. Still I forced myself to act cheerfully and was determined not to be hopeless. Little by little, however, indifference toward events, then toward people, and now toward the beauty of nature, has crept upon me.

I have spoken to Dr. Berlin about this noise and described it as a steady sound of falling rain which prevented my falling asleep, to which she replied, "Well, we do fall asleep even if it rains hard, and so will you." I do not care to talk with other physicians, as I have made a study of brain trouble more than anything else and can therefore advise myself. Besides, talking about it increases the nervous irritation. So please take this as it is written, in cool reason—it is an inevitable condition which must be braved.

Less than three years were left to test her fortitude. She grew steadily weaker and on May 12, 1902, her release came. After a night of restlessness and intense discomfort she fell asleep, never waking again but passing at sunset into the Silence.

On a beautiful afternoon, the closing scene was laid in the chapel of the Forest Hills Crematory, and the details were as she had arranged. She had requested that no flowers should be used—she who so loved Nature and all the lovely growing things—and in this her friends respected her wishes. But they could not be denied the tribute of green palms and wreaths of laurel.

There was no music, no service in the ordinary terms. Her older friend—William Lloyd Garrison—having gone before, his son of the same name and her younger friend, made a short introductory address. And then Mrs. Emma E. Butler, secretary of the board of directors of the Hospital, read the farewell letter which Dr. Zakrzewska had written for the occasion:

During my whole lifetime, I have had my own way as much as any human being can have it without entirely neglecting social rules or trespassing upon the comfort of others more than is necessary for self-preservation.

And now, upon this occasion, I wish to have my own way in taking leave of those who shall come for the last time to pay such respect as custom, inclination and friendship shall prompt, asking them to accept the assurance that I am sorry to pass from them, this time never to return.

While these words are being read to you, I shall be sleeping a peaceful, well-deserved sleep—a sleep from which I shall never arise. My body will go back to that earthly rest whence it came. My soul will live among you, even among those who will come after you.

I am not speaking of fame, nor do I think that my name, difficult though it be, will be remembered. Yet the idea for which I have worked, the seeds which I have tried to sow here and there, must live and spread and bear fruit. And after all, what matters it who prepared the way wherein we walk? We only know that great and good men and women have always lived and worked for an idea which favored progress. And so I have honestly tried to live out my nature—not actuated by an ambition to be somebody or to be remembered especially, but because I could not help it.

The pressure which in head and heart compelled me to see and to think ahead, compelled me to love to work for the benefit of womankind in general, irrespective of country or of race. By this, I do not wish to assert that I thought of all women before I thought of myself. Oh, no! It was just as much in me to provide liberally for my tastes, for my wishes, for my needs. I had about as many egotistical wants to be supplied as has the average of womankind.

To look out for self and for those necessary to my happiness, I always considered not only a pleasure but a duty. I despised the weakness of characters who could not say "No" at any time, and thus gave away and sacrificed all their strength of body and mind, as well as their money, with that soft sentimentality which finds assurance in the belief that others will take care of them as they have taken care of others.

But, in taking leave, I cannot pass by those who, in every possible way in which human beings can assist one another, have assisted me by giving me their true friendship. Of my earliest career in America, Dr. Elizabeth Blackwell has been the most powerful agent in strengthening what was weak in me; while shortly afterward, my acquaintance with Miss Mary L. Booth fed the enthusiasm kindled by Dr. Blackwell and strengthened me in my uphill path. The friendship of these two women formed the corner stone upon which I have built all my life long.

To many valuable friends in New York I owe a deep gratitude, and especially to Mrs. Robert G. Shaw of Staten Island. In Boston, I leave a great number of friends, without whom I never could have accomplished anything and who have developed my character as well as faculties dormant within me of which I was unaware. It is the contact with people of worth which develops and polishes us and illuminates our every thought and action.

To me the most valuable of these early friends were Miss Lucy Goddard, Mrs. Ednah D. Cheney, Mrs. George W. Bond, Mrs. James Freeman Clarke, Mrs. George R. Russell, Dr. Lucy E. Sewall and Dr. Helen Morton—not that I give to them a place higher than to others, but because I am fully conscious how deeply they affected my innermost life and how each one made its deep imprint upon my character.

I feel that whatever work may be ascribed to my

hand could not have been done without them. Although I could not number them in the list of other friends who, in a special sense, formed a greater part of my life's affections, still I owe to each and every one a great debt. And I wish now, whether they be still alive or in simple tribute to their memory, to tell them of my appreciation of their kindness.

To those who formed the closer family circle in my affections—Mr. Karl Heinzen, Miss Julia A. Sprague, and my sisters—I have tried to show my gratitude during the whole of my life, on the principle of Freiligrath's beautiful poem:

> O Lieb, so lang du lieben kannst;
> O Lieb, so lang du lieben magst;
> Die Stunde kommt, die Stunde kommt,
> Wo du an Grabern stehst und klagst.

And now, in closing, I wish to say farewell to all those who thought of me as a friend, to all those who were kind to me, assuring them all that the deep conviction that there can be no further life is an immense rest and peace to me. I desire no hereafter. I was born; I lived; I used my life to the best of my ability for the uplifting of my fellow creatures; and I enjoyed it daily in a thousand ways. I had many a pang, many a joy, every day of my life; and I am satisfied now to fall a victim to the laws of nature, never to rise again, never to see and know again what I have seen and known in my life.

As deeply sorry as I always have been when a friend left me, just so deeply sorry shall I be to leave those whom I loved. Yet I know that I must submit to the inevitable, and submit I do—as cheerfully as a fatal illness will allow. I have already gone in spirit, and now I am going in body. All that I leave behind is my memory in the hearts of the few who always remember those whom they have loved. Farewell.

*   *   *   *   *

Perhaps she is right. Perhaps in the ordinary egoistic sense in which the word is used, there is no such thing as Immortality. Nevertheless—*the spirit of Marie E. Zakrzewska still lives.*

AFTERWORD

THE personal quest of Marie E. Zakrzewska is ended. The land of dispossession and refusal has been penetrated by many small parties under her and other leadership, and many outposts have been established and are being valiantly held.

But the battle which she faced and fought is not ended. It remains for all lovers of justice to sustain the impulsion which carried her on and so to continue the fight till the truth of her watchword, "Science has no sex," is acknowledged. Then, and only then, will her life's work be fulfilled.

In medicine, many doors of opportunity have been opened as the result of her life and the lives of her sister pioneers. But as with her and with them, the struggle persists around the hospitals. Many if not most of the great medical schools are now open to women but to-day, even as in Dr. Zakrzewska's day, the attainment of the degree of M.D. is only the beginning of medical knowledge.

Opportunities for hospital study and training are needed not only for the subsequent year of interneship, but as a constant resource all through the professional life. With a few exceptions, these opportunities are not yet open to women, and women are to-day hampered by this exclusion even more than they were in the past.

With the modern expansion of the science and art of medicine and the increasing elaboration of the required appliances and methods of examination, hospitals have become great centers of laboratory and clinical investigation and research. And the physician who is not able to form contact with some such center is crippled and is compelled to do his work either imperfectly or at the cost of tremendous additional strain.

This is the reason why we have just said that the opening of all hospital opportunities to women on equal terms with men is yet more imperative to-day than it was when Dr. Zakrzewska made such valiant battle for her sisters.

At the same time, when women seem to have attained opportunities, they still find it necessary to remember Dr. Zakrzewska's distrust and fear of beguilement, to remain on guard and to take all possible steps to keep secure all that has been so painfully achieved.

Even among nonmedical students and in circles that are supposed to be the most broadly educated, here and there the tolerances and amenities of civilized life develop slowly. Thus as late as October 20, 1921, the students of the University of Cambridge (England) express their disapproval of even "limited membership" for women by the old, worn-out methods of mobbing and rioting—battering down and smashing the valuable memorial gates of the women's college, Newnham. The arrival of the police prevented their further progress there, but at Peile Hall, they reached the doors and tried to force entrance into the college itself, which further outrage was again prevented by the police.*

In 1922 the London Hospital decided to exclude women from the classes and services to which they had been admitted since 1908. The story has a familiar sound— ". . . the chairman emphasizes the fact that the step has not been brought about by any failure of the women students . . . who have done very well in every way, in work, in conduct, and in discipline."†

Notwithstanding all the handicaps imposed on woman, she has demonstrated that "science has no sex." Do not her opponents now need to demonstrate that they themselves are worthy followers of science by accepting truth wherever it may be found and by rendering impartial justice to every one?

As some of these pages are being written (June 21, 1921), Madame Marie Curie is in Boston.

The morning papers report that she was yesterday given a reception by Harvard University. President Lowell presided, and in his address he ranked Madame Curie with "Sir Isaac Newton and other epoch-making discoverers." He then introduced Professor Richards of the Department of Chemistry, who said, "The discovery of Madame Curie gave the world new ideas concerning the structure of the universe, and opened a new path of thought to scientists."

The highest mark of distinction which a college or university can bestow upon a person whom it de-

---

* Boston *Herald*, October 21, 1921.

† Boston *Evening Transcript*, March 30, 1922, quoting the Springfield *Republican*.

sires to honor is an honorary degree. At its Commencement, three days later, Harvard did not confer an honorary degree on Madame Curie. Would it have conferred one on Sir Isaac Newton?

Is scholarship, then, the ideal of a college or university? Or is it scholarship which happens to be attained by a sex?

But humanity is neither male nor female: it is both. And both possess all human faculties *plus* the specialized qualities of the sex of the individual. The nonrecognition of this basic fact impedes the progress of the race. And the subjection of either sex to the other impedes both.

Hence, an appeal for justice to women, such as is embodied in this life of Marie E. Zakrzewska, is equally an appeal for justice to men. The man who would hold woman in subjection is himself held in subjection. For

"The woman's cause is man's: they rise or sink
Together, dwarf'd or godlike, bond or free:
For she that out of Lethe scales with man
The shining steps of Nature, shares with man
His nights, his days, moves with him to one goal,
Stays all the fair young planet in her hands—
If she be small, slight-natured, miserable,
How shall men grow?"

NOTES

1. This statement and related ones throughout the auto-biographical chapters are the only references to her family history made in this connection by Dr. Zakrzewska.

A "Memoir of Dr. Marie Elizabeth Zakrzewska, issued by the New England Hospital for Women and Children, Boston, 1903," quotes her as writing to a friend, "I am in reality as family-proud as any aristocrat can possibly be, but I prefer to be remembered only as a woman who was willing to work for the elevation of Woman." This Memoir further says:

The Polish family of Zakrzewski of which her father and grandfather were in the line of direct descendants, is one of the most ancient in Europe and traces its history back to 911. It is named among the most powerful aristocratic "republican families of agitators" of Poland, and fell with Poland's downfall.

The princely family property—which consisted according to some accounts of ninety-nine villages—was confiscated, the main portion falling into Russia's hands in 1793. At that time Marie's grandfather saved his life by flight beyond the border, having seen his father fall on the field of battle and his mother and other members of the family perish in the flames of their castle.

Writing of the family history, a brother of Marie states: "Ludovico was the name written under the coat of arms which I often held in my hands as a boy, and Ludwig was the name borne by every eldest son of the family until 1802. When our father was born on November 11—St. Martin's Day—his mother, a good Catholic, added Martin to the name of Ludwig." His father (Marie's grandfather) was, however, the first one of the Zakrzewski family to leave the Catholic church. He became not only a Protestant but a very liberal thinker.

The family history on the mother's side is traced back only to the middle of the eighteenth century.

Marie Elizabeth Sauer, the great-grandmother of Marie, for whom she was named, was a Gypsy Queen of the Lombardi family. She was said to be "the most lovely of women, very beautiful and energetic." Her father was a surgeon and was attached to the army of Frederick the Great during the Seven Years' War. His daughter accompanied him in his work as assistant surgeon. Among those whom she attended was a Captain Urban. He had been wounded in the chest and she removed the ball. Upon his recovery they were married, much to the delight of her father, as Captain Urban belonged to the same Gypsy tribe of the Lombardi. Nine children were born to them, five daughters and four sons. They were all of unusual size, the daughters almost six feet tall, with hair flowing down to their feet; the sons seven feet tall and of perfect stature. Marie's grandmother was the middle one of these nine children, and became a veterinary surgeon. She had three daughters one of whom was the mother of Marie.

2. "The undersigned, Secretary of Legation of the United States of America, certifies that Miss Marie Elizabeth Zakrzewska has exhibited to him very strong recommendations from the highest professional authorities of Prussia, as a scientific, practical, experienced *accoucheuse* of unusual talent and skill. She has been chief *accoucheuse* in the Royal Hospital of Berlin, and possesses a certificate of her superiority from the Board of Directors of that institution. She has not only manifested great talent as a practitioner but also as a teacher; and enjoys the advantage of a moral and irreproachable private character. She has attained this high rank over many female competitors in the same branch; there being more than fifty

in the city of Berlin who threaten by their acknowledged excellence to monopolize the obstetric art.

THEO. S. FAY.

Legation United States, Berlin, Jan. 26, 1853.

(SEAL)

Upon inquiry I find that instead of fifty there are one hundred and ten female *accoucheuses* in Berlin.

THEO. S. FAY.

3. Apparently Dr. Zakrzewska had no information as to the details of raising the money which was loaned to her for defraying her living expenses while at the medical college.

In *Glances and Glimpses,* the source of such financial assistance is suggested by Dr. Harriot K. Hunt, who visited Cleveland in 1854. She speaks of the first Medical Loan Fund Association. She also speaks of the Ohio Female Medical Education Society, and quotes from the constitution of this latter an article referring to the repayment of loans.

Dr. Hunt further speaks of traveling to other towns in Ohio, lecturing on the study of medicine by women, and "establishing loan fund associations auxiliary to the Cleveland association." She particularly mentions Elyria (where Mrs. Severance also spoke), Tiffin, Columbus, Cincinnati, and Yellow Springs.

4. Elsewhere, Dr. Zakrzewska says:

In the beginning of the first winter I was the only woman; after the first month another was admitted; and during the second winter there were three besides myself who attended the lectures and graduated in the spring.

5. This attitude of the clerical profession, persisting at least as late as 1857, is also referred to by Professor Joseph

P. Remington in the report of an address published in the *American Journal of Pharmacy,* January, 1911.

6. Speaking of the visit made to Cleveland at this time, Dr. Hunt states in *Glances and Glimpses:*

In December, 1854, I started for Ohio, being desirous to understand the medical question in that State. . . . I had only heard that Marie was a student at the Cleveland College; but when I met her I felt that here was a combination of head and heart which was as uncommon as it was beautiful. . . . Further acquaintance has but deepened my interest in Marie, and Dr. Blackwell of New York must feel it a privilege to have been the means of her introduction at Cleveland as a medical student, where her noble bearing and scientific mind are perceived and acknowledged by the faculty. . . .

I attended lectures one day on a class of diseases peculiar to women, and not one shade of levity or impropriety diminished the interest of the occasion. Men and women studying together at a medical college of high standing was prophetic. I spoke with the professor after the lecture and he remarked, "We are more democratic in Ohio than you are in Massachusetts." I felt like hanging my head. The Athens of America was eclipsed by a younger sister; yet I rejoiced greatly that as the elder was unprepared to advance, the junior tripped her up triumphantly, stepped over her, and took the first prize.

. . . I thought it best to visit the towns in the northern part of Ohio and try to elicit interest in the medical question by establishing loan fund associations.

7. Mary L. Booth later earned a reputation as historian and as translator, and was the editor of *Harper's Bazar* from its beginning in 1867.

8. The first Board of Directors (nineteen in number) was made up almost entirely of women who were serving on the Board of Lady Managers for the Clinical Department of the New England Female Medical College in 1861-1862,

the last year of Dr. Zakrzewska's connection with that college. Her resignation at the end of that year caused that department to be discontinued and the services of the Lady Managers to be no longer in request by the college.

To the number of Lady Managers who transferred their interest to the new Hospital were added on the Board of Directors several men, one being the former leading trustee of the college, Hon. Samuel E. Sewall.

This historic first Board of Directors was finally constituted as follows:

Mrs. Mary C. E. Barnard
Miss Sarah P. Beck
Geo. Wm. Bond
Mrs. Louisa C. Bond
Mrs. Ednah D. Cheney
Mrs. Anna H. Clarke
Miss Mary J. Ellis
Mrs. Lucretia G. French
Miss Lucy Goddard
Fred. W. G. May
Mrs. Joanna L. Merriam
Mrs. Mary A. S. Palmer
Thomas Russell
Mrs. Caroline M. Severance
Samuel E. Sewall
John H. Stephenson
James Tolman
Mrs. Mary G. White
Dr. Marie E. Zakrzewska

9. Later, Dr. Mary E. Breed, who was graduated from the New England Female Medical College and had been a student under Dr. Zakrzewska at the New York Infirmary, became resident physician, and Miss Anita E. Tyng and Miss Lucy M. Abbott, who had been her students at the New England Female Medical College, were student assistants. Dr. John Ware consented to serve as consulting physician and Dr. Samuel Cabot as consulting surgeon.

10. Karl Heinzen is thus described by the Boston *Evening Transcript:*

He was a native of Prussia and came to America in January, 1848, as an exile, having been banished from Germany on account of a book which he published on the *Civil Service of the Prussian Government,* which showed that, instead of the promised constitutional government, a complete net of absolutism was extending over every province of Prussia.

On the breaking out of the revolution of 1848 in France and Germany, he left America in May to participate in the movement in Europe; after its suppression he was again exiled, going first to Switzerland and afterwards to England. But in 1850 he again came to America which has since been the scene of his labors.

On his arrival he found almost the entire German population in the Democratic and pro-slavery party; he therefore established here the first anti-slavery German newspaper. This exposed him to severe persecutions by the Democrats, so that his life was threatened in New York City and in Toledo, Ohio.

He was also the first among the German-Americans to advocate woman suffrage.

Since 1858 he has lived in Boston, and during this time he has stood on terms of firm friendship with William Lloyd Garrison who frequently translated Mr. Heinzen's articles for the *Liberator*.

Mr. Heinzen was the most radical thinker whom the Germans in America possess. Besides editing for more than twenty-five years a newspaper, *The Pioneer*, he has published a number of valuable books on political, philosophical and social subjects.

11. Dr. Tyng had been a student at the New England Female Medical College under Dr. Zakrzewska, later a resident student at the New England Hospital and then a graduate of the Philadelphia medical school—this school now becoming established on a more stable foundation and having changed its name from the Female Medical College of Pennsylvania to the Woman's Medical College of Pennsylvania.

12. Dr. Thompson was a graduate of the New England Female Medical College, studying for two years under Dr. Zakrzewska. Later she received an honorary degree

from the Woman's Medical College of Pennsylvania. The Chicago Hospital for Women and Children which she founded was afterwards named the Mary Thompson Chicago Hospital for Women and Children.

In an affectionate letter to Dr. Zakrzewska in later years, Dr. Thompson rallies this former teacher on her frank remarks when trying to goad the students of the New England Female Medical College to better work, saying:

I wished to tell you of our work here that you might know that we are doing something more than "the ordinary run of nurses," I having heard it remarked in times past that that was all we would amount to. That did not stimulate me in the least to this kind of work. But I will tell you what did—it was the actual love of surgery and the witnessing many men operate when I felt that I could do quite as well as they did. Since writing you, my third case of ovariotomy has done well.

13. Dr. Buckel was graduated in Philadelphia and then served under Dr. Zakrzewska as resident student at the New York Infirmary. During the last two years of the Civil War she rendered efficient service in the United States military hospitals of the Southwest, earning the soubriquet of "The Little Major." *The Survey*, May 17, 1913, says: "She selected and supervised the nurses, kept records in the absence of clerks, wrote letters for sick soldiers, obtained furloughs for convalescents, and comforted the dying." In the year 1865-1866, she succeeded Dr. Ruth A. Gerry as assistant physician at the New England Hospital, the latter returning to the practice which she had already started at Ypsilanti, and beginning to share in the long fight for the admission of women to the University of Michigan.

14. After receiving her degree of M.D. at Berne, **Dr.**

Sophia Jex-Blake returned to Great Britain and was largely instrumental in establishing the London School of Medicine for Women and in obtaining hospital facilities for it. She has reported her experience in *Medicine as a Profession for Women* and in *Medical Education of Women*. Charles Reade makes extensive use of both of these articles in writing his novel *The Woman Hater*.

15. Dr. Morton was a classmate of Dr. Sewall when both were students of Dr. Zakrzewska at the New England Female Medical College. She had spent four years in study at the Paris Maternité during the last two of which she had served as assistant teacher.

She returned to Boston in 1867 to begin the practice of her profession. She then became connected with the New England Hospital, her first appointment being on the staff of the Dispensary. Here she became the successor of Dr. Zakrzewska, the latter resigning from this branch of the work and leaving it entirely to the constantly growing number of younger medical women.

16. (p. 355) There are two great causes of sickness in our lying-in wards. First, mental distress during pregnancy, caused by poverty or neglect; second, the exposure and fatigue which many endure before coming to us.

One young girl, late last fall, had been sleeping for a week in outhouses. Another came in the cold winter weather, after wandering in a bewildered condition in the streets with wet skirts and no stockings, searching for some place of shelter in her distress. Another when she entered was very sick with acute pleurisy and pneumonia, so that even before her delivery her life was threatened. Several cases of intermittent fever and one of typhus fever were admitted under such circumstances that we could not avoid taking them without being guilty of inhumanity. Two women in a comatose condition from puerperal convulsions were also taken in. One of these last was restored to health, while the other never recovered consciousness.

We have taken in several babies who were so poisoned
with patented nostrums that only the most vigorous treatment with antidotes could rouse them, and weeks of the
most assiduous nursing were necessary to restore their en-
feebled vitality.

Some of you saw in one of the wards the wretched little
creature who was brought by its mother to us in a comatose state, with the skin drawn loosely over its bones and
its half-closed glassy eyes sunk deeply in their sockets.
This child had been boarded out by its mother while she
worked at service, and it had been gradually declining until
at the age of three and one-half months, it weighed but
seven and one-half pounds.

This was an extreme case, but frequently a practiced
eye will detect the same process going on. Often when I
am called to a sick child, I recognize in the ashy hue, sunken
eyes and other well-known symptoms, the work of some
"soothing syrup" or other equally pernicious drug. Pitiful indeed is the fate of babies deprived of their natural
guardians and subjected to the influence of these infamous
nostrums.

Can we not find some means to secure to infants a
mother's care and love for at least the first year of their
lives, by furnishing these mothers with some honest means
of support, and thus saving both mothers and children? I
leave this important question for you to consider, for even
if it is not strictly part of our work, it is a sequel to one
department of our Hospital.

A young woman, who in her childhood lost her mother
and whose stepmother not only kept a house of ill-fame
but sent this daughter to another, has now a beautiful baby
to which she is so strongly attached that, in spite of the
evil influences of all her past life, she is willing to do even
the hardest work for the sake of keeping her baby with her.
Yet, only a few evenings ago she came, with her blue-
eyed baby sweetly smiling in the soft wrappings provided
by its fond mother, and said that she must give it up.
"Nobody." she said, "would take *her* with her baby," and

I saw the hard look in her eyes and the bitter smile that made me tremble for her future, though I am confident that she had the will and the strength to earn her living honestly.

Last winter we were called to attend a woman in a difficult and complicated labor. She lived in a dark basement with floor wet and broken, the scanty bedcovering eked out by her husband's old coat (which he himself needed) and the small pile of coal on the floor being the only comforts visible except the stove. Cold, faint and hungry, this woman had suffered for hours. When she was safely delivered, public charity could not make her comfortable—it was private benevolence that gave her blankets, sheets, clothing and care.

Another case of recent occurrence shows how insufficient is the law to take care of the sick. A woman in one of the worst localities in the city who was beaten by her drunken husband and turned out of doors, was seized with premature labor in the streets and found her way into the house of a neighbor. This neighbor, Mrs. M., who was nearly blind, supported by her daily earnings herself and an interesting little boy whom she had taken from the city crier's to nurse and whom she had kept with her rather than send him to Tewksbury.

Mrs. M. allowed the woman to stay, and on the third day I was sent for and found her in an almost dying condition. It was late Saturday evening, and there was neither food nor fuel in the house. The woman was too ill to be removed, no aid could be obtained from the city before Monday, and then the legal allowance would be only two dollars in groceries and one dollar in money. Clothing, a bed and a nurse were absolutely needed. These were provided by private charity and the woman recovered, though it was said that three different physicians who were called in by the neighbors had declined to attend her as they considered it useless under such adverse circumstances to attempt to save her.

The first time this woman stepped out of doors she

walked from the North End to the Hospital to see if we could not get work for her. Her husband, who had been released from the jail where he had been kept awaiting the result of her illness, had visited her and told her he should do nothing more for her. Also, Mrs. M., who had given her shelter, was about to be turned out of her rooms because she had not been able to work as usual to earn her rent.

It is true that all these sufferers were drunkards, but I mention their cases to show how the Hospital leads us into every path of reform.

In order to accomplish permanent good, it is necessary to remove the causes of evil. For this reason, we are deeply interested in every effort to dispel ignorance, promote temperance, and banish licentiousness and other vices, for all these have a direct influence on health or disease. We frequently find it necessary not only to watch over the individual case of illness but to see that the whole tenement is cleaned and ventilated; or, when this is impossible, we sometimes succeed in removing the whole family to a more healthful locality away from their old associates and the low, drinking saloons.

Thus it will be seen that our students have a large field of labor open to them—every woman whom we help to educate not only adds one to the band of workers but strengthens our position and enlarges our means of usefulness. Hence, it is all-important that we gain every possible advantage for our students, and it is hard to see denied to them the valuable opportunities so freely offered to young men in this city, for we feel that the very best America affords comes far short of our wants.

17. The new Hospital is described in the annual report:

Although within the bounds of the city, thus giving the advantages of water, gas and the other conveniences of city life, the land is very high and commands an extensive and beautiful view of Jamaica Plain, Roxbury and Brookline.

It is also easily accessible both by horse and steam cars, and seems to combine all the important requisites of good air, light and easy access at a moderate price.

The beautiful exterior of the building is due to the taste and skill of our architects, Messrs. Cummings and Sears, who have successfully grappled with the problem of designing a hospital which shall be beautiful in proportion, form and color, and so contribute to the pleasure of all connected with it, without sacrificing either interior comfort or economy of means.

The excellence of the interior arrangements, especially of the wards and the nurses' rooms (which differ from those of any hospital known to the Committee), is due to the Women Physicians who, having learned from long experience the needs of their patients, have striven to meet them by arrangements at once simple and ingenious.

Our first object was to secure an entire isolation of the lying-in patients from those of the medical and the surgical wards, so as to guard against all possible danger of infection passing from one to the other. This has been effected by a separate house, called the "Maternity Cottage" for the lying-in patients.

In this building, the two stories are so arranged that one can be thoroughly cleansed and aired while the other is in use. Our plan contemplates a second similar building as soon as our means will enable us to construct it. Then, in case of any threatened danger, one house can be entirely isolated, while all new patients are taken to the other. In this way, we can increase our Lying-in Department to any desirable extent without incurring the dangers attendant upon large hospitals.

The next consideration was to get as much sunlight as possible into the patients' rooms and to give the nurses, who are all human beings and need to be cared for as well as others, good airy rooms in which to take their rest when rest is possible to them. For this reason, all the medical wards have been placed on the back of the house, which looks nearly south.

Each ward consists of two rooms—one for two beds and one for four—with a nurse's room between. The nurse can thus often have the benefit of the solitude and quiet of her own room and yet be so close to her patients that nothing can escape her notice. A bathroom, also enjoying the sunshine, separates the two wards and can be used by the patients of either. These light, airy, sunny wards with their open fireplaces seem more like the rooms of a pleasant home than the dreary apartments of a hospital.

The house does not square exactly with the points of the compass, and the northern side is touched by the sun during some part of the day, thereby securing it from dampness. The eastern surgical ward projects beyond the other part of the house, and so gains a southern window for light and cheerful sunshine. A similar projection on the western side makes a pleasant parlor for the patients.

The rest of this side of the house is occupied by the patients' admission room, tea kitchen, etc., in which sunshine is not so important.

The Children's Ward, in the upper story, is a new feature of which we have long felt the want. It is large, airy and convenient.

The furniture of the wards was mainly provided by individuals and by various churches and societies in the city and vicinity. The wards were named after the donors, who promised to keep them in order and in repair, the names to be retained as long as the rooms were thus sustained.

18. Dr. Dimock had been a student in the Hospital in 1867. As was the case with several other students, she thus at the beginning of her medical life came under the teachings of Dr. Zakrzewska. We may judge of the trend of these teachings from what Dr. Zakrzewska writes elsewhere as to her advice to Dr. Sewall when the latter wished to begin the study of medicine. She says:

"I advised her to lay a foundation by first studying

natural history—biology, comparative physiology and microscopical anatomy." And we are already familiar with the convictions of Dr. Zakrzewska that Europe at that time offered both to men and women better opportunities for a medical education than did the United States.

Susan Dimock differed from these other students in that she had more initiative, or more self-dependence, or less fear of circumstance and convention, or some other temperamental quality. Or perhaps it was the financial situation—that great lion in the path of women not trained in self-support—that she felt she could control, through Dr. Zakrzewska and other friends.

At any rate, the resulting reaction of Dr. Zakrzewska's teaching upon this temperament was such that Susan Dimock decided to go abroad for her entire medical course, to study there and to be graduated there—almost the first American woman to take such a radical step, and one of a lengthening procession of women from many countries who were driven into temporary exile by their ambition to qualify themselves for their chosen profession, having found the best opportunities at home reserved for the exclusive use of their brothers.

She entered the University of Zurich, and after completing the required five years of study, received her degree, returning to Boston as the new building of the Hospital was in course of erection. She had paid particular attention to surgery and was intending to specialize in that branch.

19. Dr. Keller was a graduate of the Woman's Medical College of Pennsylvania and she had been attending physician at the Woman's Hospital in Philadelphia. She had also had considerable surgical experience in hospital and private practice.

20. The New England Hospital Medical Society, later the New England Women's Medical Society.

21. Dr. Call was a student of the Hospital and later was graduated at the head of her class in the University of Michigan. She then spent a year studying in Europe before beginning work at the Dispensary.

22. The twin sisters, Drs. Augusta and Emily Pope, after being graduated at the New England Female Medical College, went to Europe to study for an additional year, becoming connected with the Dispensary on their return. Both later received an honorary degree of M.D. from the Woman's Medical College of Pennsylvania.

23. Among the internes whose address in India was, unfortunately, not for long, was the charming Dr. Anandabai Joshee, the first Hindoo woman to seek medical education in America, and who had been graduated at the Woman's Medical College of Pennsylvania.

Coming to Boston in the summer of 1886, she served only a short time when her health failed. She returned to India to become physician in charge of the Female Ward of the Albert Edward Hospital in Kolhapur, but she died from tuberculosis a few months later, before reaching her twenty-second birthday.

24. Dr. Clarke was a member of the board of trustees of the New England Female Medical College when Dr. Zakrzewska became a member of the faculty. He resigned this trusteeship when she resigned from the faculty, and his wife, Mrs. Anna H. Clarke, became a member of the board of directors of the New England Hospital which was founded immediately thereafter.

Mrs. Clarke remained a member of the board of directors until her death in 1897. Their daughter, Miss Lilian Freeman Clarke, was always interested in the Hospital and, as already stated, she assisted in organizing in connection with the Maternity the first hospital social service work in America.

25. (p. 467)

1. John Ware.	15. James R. Chadwick.
2. Samuel Cabot.	16. Geo. F. Jelly.
3. Walter Channing.	17. J. J. Putnam.
4. Henry I. Bowditch.	18. Maurice H. Richardson.
5. E. C. Rolfe.	19. Clarence J. Blake.
6. Edward Jarvis.	20. F. B. Mallory.
7. Edward H. Clarke.	21. Vincent Y. Bowditch.
8. Francis Minot.	22. W. F. Whitney.
9. B. Joy Jeffries.	23. G. A. Leland.
10. Reginald H. Fitz.	24. F. C. Shattuck.
11. C. H. Osgood.	25. C. F. Withington.
12. G. G. Tarbell.	26. J. E. Goldthwait.
13. Arthur T. Cabot.	27. Richard C. Cabot.
14. W. W. Gannett.	

26. In 1910, the Children's Department obtained a building of its own in the Kimball Cottage. This was named for Miss Helen Kimball and for her father, Moses K. Kimball, who was a staunch supporter of the Hospital. Mrs. Cheney became president in 1887, upon the resignation of Miss Lucy Goddard, the first president, and continued in office till 1902 when she resigned and was succeeded by Miss Kimball.

27. An interesting note in connection with the new Surgical Building was the receipt through Dr. Zakrzewska of a contribution of five hundred dollars towards its construction, from one of her classmates at the Cleveland Medical College, Dr. Cordelia A. Greene, then established at Castile, N. Y.

BIBLIOGRAPHY

BLACKWELL, ELIZABETH, M.D., *Pioneer Work in Opening the Medical Profession to Women.*

CHADWICK, JAMES R., M.D., ''The Study and Practice of Medicine by Women'' (*International Review,* October, 1879).

DALL, MRS. CAROLINE H., *A Practical Illustration of Woman's Right to Labor, or A Letter from Marie E. Zakrzewska, M.D., late of Berlin, Prussia,* 1860.

GREGORY, SAMUEL, *Man-Midwifery.*
Reports of the Boston Female Medical School; the Female Medical Education Society; and the New England Female Medical College.

HUNT, DR. HARRIOT KEZIA, *Glances and Glimpses,* 1856.

JEX-BLAKE, SOPHIA, M.D., *Medicine as a Profession for Women; Medical Education of Women.*

LIVERMORE, MRS. MARY A., *The Business Folio,* Boston, March, 1895.

NEW ENGLAND HOSPITAL FOR WOMEN AND CHILDREN, Memoir of Marie E. Zakrzewska, M.D., 1903.

PUTNAM-JACOBI, MARY, M.D., ''Women in Medicine'' (*Woman's Work in America,* 1891).

READE, CHARLES, *The Woman Hater.*

SIMS, J. MARION, M.D., *The Story of my Life,* 1884.

INDEX

(I)

THE END

American Women: Images and Realities

An Arno Press Collection

[Adams, Charles F., editor]. **Correspondence between John Adams and Mercy Warren Relating to Her "History of the American Revolution," July-August, 1807.** With a new appendix of specimen pages from the **"History."** 1878.

[Arling], Emanie Sachs. **"The Terrible Siren": Victoria Woodhull, (1838-1927).** 1928.

Beard, Mary Ritter. **Woman's Work in Municipalities.** 1915.

Blanc, Madame [Marie Therese de Solms]. **The Condition of Woman in the United States.** 1895.

Bradford, Gamaliel. **Wives.** 1925.

Branagan, Thomas. **The Excellency of the Female Character Vindicated.** 1808.

Breckinridge, Sophonisba P. **Women in the Twentieth Century.** 1933.

Campbell, Helen. **Women Wage-Earners.** 1893.

Coolidge, Mary Roberts. **Why Women Are So.** 1912.

Dall, Caroline H. **The College, the Market, and the Court.** 1867.

[D'Arusmont], Frances Wright. **Life, Letters and Lectures: 1834, 1844.** 1972.

Davis, Almond H. **The Female Preacher, or Memoir of Salome Lincoln.** 1843.

Ellington, George. **The Women of New York.** 1869.

Farnham, Eliza W[oodson]. **Life in Prairie Land.** 1846.

Gage, Matilda Joslyn. **Woman, Church and State.** [1900].

Gilman, Charlotte Perkins. **The Living of Charlotte Perkins Gilman.** 1935.

Groves, Ernest R. **The American Woman.** 1944.

Hale, [Sarah J.] **Manners; or, Happy Homes and Good Society All the Year Round.** 1868.

Higginson, Thomas Wentworth. **Women and the Alphabet.** 1900.

Howe, Julia Ward, editor. **Sex and Education.** 1874.

La Follette, Suzanne. **Concerning Women.** 1926.

Leslie, Eliza . **Miss Leslie's Behaviour Book: A Guide and Manual for Ladies.** 1859.

Livermore, Mary A. **My Story of the War.** 1889.

Logan, Mrs. John A. (Mary S.) **The Part Taken By Women in American History.** 1912.

McGuire, Judith W. (A Lady of Virginia). **Diary of a Southern Refugee, During the War.** 1867.

Mann, Herman . **The Female Review: Life of Deborah Sampson.** 1866.

Meyer, Annie Nathan, editor.**Woman's Work in America.** 1891.

Myerson, Abraham. **The Nervous Housewife.** 1927.

Parsons, Elsie Clews. **The Old-Fashioned Woman.** 1913.

Porter, Sarah Harvey. **The Life and Times of Anne Royall.** 1909.

Pruette, Lorine. **Women and Leisure: A Study of Social Waste.** 1924.

Salmon, Lucy Maynard. **Domestic Service.** 1897.

Sanger, William W. **The History of Prostitution.** 1859.

Smith, Julia E. **Abby Smith and Her Cows.** 1877.

Spencer, Anna Garlin. **Woman's Share in Social Culture.** 1913.

Sprague, William Forrest. **Women and the West.** 1940.

Stanton, Elizabeth Cady. **The Woman's Bible** Parts I and II. 1895/1898.

Stewart, Mrs. Eliza Daniel . **Memories of the Crusade.** 1889.

Todd, John. **Woman's Rights.** 1867. [Dodge, Mary A.] (Gail Hamilton, pseud.) **Woman's Wrongs.** 1868.

Van Rensselaer, Mrs. John King. **The Goede Vrouw of Mana-ha-ta.** 1898.

Velazquez, Loreta Janeta. **The Woman in Battle.** 1876.

Vietor, Agnes C., editor. **A Woman's Quest: The Life of Marie E. Zakrzewska, M.D.** 1924.

Woodbury , Helen L. Sumn er. **Equal Suffrage.** 1909.

Young, Ann Eliza. **Wife No. 19.** 1875.

Date Due